RAW FOOD WORKS

COMPILED AND EDITED BY
DIANA STORE

www.rawfoodworks.org

Published by Rawsuperfoods.com

Raw Food Works
Diana Store

ISBN/EAN: 978-90-813376-2-5
Title: Raw Food Works
Subtitle: Leading Experts Explain Why
Author: Diana Store

Published by:
www.rawsuperfoods.com
Raw Superfoods
Tobias MC Asserstraat 1 bg
1063 NB Amsterdam
The Netherlands

Info@rawsuperfoods.com
www.rawsuperfoods.com

Tel: 0031 20 4038844
Fax: 0031 20 4038814

Editorial assistant: Carol Harper
Editorial assistant: David Wiley
Cover Design: Kiryl Lysenka
Book Design: Sean and Kelly Smith
Total Book Design: Diana Store

For substantial discounts on bulk ordering please contact the publisher through:

www.rawfoodworks.org
www.rawsuperfoods.com

ACKNOWLEDGEMENTS

This book was truly created through a team effort that took countless hours of discussions, writings, and revisions. It could not have been created alone.

I would like to acknowledge each and every author who contributed to this book, whose inspiring wisdom and words may serve us all.

I would particularly like to thank Brian and Anna Maria Clement, who hosted the International Living Foods Summit meetings, from which the outline of this book originated. I would further like to thank Gabriel Cousens, whose initial encouragement for the idea of the book helped plant the seed for its growth.

In addition to all of the contributors to the book, I am indebted to the production team for their professional support in bringing the project to timely fruition.

Many special thanks are extended to my family and friends, who have provided valuable support throughout the book's process.

This book is dedicated to all those who are willing to take responsibility for their own great health

"This beautiful book that contains the golden guidance of many brilliant experts is the story of my life. In 1975, at the age of 31—a single Mom without energy, and with much sadness and stress--I discovered the possibility of raw food and found a new person inside myself. I found glowing health, vitality, persistence, purity, and a deep connection to my spiritual nature that I never knew existed. My body transformed from lumpy and dumpy to slender and shiny. Whether raw food becomes your life path or a method of healing that will not fail you, it is a life-enhancing, life-saving choice you must now know about and always be able to use. Believe these teachers when they tell you that raw food will heal you. Raw food will make you feel young no matter what your age. Raw food will show you how beautiful you truly are. My admiration, love and gratitude are boundless for Diana Store and for the dedicated wisdom teachers who have contributed to this valuable work. Try what they recommend! You absolutely deserve to experience the fun and fantastic feeling that raw food brings into your life!"

Marilyn Diamond
Co-author Fit for Life

TABLE OF CONTENTS

Introduction - Diana Store...1

Part 1: The Optimum Diet For Health And Longevity 5

1. Vegan 2.0 - Everyone@Plant-Based - David Rainoshek MA.....................7

2. Organics For Life - Cherie Soria...35

3. Enzymes - Viktoras Kulvinskas MS...43

4. The Principle Of 80% Raw - Brian Clement PhD, NMD, LNC.....................57

5. Deep Food - Accessing Nutrient Density From The Ground Up -
   David Rainoshek MA and Katrina Rainoshek.................................63

6. God Sleeps In Stone: The Power Of Minerals To Improve Health -
   David Wolfe...83

7. High Water Content Foods And The Necessity For Proper
   Hydration - Dorit..95

8. The Value Of Raw Vegetable Juices - Rev. George Malkmus....................103

9. Chlorophyll Rich Green Foods In Three Parts................................111

   The Miracle Powers Of Chlorophyll - Victoria Boutenko....................111

   The Healing Power Of Wheatgrass - Jill Swyers............................114

   Primordial All Organic AFA - Michael Saiber
   and Tamera Campbell...117

10. The Importance Of Essential Fatty Acids - Rick Dina DC...................123

11. The Key Of Low Sugar Consumption -
    Brian Clement PhD, NMD, LNC...131

12. The Body's Need For Adequate Salt - Jameth Sheridan ND...................137

13. Enlightened Eating With Calorie Prudence - David Rainoshek MA............145

14. Detoxification And Healing - Brenda Cobb.................................165

15. Superfoods And Supplements - Jameth Sheridan ND.........................173

16. The Importance Of Vitamin B12 -
    Gabriel Cousens MD, MD(H) and Brian Clement PhD, NMD, LNC......189

17. Dark Field Microscopy - Anna Maria Clement PhD, NMD, LNC..................203

18. How To Make The Change Easily, Joyfully And Successfully -
    Karen Knowler..213

19. Its Not Just What You Eat - Lifestyle And Beyond -
    Jameth Sheridan ND..221

Part 2. The Principles In Practice..231

Healing Diabetes Requires A Shift In Consciousness -
    Gabriel Cousens MD, MD(H)..233

Afterword. Getting On Track And Staying On Track -
    Walter Urban PhD..263

INTRODUCTION

Diana Store

What now makes up the mainstream understanding of what a raw food diet is has its roots in a century-long history of alternative healing and lifestyle movements, coming from European fasting spas to Californian "Nature Boys", the Natural Hygiene philosophy, the Living Foods lifestyle developed by Ann Wigmore in the 1960s, to the present-day burgeoning Raw culture, with an abundance of high-quality resources, including books, superfoods, retreats, festivals, films, and restaurants, all with a focus on a Raw and Living Foods Diet and Lifestyle.

As a growing number of people have become interested in this diet and lifestyle in recent years, it was found that the teachings being disseminated from the disparate corners of this still-young movement did not always correspond with each other. A lack of consensus among teachers often created confusion for individuals seeking to get onto the best dietary path and claim the promised benefits. The differences of opinion became so incredibly obvious at one international gathering (The Fresh Network Festival, UK, 2004), it was decided that the leading raw food teachers would come together and discuss, from a scientific basis, what the main and essential points of a nutritionally sound raw-food approach to diet should be.

As "the father of live foods" Viktoras Kulvinskas put it in his announcement of the event:

"Every great movement that has effectively weathered the ages and enriched the world's cultures has organized and together formulated a concise, clear, and passionate message. As a senior member of our important group, I feel that it is time to gather at a round table and enhance our mission of helping a suffering humanity. To do this we must establish and strengthen our vital community. Together, we can explore and create a dynamic system of health that is rivaled by none other. This will be accomplished by respecting everyone's core beliefs, yet unifying our voice. Everyone from healthy, young athletic individuals to catastrophically ill sufferers must be addressed in a way that would best assist them in their progression to greater health."

The first International Living Foods Summit took place in January 2006 at West Palm Beach, Florida attended by 25 teachers from eight different countries, with a combined personal experience of over 434 years following a vegan or raw food lifestyle. This meeting and a second Summit the following year produced a Statement of the key principles for an Optimum Diet for Health and Longevity. This has mostly recently been tweaked during the recent Summit of May 2009. The Statement represents a consensus of agreement between all the teachers who participated in creating it. Please note a few additional notable colleagues were welcomed to join in the creation of this book, who did not attend a Summit or contribute directly to writing the Statement.

The aim of Raw Food Works is to offer a more elaborate explanation of all the points covered, to present the different facets of a successful raw-food diet in a balanced way, and to present via a collective effort a state-of-the-art document about what WORKS.

I welcome you to step into the world of raw and living foods and watch your life transform!

INTERNATIONAL LIVING FOOD SUMMIT
Vibrant Health Through Plant-Based Nutrition

These historic summits were held at the Hippocrates Health Institute in West Palm Beach, Florida on January 14, 2006, April 28, 2007 and May 2, 2009. The summits convened to unify the leadership in the Living Food Movement, establishing scientifically based common standards for optimum health.

Leaders from eight countries (with a combined total of over 600 years following this lifestyle) agreed on the following standards:

The Optimum Diet for Health/Longevity:
- Vegan (no animal products of any kind, cooked *or* raw)
- Organic
- Whole Foods
- High in nutrition such as vitamins, antioxidants, and phytonutrients
- Highly mineralized
- Contains a significant quantity of chlorophyll-rich green foods
- Contains adequate complete protein from plant sources
- Contains a large proportion of high-water-content foods
- Provides excellent hydration
- Includes raw vegetable juices
- Contains all essential fatty acids, which can be obtained from naturally occurring plant sources
- Is at least 80% raw (the remaining to be Vegan, whole food, and organic)
- Has moderate yet adequate caloric intake
- Contains only low to moderate sugar and exclusively from whole-food sources (fruitarianism is *strongly discouraged*)
- Contains adequate amounts of unprocessed salts, as needed (depending upon your constitution)
- Is nutritionally optimal for both detoxification and rebuilding

We also agree that:
• Eating local, ripe, seasonally available foods as appropriate is adviseable.

• Deficiencies of both Vitamin B-12 and Vitamin D are common issues for mental and physical health, for anyone on any diet. Plant-based supplementation of Vitamin B-12 is imperative. Adequate Vitamin D levels can be maintained with sufficient sun exposure. When exposure is inadequate, take appropriate levels of plant based Vitamin D supplementation.

• The addition of enzyme-active superfoods and whole-food supplements is also advised.

• Caffeinated and/or addictive substances *(even in their raw form)*, such as cocoa/chocolate, coffee, caffeinated teas, and alcoholic beverages are highly discouraged.

• This way of eating can be further optimized by tailoring it based on *individual needs* (within the principles stated).

• Benefits derived by following these principles are proportional to how well they are followed.

• We will remain open-minded, and this information will be updated and expanded upon if necessary, as new research becomes available.

• Diet is a critical part of a healthy lifestyle, yet not the entire picture. A full-spectrum, health-supportive lifestyle is encouraged. This includes physical exercise, exposure to sunshine, as well as psychological health. Avoiding environmental toxins and toxic products is essential. Paramount is pure water (for consumption and bathing), the use of natural fiber clothing, and non-toxic personal-care products. Also consider healthy options in home furnishings/building materials and related items.

All participating leaders agree that eating according to the International Living food Summit Guidelines will significantly address the urgent issues of health, environmental sustainability, world hunger, and a compassionate respect for all life.

The following leaders support these principles:
(listed in alphabetical order)

Fred Bischi, PhD – USA; Tamera Campbell – Vision – USA; Rajaa Chbani – Pharmacie L'Unite – Morocco; Katharine Clark, RN, CMT, CCT - USA Gabriel Cousens, MD, MD(H) – Diplomat American Board of Holistic Medicine – USA; Brenda Cobb – Living Foods Institute – USA; Anna Maria Clement, CN, NMD, PhD – Hippocrates Health Institute – USA; Brian Clement, CN, NMD, PhD – Hippocrates Health Institute – USA; Karin Dina, DC – RawFoodEducation.com – USA; Rick Dina, DC – RawFoodEducation.com – USA; Carole Dougoud – Institute Haute Vitalite – Switzerland; Dorit – Serenity Spaces - USA/Israel; John Eagle Freedom – Health City USA; Kare Engstrom – Dietician - Sweden; Laura Gonzalez – GWAH Healing Institute – USA; Jane Holmes – Living Foods Institute – USA; Elizabeth Kapadia, DN – GWAH Healing Institute – USA; Viktoras Kulvinskas – "Grandfather" of the Living Foods Movement – USA; Dan Ladermann - Living Light International – USA; Marie Christine; Lhermitte – Chemin du mas Magnuel - France; George Malkmus – Hallelujah Acres – USA; Rhonda Malkmus – Hallelujah Acres – USA; Paul Nison – The Raw Life – USA; Katrina Rainoshek – JuiceFeasting.com – USA; David Rainoshek – JuiceFeasting.com – USA; Claudine Richard – Naturopath – France; Michael Saiber – Vision – USA; Cherie Soria – Living Light International – USA ; Jameth Sheridan, ND – HealthForce Nutritionals – USA; Diana Store – RawSuperfoods.com – UK/The Netherlands; Jill Swyers – Living Foods For Health – UK/Portugal; Walter J. Urban, PhD – USA - Costa Rica

PART I

The Optimum Diet
For Health and Longevity

Part 1

1

Vegan 2.0: Everyone@ Plant-Based

David Rainoshek, MA

Vegans in Hummers do more for reducing greenhouse gasses than do meat-eaters who cruise around in hybrids or collect recyclable soda cans.[1] A recent clinical trial showed that a prudent vegan diet can reverse heart disease 100% of the time.[2] Folks accessing a plant-based diet have higher IQs,[3] lower blood pressure,[4] lower cholesterol,[5][6] reduced mortality,[7] healthier weight,[8] and a reduced chance of developing diabetes at any age (and can even heal their diabetes).[9][10] A plant-based diet reduces the personal risk and societal rates of Alzheimer's,[11][12] stroke,[13] breast cancer,[14] colon cancer,[15] prostate cancer,[16] arthritis, multiple sclerosis (MS),[17] osteoporosis,[18] and kidney disease.[19][20] Plant-based can even improve your sex life and save you lots of money on your car insurance.

Yes, it's all true except the car insurance, and the reason it is true is because plant-based is far enough up what I call The Spectrum of Diet™, which is a basic stages conception encompassing every dietary methodology in Westernized nations. *(see below)*

The new activism
It is important to recognize the kind of new activism we are practicing now in the West in the vegan/plant-based community. For many generations, activism looked like letter writing, marches, chanting/yelling, holding up signs – classic protest activity. Governments of the world (at least the politicians in power) are

not listening to this kind of activism. We need something of significant, lasting impact that *we can all do* so that individuals feel empowered. The way you live your life on a day-to-day basis can have the impact that you desire, or as M.K. Gandhi said, *"you must be the change you want to see in the world".* We call this *subtle activism.*

We can probably all acknowledge that, to the greatest extent possible, our food should create as little harm and suffering as possible. Despite our global history of war and violence, humanity is overwhelmingly averse to causing harm. What is not often considered, but causes a considerable amount of suffering, is the effect food production and processing has on humanity, our economies, and the ecology of the planet. How we eat is our most fundamental interaction with the living planet. The foods we choose are an important way in which we acknowledge who we are, and in how we express our love for ourselves and all creation. Eating a plant-sourced cuisine as an act of non-violence is backed by clinical research, cross-cultural studies, decades of dietary experience by hundreds of thousands, and our world religious heritage. It acknowledges the current needs of all inhabitants on earth, including their economic viability, cultural survival and even the survival of life itself.

John Robbins, author of *The Food Revolution,* said we have the opportunity to vote three times a day. In 2009, the US is projected to spend $2.9 trillion on health care,[21] and $1.3 trillion on food, 90% of which is processed. These nutrient-poor foods make the US one of the sickest of the well-fed nations in the world. A plant-sourced diet of whole foods has the potential *positively to shift $4.2 trillion dollars of the US economy each year,* making a move to plant-based the most revolutionary form of activism currently available. In addition, a global shift to vegan would make enough food available for the people of the world to be fed seven times over at current agricultural production levels, significantly reduce greenhouse gases (more than if we banned all motorized vehicles), and shift US and global economies to a more sustainable, health-promoting/protecting mode. There are many other reasons why in the pages that follow, but this provides a striking first perspective on the potential impact of veganism.

From existing to living – the Spectrum of Diet™

FAST FOOD	STANDARD AMERICAN	WHOLE FOODS	COOKED VEGETARIAN	COOKED VEGAN	RAW / LIVE VEGAN	JUICE FASTING TO JUICE FEASTING
EGOCENTRIC	SOCIOCENTRIC			WORLDCENTRIC		
SHALLOW FOODS / EXISTING <----------------------------> DEEP FOODS / LIVING						

Figure 1: The Spectrum of Diet™ in Westernized Cultures, David Rainoshek, M.A., www.JuiceFeasting.com

As we shift from left to right towards a plant-based diet, we also move from low nutrient- to high nutrient-density foods; from the creation of symptoms and disease to their transformation; dead food to vibrant, living food; maximum to minimum health care costs; below average to above average lifespan; millions dying of starvation to almost none; a *translative diet* of eating for comfort alone to a *transformative cuisine* of eating for personal growth. Research and data from nations worldwide show that moving to a plant-sourced diet means the possible prevention and elimination of overweight/obesity, heart disease, diabetes, arthritis, hypertension, depression, and constipation, just to name a few. Moving up the Spectrum of Diet™ is a transformation from a shallow narcissistic/egocentric existence of eating for oneself to an increasingly conscious, world-centric way of living.

Whole Food Vegan: the Foundation
When it comes to nutrition and eating a vegan diet, accessing and maintaining whole foods and vegan simultaneously is essential. Whole food veganism is the *foundation* of success at the next stage, raw/live vegan. Coca-Cola and french fries are all vegan, but pathological, unhealthy vegan that forgot something. In the raw/live food world, there is the widely popular, black-and-white notion that there are only two categories of food, and two only(!) – raw/live and cooked – with nothing in between. In this dichotomy, steamed vegetables are put in virtually the same category as fried chickens. According to this misguided idea, eating a 100% whole food, gluten-free, agave sweetened, fat free muffin with lots of organic berries in it, might as well be the nutritional equivalent of eating regular doughnuts, dairy ice cream, and topping it off with cookie dough! The notion that all plant-based whole foods subjected to any heat (like vegetables, grains, potatoes, squashes, legumes) are thus poison is hyperbole, misleading, and does a disservice to the extraordinary value of a healthy, whole foods vegan practice.

Many of us, in our understandable excitement about raw/live foods, go from junk foods to live foods, without a foundation of Whole Food veganism. When results are experienced, they are attributed to benefits of eating raw and living foods only. However, if you move through the Spectrum from junk foods and animal products to healthy, whole vegan foods like fruits, vegetables, nuts, seeds, etc, you are making bigger changes with the type of food you are eating than whether or not you're cooking it. Experience has shown when the foundation of whole foods vegan is ignored, you are likely to fail on raw foods, end up eating hardcore junk foods and/or becoming an ex-vegan. Inclusion of whole vegan foods and simultaneous jettisoning of animal products are the most important dietary foundations for success on a raw/live vegan program. These realities have always been true, but lately the game has re-organized itself at a higher, more exciting and inclusive level. Enter Vegan 2.0.

Vegan 2.0: log in
In the last 10 years, we at the plant-based levels of the Spectrum have shifted from Vegan 1.0 to Vegan 2.0. The vegan position, due to lack of a *critical amassing* of scientific data, articles, books, recipes, personal accounts and living examples (despite the dedicated and skilful effort of many teachers), has been relegated in the mind of the media and the general public. The popular image of vegans is anti-establishment political activists and eco-freak green nature lovers who still drive/live in VWs, grow (wheat)grass, wear flowers in their hair, or wax poetic about the Aquarian Age. At Vegan 1.0, proponents, as a group, lacked sufficient technology to interconnect in a way that matched what they were saying:

The true reality is that all things are interconnected, and what we eat is of fundamental importance to every aspect of existence.

Then around 1995, the Internet exploded onto the scene... and a massive potential opened up. Welcome to Vegan 2.0, where we are ordering books online, reading 35 different blog and news site feeds, watching scientific data, professional guidance, and personal accounts that stream generously from free video technology and meeting on a variety of social networking sites. In Vegan 2.0 you are totally hooked in to podcasts, your ipod is loaded with talks on nutrition and life transformation, you access cacao from Ecuador, maca from Peru, goji berries from Tibet, have tried ten different superfood powders. Your online profiles are pimped in shades of green, brown, and blue to the delight of your educated group of friends in numerous international locations and of diverse educational levels, cultural backgrounds, and persuasions. The days of *maybe* catching John Robbins' *Diet for a New America* on PBS, or ordering it on VHS (allow 6 weeks for delivery) are over – you can watch it online this minute, along with thousands of other excellent documentaries to support you on your path of complete health, not as a destination, but as an unfolding experience you can share with others internationally, instantaneously.

Finally, you have recognized that in many ways, when it comes to health and nutrition, you can find out more in a 15-minute search than those folks with the letters after their names ever knew, or the health reports in the media ever revealed. Healing has evolved into transformation, before/after pictures, and videos have become global inspirations, and health challenges have become exciting opportunities to open up to a community of people who are going on a hero's journey of self – and global – discovery. The fear (of being alone, being sick, or not getting your protein) is lifting, and in its place we are finding fascination. Vegan 2.0 is cool because everyone (not just the romantic wheatgrass Aquarians) is now invited, from teens who want to be smarter than their parents to parents who want to catch up with their kids! The invitation is global! Enter quilt-making grandparents who don't want arthritis – or global warming – or war for petroleum resources; politicians who see *significant increases* in overweight/ obesity and want better health for their nation; activists seeking an end to hunger and CEOs after better job performance and lower health insurance rates for their companies; Health practitioners who want to be more effective and parents who want healthier babies join the growing band of people who want the health that Vegan delivers.

One of the reasons it is cool is due to the challenges we face internationally. 21st Century challenges and the simultaneous rise of information technology are quickly ushering us from the ego- and sociocentric (what's best for me and those around me) to worldcentric (I eat and live as an act of love for all). Due to our recognized and obvious global interconnection and perfect storm of challenges, an exciting and new kind of activism has presented itself.

Plant-based: Current fad or perennial wisdom?
"A human being is part of the whole called by us universe, a part limited in time

and space. He experiences himself, his thoughts and feelings as something separated from the rest, a kind of optical delusion of his consciousness. This delusion is a kind of prison for us, restricting us to our personal desires and to affection for a few persons nearest to us. Our task must be to free ourselves from this prison by widening our circle of compassion to embrace all living creatures and the whole of nature in its beauty." – Albert Einstein

The history of eating a diet of plant foods, abstaining from meat eating, fasting and drinking plant juices, and using herbs to heal goes back possibly farther than recorded history. Hippocrates, the father of medicine (460–357 BC) said, *"He who does not know food, how can he understand the diseases of man?"* Genesis 1:29 is a pretty early Biblical endorsement of a plant-source diet: *"See, I give you every seed-bearing plant that is upon all the earth, and every tree that has seed-bearing fruit; they shall be yours for food."* Howard Williams' *The Ethics of Diet* outlines a long history of abstaining from flesh-eating (*kreophagy*) and eating a plant-based diet, citing more than 50 major Western thinkers such as Hesiod, Pythagorus, Plato, Socrates, Ovid, Seneca, Plutarch, Thomas More, Voltaire, Rousseau, Isaac Newton, Shelley, Leonardo DaVinci, Schopenhauer, and Albert Einstein (who is great to quote, because no one is going to be quick to argue against the intelligence that developed the General Theory of Relativity). *This is no fad*; it is rooted deeply in our cultural, spiritual, scientific, ecological, and genetic heritage. It is truly a diet and lifestyle that significantly meet the needs of our times. With that, let's look at what our bodies are best suited and designed to eat.

Our food: Do you want …. with that?
It is important to establish generally what we all need and want in our food, and what we want as a result of eating it. Later we can use these orienting generalizations to see whether the food we are eating fits the bill. Health pioneer Paul Bragg used to say, *"I want to talk with you about the most important person in the world, and that is you. You are a universe within yourself".* So what does your own personal universe require from food?

Nutritional elements
Protein (leafy greens are 20–30% protein)
Fat (including omega-3,6, and 9 fatty acids)
Carbohydrates
Minerals (numerous sources suggest we need 92 mineral elements for optimal health)
Enzymes (only live, plant-based food sources contain living enzymes)
Phytonutrients-vitamins-antioxidants-chlorophyll (plants contain hundreds or thousands of essential health-protecting/promoting phytonutrients)
Probiotics (healthy, beneficial *flora* for digestive health)
Water (cooking and processing evaporates away valuable water from our food)

When these elements are in play, we have what Dr. Richard Anderson defines as a true food[22]: "I propose that the true definition of a food is as follows: a substance that nourishes or fuels the body with life-giving forces (i.e. life-force, vitamins, minerals, enzymes, amino acids, etc.) without injury to its normal functions, thereby strengthening, energizing, and maintaining it. Food is not simply something one puts in the mouth, chews, and swallows. Food should not deplete or rob the body of its needed essence or harm it in any way."

Beyond providing the basic nutritional elements for maintenance of health and disease prevention, we can all agree that our food should not deplete the body of what it already has. Furthermore, we don't want our food to harm us from added chemicals, processing, irradiation, genetic modification, or any other modification from its health-promoting original state.

Whole foods: click!
A shift to the level of whole foods is for many of us the first time we approach foods consciously – beyond what our taste buds tell us. If not, consider your-self lucky, but either way Whole Food is an aspect of the Spectrum not to be left behind. Many of us move to whole foods because we realize *we have been screwed.* The food we have been eating at the fast food and SAD (Standard American diet) stages is lacking in essential nutrients, is chock-full of things we definitely don't want, and may be making us feel like the floor of a bathroom. So what do we incorporate, and what do we leave behind with whole foods?

Junk overboard
Perhaps even before thinking about the toxic elements in your processed food, you begin to remove and replace toxic products with more natural options in your cleaning and personal supplies – kitchen, laundry, bathroom, make-up, tooth-paste, soap. According to Randall Fitzgerald, author of *The Hundred Year Lie,* *"...we each use nine personal care products daily, containing about 126 chemi-cal ingredients."* You may get also get a water filter to remove chlorine, fluoride, PCBs, agrochemicals and industrial chemicals from your water. And you throw out the microwave in favor of not practicing any more nuclear experimentation with your food or the body that eats it.

In your cupboard, out go the refined and hydrogenated vegetable oils, iodized salt, processed white sugar, white flour, packages of McDonald's ketchup and Taco Bell mustard, Wonder Bread, Skippy peanut butter, multi-colored cake sprinkles, canned fruits in corn syrup, instant mashed potatoes, baking powder, MSG excitotoxin-laden chips, the NutraSweet and Splenda, the Fruit Loops and Count Chocula, instant coffee, food colorings, instant noodles, and the infamous Twinkies. You head to your refrigerator/freezer with a garbage bag, and toss in the frozen dinners, margarine, popsicles, salad dressings, jello, soda, instant lemonade, Jimmy Dean Chocolate Chip Pancakes and Sausage on a Stick, "en-ergy" drinks... It's a real tour of Culinary Americana, and while part of you grieves the loss, the miraculous being you truly are is glad to be taking your first strong steps out of the Dietary Matrix.

New prizes
When one pantry or refrigerator door closes, a new one opens. With Whole Food, you develop an awareness of what is in the food you are eating. Whole foods retain many of the essential nutrients your body needs. The fiber is back

– and we are not talking about bran muffins, but the natural fiber in whole fruits and vegetables. The colors in your food are now phytonutrients, the flavors are authentic, more vitamins and minerals are present, working in a positive synergy to help your body assimilate much needed nutrition.

In your kitchen you have replaced Culinary Americana with fresh fruits, vegetables, nuts, seeds, sea vegetables, cold pressed oils, and herbs. You have Celtic sea salt, Himalayan salt, miso, or gluten-free tamari. The instant dinners are still there, but now they are organic and made from whole foods – much better. You buy foods from the bulk section – whole grains, beans, and brown rice. You are more inclined to steam your foods rather than fry them, and beneficial herbal teas, instead of coffee, become good till the last drop.

Your first experience of this is a new sense of being a self-directed, autonomous person taking greater conscious control of your health. You begin to recognize that the predominant determining factors to your health are not genetics, but your environment, lifestyle, and diet. You recognize that you are what you eat. As Sam Graci says in *The Food Connection*, you ask yourself, *"Do I want* this *food to become my face, hair, energy, thinking, moods, bones, muscles, organs, or immune system?"*

Your food is more *satiating* because your body is getting more nutrition and fiber. This enables you to eat fewer calories than before, promoting healthy weight and longevity. Your digestion is better, and your bowel movements are more regular. Because your carbohydrates are not processed, you have decreased the glycemic index of your diet, which begins to limit blood sugar spikes and precipitous blood sugar crashes often experienced with white flour and sugar. You begin to leave behind the chances of developing diabetes. Whole foods are more hydrating, therefore mental function, hormone balance, immune system function, sleep, and other health realities related to hydration improve.

Health challenges begin to resolve. Moving up the Spectrum to Whole Food Vegan, people have lost tremendous amounts of weight, greatly enhanced their endurance and athletic performance, sky-rocketed their energy, and overcome cancers, heart disease, strokes, arthritis, osteoporosis, etc. Moving up the Spectrum from here will further these positive impacts, but Whole Foods Vegan is a significant step.

Who are you? – comparative anatomy

"You put a baby in a crib with an apple and a rabbit. If it eats the rabbit and plays with the apple, I'll buy you a new car." – Harvey Diamond, author of Fit for Life

Ever put sugar in the gas tank of your car? In *the late 1800s* Rudolph Diesel brilliantly designed his diesel engine to burn vegetable-based fuels, which, evidently, creates the fewest emissions, best gas mileage, least wear and tear, and hence the longest engine life. Everything that moves has a design, and fuel sources that match it, for greatest function, efficiency, and lifespan. If we are to discover what our "natural" diet is – our best fuel source – one that honors our true nature, and uncovers our greatest capacities, we need to begin at a place free of the *potentially* limited or partial perspectives of religious views (Jesus ate it, the Buddha did not eat that, the ancient folks made it this way); egocentrism (what I want); socio-centrism (what is best for my group); world-centrism (what is best for the world); Darwinism (survival of the fittest, baby); our ideas of what past cultures ate (caveman diet), and get down to who we are anatomically. Then, we will have a much better foundation and appreciation for the modern scientific data we now have on diet, health, and longevity with plant-based cuisine.

Comparative anatomy works on the simple and demonstrable fact that the biological form usually defines function. The science of comparative anatomy provides us with an indicator of *human nutrition* which was not established by culture, but is certainly that of a herbivore or frugivore, and not a carnivore or omnivore.

Figure 2 on the following page is a chart from "The Comparative Anatomy of Eating" by Dr Milton Mills, comparing the typical anatomical features of carnivores, omnivores, herbivores, and humans. Notice how closely human physical characteristics match those of herbivores.[23]

Paleontologist Richard Leakey, widely acknowledged as one of the world's foremost experts on the evolution of the human diet, sums it up well: *"You can't tear flesh by hand, you can't tear hide by hand. We don't have large canine teeth, and we wouldn't have been able to deal with food sources that required those large canines."* And even if you had large canine teeth, would you want to bite into a deer as it walks past?

Organic: Is there anything in it?
"A nation that destroys its soils destroys itself." – US President Franklin D. Roosevelt

In the United States alone in the 1990s, an average of 4.5 billion pounds of pesticides were used each year and another 700 million pounds exported. – USDA Data

Agrochemicals can affect every living organism. The most detrimental effects of pesticides, herbicides, and fungicides include cancer, nervous system disorders, birth defects, alterations of DNA, liver or kidney, lung, and reproductive problems, and an overall disruption of ecological cycles of the planet. Pesticide usage is a major public health problem worldwide. For a deeper understanding of the importance of organic foods, please see chapter two. With increased nutrients in hand, additives and toxins jettisoned, and a recognition that maybe our bodies are not so well designed to eat animal products, what do things look like?

Vegan: the territory
"There is no disease, bodily or mental, which adoption of a vegetable diet and pure water has not infallibly mitigated, wherever the experiment has been fairly tried." – Percy Bysshe Shelley (1792-1822), English poet

Comparative anatomy chart (Figure 2)

Feature	Carnivore	Herbivore	Omnivore	Human
Facial Muscles	Reduced to allow wide mouth gape	Well-developed	Reduced	Well-developed
Jaw Type	Angle not expanded	Expanded angle	Angle not expanded	Expanded angle
Jaw Joint Location	On same plane as molar teeth	Above the plane of the molars	On same plane as molar teeth	Above the plane of the molars
Jaw Motion	Shearing; minimal side-to-side motion	No shear; good side-to-side, front-to-back	Shearing; minimal side-to-side	No shear; good side-to-side, front-to-back
Major Jaw Muscles	Temporalis	Masseter and pterygoids	Temporalis	Masseter and pterygoids
Mouth Opening vs. Head Size	Large	Small	Large	Small
Teeth: Incisors	Short and pointed	Broad, flattened and spade shaped	Short and pointed	Broad, flattened and spade shaped
Teeth: Canines	Long, sharp and curved	Dull and short or long (for defense), or none	Long, sharp and curved	Short and blunted
Teeth: Molars	Sharp, jagged and blade shaped	Flattened with cusps vs. complex surface	Sharp blades and/or flattened	Flattened with nodular cusps
Chewing	None; swallows food whole	Extensive chewing necessary	Swallows food whole and/or simple crushing	Extensive chewing necessary
Saliva	No digestive enzymes and Acidic	Carbohydrate digesting enzymes And Acidic	No digestive enzymes	Carbohydrate digesting enzymes And Acidic
Blood	Acidic	Alkaline		Alkaline
Urine	Acidic	Alkaline	Acidic	Alkaline
Stomach Acidity	Less than or equal to pH 1 with food in stomach	pH 4 to 5 with food in stomach	Less than or equal to pH 1 with food in stomach	pH 4 to 5 with food in stomach
Stomach Capacity	60% to 70% of total volume of digestive tract	Less than 30% of total volume of digestive tract	60% to 70% of total volume of digestive tract	21% to 27% of total volume of digestive tract
Length of Small Intestine	3 to 6 times trunk length	10 to 12+ times trunk length	4 to 6 times trunk length	10 to 12 times trunk length
Colon	Simple, short and smooth, no fermentation	Long, complex; may be sacculated, may ferment	Simple, short and smooth, no fermentation	Long, sacculated, may ferment
Liver	Can detoxify vitamin A	Cannot detoxify vitamin A	Can detoxify vitamin A	Cannot detoxify vitamin A
Liver	Contains *uricase*, an enzyme used to break down uric acid	Low tolerance for uric acid		Low tolerance for uric acid
Kidney	Extremely concentrated urine	Moderately concentrated urine	Extremely concentrated urine	Moderately concentrated urine
Nails	Sharp claws	Flattened nails or blunt hooves	Sharp claws	Flattened nails
Thermostasis	Hyperventilation (via the mouth)	Perspiration (via the skin)	Hyperventilation (via the mouth)	Perspiration (via the skin)

Figure 2: Comparative Anatomy Chart adapted from *The Comparative Anatomy of Eating* by Milton R. Mills, M.D., and *The Sunfood Diet Success System* by David Wolfe

Eating a plant-based diet greatly reduces your risk of preventable diseases, adding "years to your life and life to your years." We are going to get down to the scientific nitty gritty on why we don't eat animals, but first let's step back and take a much larger view of why this is generally such an unhealthy practice by looking at the nature of physical reality. When it comes to your food, you want as few possibilities for screw-ups as possible while still receiving all the nourishment you require. Spinach does not get cancer, but livestock do. Eating complex organisms like animals means a greater likelihood that you are going to ingest things that create chaos instead of order in your own complex system. The further you move up the protein chain, the more concentrated environmental toxins become. If there is toxicity in their air, water, and/or food environment—chemicals, pesticides, herbicides, larvicides, fungicides, detergents, bleaches, solvents—these toxins accumulate in the animal. Dairy products contain five times as many pesticides as commercial fruits and vegetables. Flesh foods, such as fish or chicken, contain 15 times as many pesticide residues as commercial fruits and vegetables.[24] The Environmental Protection Agency estimates that fish can accumulate up to *nine million times* the level of PCBs than the water they live in. Animals are a major source of pesticide exposure.[25]

A study published in the *Diet and Nutrition Letter* of Tufts University reported that the more fish pregnant mothers ate, the more their babies showed abnormal reflexes, general weakness, slower responses to stimuli, and signs of depression.[26] In a follow-up study there was a definite correlation between the amount of fish the mothers ate and the child's brain development, even if fish was eaten only once a month. The more fish the pregnant mothers ate, the lower the verbal IQ of the children was.[27] These children also had lower SAT scores 17 to 18 years later. Children, usually the most sensitive to toxins, are prime indicators of what may be happening to adults on a more subtle level. In short, we want to eat simpler food, lower on the food chain that does not have as many opportunities to gather toxins, or contain chaos-creating elements. In the move up the Spectrum of Diet, people typically drop meat first, then dairy, so let's begin there. Then we will get into the scientific research and cross-cultural data.

General downsides of eating meat
First, let it be said that we cannot qualify meat as "not food". Many cultures throughout human history up to the present day have used meat as an important part of their diet. The authors grew up on it. It is food and can be used for food. We are not demonizing meat-eating – *we are going to put it in proper context vis-à-vis human, ecological, economic, and social health*, and illustrate conclusively why those wanting excellent health are compelled to move beyond meat and dairy.

We need to move beyond meat because of the associations with:

- Uric acid from protein metabolism, leading to osteoporosis, arthritis, gout, kidney stones, acid/alkaline imbalance
- Very low in calcium versus phosphorus
- Toxic iron
- No fiber (constipating)
- High in saturated fat & cholesterol
- Increased heart disease, diabetes, strokes, cancers, inflammatory disease
- High exposure to hormones and antibiotics used in farming industry
- High exposure to agrochemicals, industrial chemicals, heavy metals

General downsides of eating dairy

Dairy is a tough one for many of us to move beyond, and it's not the milk – *it's the cheese*. Whether raw or pasteurized, there are opioids called *casomorphins* in cows' milk that make it very addictive. According to Dr. Neal Barnard, MD, President of the Physician's Committee for Responsible Medicine, the strongest morphinogenic compound in dairy is as powerful as 1/10th the power of pure morphine. When it comes to nutrition, the risks and results of eating dairy products are less than desirable, and include increased heart disease, cancers, overweight, asthma, osteoporosis, diabetes, and allergies. John McDougall lays this out clearly in his talk *"On the Perils of Dairy Products"*, and Robert Cohen is straight to the point in his interview, *"Milk: The Deadly Poison."* According to Michael Anderson in his excellent video, *Eating, "Drinking three glasses of milk a day is the artery-clogging equivalent of eating 21 slices of bacon. A pint of ice cream is the equivalent of 24 slices of bacon."*

That's just gross. One cubic centimeter (cc) of commercial cow's milk is allowed to have up to 750,000 somatic cells ("pus") and 20,000 live bacteria before it is unfit for sale. This equals a whopping 20 million live, squiggly bacteria and up to 750 *million* pus cells per liter. Besides pus cells and blood, normal now in milk produced with machines, milk is also high in pesticides, herbicides, antibiotics, hormones, radioactive iodine, and disease factors such as mad cow prion and bovine leukemia virus.

Casein. Another problem with milk is that 87% of the protein in milk is *casein*, which is a known carcinogen. Casein is a powerful binder, a polymer used to make plastics, and a tenacious glue. *Caseinate* is the main component in Elmer's glue, and a lot of home furniture is held together with it. So too is the label affixed to a bottle of beer. If you are a beer drinker, good luck trying to scrape that label off.

Why we need to move beyond dairy:

- Dairy is highly allergenic and mucus forming, and contributes to asthma
- Most people are lactose intolerant
- Milk is for babies
- Addictive casomorphins
- *Promotes* osteoporosis, heart disease, diabetes (Type-1 and Type-2)
- Concentrates environmental toxins
- High in the cancer-promoting protein, casein

- Highly constipating
- Eating the animals own metabolic wastes (endogenous)

Meat and dairy: health challenges and biological data
"People occasionally stumble across the truth, but most of them pick themselves up and hurry off as if nothing ever happened." – Winston Churchill

Overweight/Obesity
According to T. Colin Campbell, PhD, numerous studies have shown that vegetarians and vegans are slimmer than their meat-eating counterparts. People in these studies who are vegetarian or vegan are anywhere from five to 30 pounds slimmer than their fellow citizens.[28, 29, 30, 31, 32, 33, 34] If you are overweight or obese, this condition generally goes hand in hand with the other conditions we are about to discuss that are promoted by eating animal products.

Diabetes
A quarter pound of beef raises insulin levels in diabetics as much as a quarter pound of straight sugar. – Diabetes Care 7, 1984, p. 465
Cheese and beef elevate insulin levels higher than "dreaded" high-carbohydrate foods like pasta. – American Journal of Clinical Nutrition 50, 1997, p. 1264
A single burger's worth of beef, or three slices of cheddar cheese, boost insulin levels more than almost two cups of cooked pasta. – American Journal of Clinical Nutrition 50, 1997, p. 1264

Meat and dairy are *diabetogenic*. Let's look briefly at meat and dairy in particular, and why the scientific data confirm that they are diabetes-causing foods. Studies have shown that Seventh-Day Adventist men who ate meat six or more days a week had 3.8 times greater risk of having diabetes mentioned on their death certificates compared with Seventh-Day Adventists who were lacto-ovo-vegetarians.[35] This would not be unexpected, as meat contains considerable cholesterol and saturated fat, resulting in a higher risk of atherosclerosis, the major cause of death among diabetics. The unexpected finding was that 20 years prior, at the outset of the study, those who were non-diabetic were more apt to get diabetes if they were in the habit of consuming meat.

ASSOCIATION OF COW'S MILK CONSUMPTION AND INCIDENCE OF TYPE 1 DIABETES IN DIFFERENT COUNTRIES

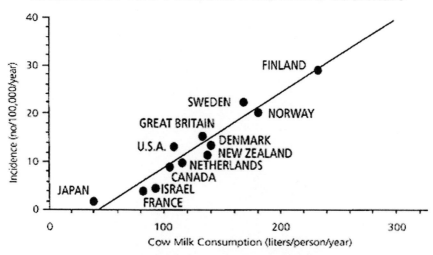

Figure 3: Association of Cow's Milk Consumption and Incidence of Type-1 Diabetes in Different Countries from *The China Study* by T. Colin Campbell

Another study in Finland showed that the consumption of cow's milk increased the rate of Type-1 diabetes by 500–600%.[36] The overall results strongly suggest that cow's milk, especially in children who are genetically susceptible and who are weaned before three months, significantly increases the risk of developing Type-1 diabetes. For more excellent information on diabetes and diet, please see Section Two of this book.

Heart disease
"Ninety to ninety-seven percent of heart disease, the cause of more than one half of the deaths in the United States, could be prevented by a vegetarian diet." – *1961 Journal of the American Medical Association.*[37]

One of the most famous plant-based heart disease reversal studies was conducted by Harvard graduate Dr. Dean Ornish in his Lifestyle Heart Trial. His 28 patients ate an almost 100% plant-based diet for a year, with the exception of egg whites and one cup a day of non-fat dairy. Patients exercised for three hours a week, and met as a group with Dr. Ornish for support. No drugs or surgeries were involved. The results? Dr. Ornish's patients' LDL (bad) cholesterol dropped 40%. The frequency, duration, and severity of their chest pain decreased dramatically. On angiograms, artery shrinkage could be seen in a whopping 82% of his patients, with no surgical intervention or drugs. Dr. Ornish's program has been so successful, dozens of insurance providers in the US cover the costs for their patients.

This success was duplicated by Dr. Caldwell B. Esselstyn of the Cleveland Clinic. Dr. Esselstyn's study[38] showed the reversal of cardiovascular disease with a 100% success rate among patients who followed a vegan diet with *no cooked oil.*[39] If you, or a friend or loved ones, have cardiovascular disease, the next two figures below may be the most important things you see in your life, and are resounding evidence of the need for a diet of plant foods.

**CORONARY ARTERY BEFORE AND AFTER
CONSUMING PLANT-BASED DIET**

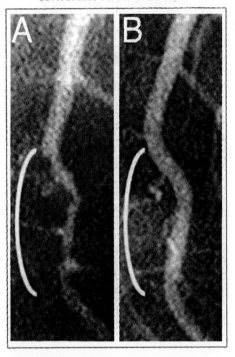

Figure 4: Coronary angiograms of the distal left anterior descending artery before (A) and after (B) thirty-two months of a plant-based diet without cholesterol-lowering medication, showing profound improvement from Dr. Caldwell B Esselstyn, www.HeartAttackProof.com

What you are seeing on the right side is the opening of a coronary artery after 32 months on a plant-based diet. Yet heart disease is one of our leading causes of death in Westernized nations. The second figure supporting the case for diet as the underlying cause or prevention for heart disease is found in *Eat to Live* by Dr. Joel Fuhrman.[40]

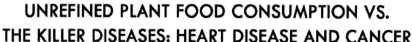

UNREFINED PLANT FOOD CONSUMPTION VS.
THE KILLER DISEASES: HEART DISEASE AND CANCER

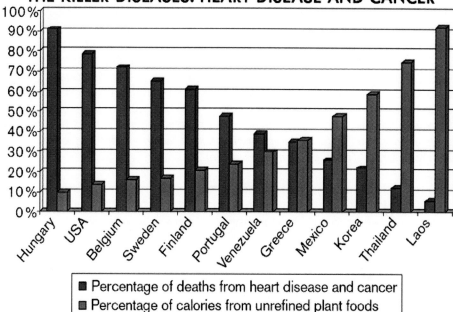

■ Percentage of deaths from heart disease and cancer
■ Percentage of calories from unrefined plant foods

Figure 5: Unrefined plant food consumption and the killer diseases: heart disease and cancer. Source: *Eat to Live* **by Dr. Joel Fuhrman, MD www.DrFurhman.com**

Populations with low death rates from the major killer diseases are populations that consume more than 75% of their calories from unrefined plant foods, and almost never have overweight members. According to Dr. Joel Fuhrman, this is at least ten times more unrefined plant-based foods than the average American consumes.[41]

Breast and prostate cancer

According to a study cited in the journal *Cancer*, men who drank three or more glasses a day of whole milk had a 2.49 times increase in prostate cancer.[42] A 2001 Harvard review of the research put a finer point on it:

Twelve of ... fourteen case-control studies and seven of ... nine cohort studies [have] observed a positive association for some measure of dairy products and prostate cancer; this is one of the most consistent dietary predictors for prostate cancer in the published literature. In these studies, men with the highest dairy intakes had approximately double the risk of total prostate cancer, and up to a fourfold increase in risk of metastatic or fatal prostate cancer relative to low consumers.[43]

Insight into this cancer and dairy food connection is provided by the life-long work of T. Colin Campbell, PhD from Cornell University, who did a 27-year study,

The China Study, jointly arranged by Cornell, Oxford, and the Chinese Academy of Preventive Medicine. It involved 6,500 persons in China and investigated the role of protein in promoting cancer. They found one protein that consistently and strongly promoted cancer: the casein in cow's milk. **Casein is 87% of the protein in dairy, and it promotes all stages of the cancer process.** *What were the safe proteins they found in their study? Those from plant sources.* In fact, their research found that the people who ate the most plant-based foods were the healthiest and tended to avoid chronic disease. More importantly, they discovered through the findings of other researchers and clinicians worldwide, as we have, that *"the diet that has time and again been shown to reverse and/ or prevent [diseases caused by animal protein consumption] is the same whole- foods, plant-based diet found to promote optimal health."* According to T. Colin Campbell, PhD, *"The findings are consistent."*

The chart below illustrates that the lowest rates of breast and prostate cancer are consistently in China and Japan, where dairy and animal meat is rarely eaten.

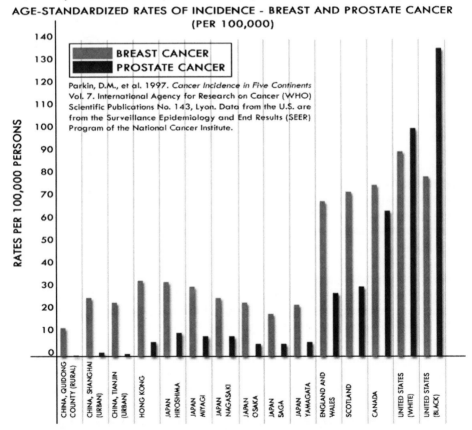

Figure 6: Age-Standardized Rates of Incidence: Breast and Prostate Can- cer. Data Source: The No Dairy Breast Cancer Prevention Program by Dr. Jane Plant, Ph.D

As Jane Plant, PhD remarks in *The No Dairy Breast Cancer Prevention Program*:

"The Japanese cities of Hiroshima and Nagasaki have similar rates of breast cancer: and remember, both cities were attacked with nuclear weapons, so in addition to the usual pollution-related cancers, one would also expect to find some radiation-related cases. If, as a North American woman, one was living a Japanese lifestyle in industrialized, irradiated Hiroshima, you would slash your risk of contracting breast cancer by a half to a third. The conclusion is inescapable. Clearly, some lifestyle factor not related to pollution, urbanization, or the environment is seriously increasing the Western woman's chance of contracting breast cancer." [44]

Dr. Plant continues:
"We know...the huge difference in breast and prostate cancer rates between Eastern and Western countries, isn't genetic. Migration studies show that when Chinese or Japanese people move to the West, within one or two generations their rates of incidence and mortality from breast and prostate cancer approach those of their host community." [45]

Osteoporosis

Osteoporosis is significantly higher in meat eaters and women who drink three or more glasses of milk per day. Research suggests that the higher amounts of protein create an acidity that forces the bones to give up calcium to neutralize the acidity. According to Dr Neal Barnard, *"Animal proteins are high in sulfur containing amino acids. These acidic protein-building blocks tend to leach calcium from the bones, and that calcium passes through the kidneys and into the urine."* [46] Citing a 1980 study in the journal *Clinical Orthopedics and Related Research,* Mark Hegsted of Harvard University points out that people in the US and Scandinavian countries consume more dairy products than anywhere else in the world, yet have the highest rates of osteoporosis. [47] A 1985 study in *The American Journal of Clinical Nutrition* suggests that dairy products offer no protection against osteoporosis. [48]

The bottom line is that calcium deficiency is not a threat to someone eating a plant-source-only cuisine. Inadequate calcium intake appears not to be a problem at all. According to C.R. Patterson in the *Postgraduate Medical Journal* in 1978, *"In Western countries the usual calcium intake is of the order of 800-1000 mg/ day; in many developing countries figures of 300-500 mg/day are found. There is no evidence that people with such a low intake have any problems with bones or teeth. It seems likely that normal people can adapt to have a normal calcium balance on calcium intakes as low as 150-200 mg/day and that this adaptation is sufficient even in pregnancy and lactation."* [49]

One of our very best sources of calcium is leafy greens. In The Sunfood Diet Success System, David Wolfe writes, *"The body best assimilates calcium when both magnesium and manganese are present together. Green leafy vegetables are high in magnesium, manganese, and silicon. One to two pounds of whole or juiced green-leafy vegetables will be adequate."* [50] Our best high-calcium foods are sesame seeds, dulse, Irish moss, kelp, and leafy greens, as well as most seeds, nuts, and grains.

Allergies and lactose intolerance

Cow's milk is the number one cause of food allergies among infants and children, according to the American Gastroenterological Association.[51] Most people begin to produce less lactase, the enzyme that helps with the digestion of milk, when they are as young as two years old. This reduction can lead to lactose intolerance.[52] Millions of Americans are lactose intolerant, and an estimated 90% of Asian Americans and 75% of Native- and African Americans suffer from the condition, which can cause bloating, gas, cramps, vomiting, headaches, rashes, and asthma.[53] Studies have also found that autism and schizophrenia in children may be linked to the body's inability to digest the milk protein casein; symptoms of these diseases diminished or disappeared in 80% of the children who were switched to milk-free diets.[54] A UK study showed that people who were suffering from irregular heartbeats, asthma, headaches, fatigue, and digestive problems *"showed marked and often complete improvements in their health after cutting milk from their diets."*[55] Research cited by Robert Cohen, author of *Don't Drink Your Milk,* states that there is up to a gallon of extra mucus in the body created by drinking dairy.

Where do you get your ....?

What is probably dawning on you is that more important than, "Where do you get your _____?" is the question, "Where do you get your information?" Agribusiness, pharmaceutical and medical organizations, the media who advertise them and the companies that sell their products have gone to great lengths since the early 1900s to craft social policies, practices, and personal opinion away from a plant-based diet. Following is some good information and resources on how to answer common questions in your own mind, and those that may arise from well-meaning family, friends, co-workers, and even health professionals.

The benefits of a plant-based diet is professionally recognized by the American Dietetic Association (ADA), the world's largest organization of professional dieticians which published the following statements in June 2003 on a vegetarian diet and lifestyle:[56]

Vegetarians have been reported to have lower body mass indices than non-vegetarians, as well as lower rates of death from ischemic heart disease; vegetarians also show lower blood cholesterol levels; lower blood pressure; and lower rates of hypertension, Type-2 diabetes, and prostate and colon cancer. Well-planned vegan and other types of vegetarian diets are appropriate for all stages of the life cycle, including during pregnancy, lactation, infancy, childhood, and adolescence. Vegetarian diets offer a number of nutritional benefits, including lower levels of saturated fat, cholesterol, and animal protein, as well as higher levels of carbohydrates, fiber, magnesium, potassium, folate, and antioxidants such as vitamins C and E and phytochemicals....

It is the position of the American Dietetic Association and Dietitians of Canada that appropriately planned vegetarian diets are healthful, nutritionally adequate and provide health benefits in the prevention and treatment of certain diseases.

Protein: no question

Vegans get their dietary protein from the most abundant protein source on the planet: plants. Plant protein, such as greens, builds animals such as buffalo, elephants, gorillas and giraffes into some of the largest animals on earth. If you are eating sufficient Whole Food vegan calories, you are getting ample protein. Proteins are constructed as long chains of hundreds or thousands of amino acids, of which there are 15–20 different kinds. Some amino acids can be made by the body from other aminos, but eight essential amino acids must be provided by food.

Protein combining

Fortunately, this is a non-issue. In their Position Paper on Vegetarian Diets, The American Dietetic Association states:

"Plant protein can meet requirements when a variety of plant foods is consumed and energy needs are met. Research indicates that an assortment of plant foods eaten over the course of a day can provide all essential amino acids and ensure adequate nitrogen retention and use in healthy adults, thus complementary proteins do not need to be consumed at the same meal."

How much?

We need between 25–35 grams of uncooked plant protein per day. The Journal of Clinical Nutrition states that we need approximately 2.5% of our total calories to be protein. This is approximately 18 grams of protein per day. The World Health Organization suggests 4.5% of our calories, or about 32 grams per day. According to Chittenden's extensive studies on soldiers and athletes, 30–50 grams per day is a sufficient window for maximum physical performance.[57] Human mother's milk has about 1.4% of its calories as protein, and that is for a growing baby. During pregnancy, a mother's body requires more protein, and during the developmental years through age 20, protein needs shift, striking above the adult average from ages 10–20.

The risk we are running in the Westernized world is eating *too much protein*, specifically animal protein. The overeating of animal protein is behind many Western diseases, such as heart disease, diabetes, cancers, kidney damage, osteoporosis, schizophrenia, arthritis, premature aging and shorter life expectancy. If you are just getting into plant-based foods, remember that when you think you are craving high-protein meat, you are probably hungry for *fat*, not protein, hence many vegans use nuts for protein.

Where do you get it?

Legumes (30–50% protein)
Soybeans
Tempeh
Tofu
Lentils
Chickpeas

Kidney beans
Black beans
Peas, etc.
(Note: raw legumes not recommended)

Green Vegetables (15–30% protein)
Spinach
Watercress
Arugula
Kale
Broccoli
Brussels sprouts
Collard greens
Parsley
Sea vegetables (Kelp, Nori, Dulse, Arame, Wakame, Hijiki, Kombu)

Superfoods (up to 65% protein)
Spirulina
Klamath Lake blue-green algae.
Chlorella
Bee pollen
Powdered grasses
Green superfood powder concentrates

Nuts and Seeds
Hemp seeds, flax seeds, chia seeds, pumpkin seeds, sunflower seeds, walnuts, almonds, sesame seeds, cashews, filberts, brazil nuts

Iron
According to Dr Gabriel Cousens, *"Close to 57% of meat eaters are deficient in iron. Vitamin C in fruits and vegetables naturally amplifies the assimilation of iron, which may explain why vegetarians have less iron deficiency than meat eaters."*[58]
Iron is toxic from both animal products and supplements. Iron is an oxidant (it increases free radical activity in the body). Excess iron is also strongly associated with heart disease. There is no toxicity of iron from whole plant sources, as it is only absorbed when needed. Plant sources include: spirulina, dulse, kelp, black cherries, blackberries, raisins, leafy greens, and chlorophyll. For more on chlorophyll, which is excellent for improving iron levels, please see chapter nine.

B-12
This is an important topic. We have a whole chapter devoted to this subject in this book, so for more up-to-date goodies on this topic, see chapter sixteen. Briefly, vitamin B-12 deficiency is not a vegan-specific issue. Non-vegans can, and regularly do, become ill due to B-12 deficiency. Fringe, limited vegan diets (such as strict fruitarian) are often deficient in B-12. This does not apply to sensible veganism. The bottom line is that everyone has the potential to be B-12 deficient, vegan or not. Take the easy, vegan steps to prevent this avoidable health challenge, as discussed in chapter sixteen.

Vitamin D: clever vegans

In June 2007, The American Journal of Clinical Nutrition released astounding results of a clinical trial in which the effect of administering 1,000 IU/day of vitamin D (with calcium) was evaluated in 1,180 women. After only four years, they found an astounding 77% reduction in cancer incidence in the group receiving vitamin D compared with placebo. According to William Faloon of Life Extension Magazine, *"We have identified 89 studies that describe how greater vitamin D levels reduce cancers of the breast, prostate, colon, esophagus, pancreas, ovary, rectum, bladder, kidney, lung and uterus, as well as non-Hodgkin's lymphoma and multiple myeloma."*[59]

Where do we get this miracle Vitamin? The best source is the sun. If you are fair skinned, 15–20 minutes a day of sunlight will do you. If your skin pigment is darker, however, you do not get anywhere near the level of vitamin D from the sun, and this is why such high levels of breast and prostate cancer are seen among people of color living in northern climates. Therefore, if you have dark skin, you need more sun, or vitamin D from plant sources and/or plant-based vitamin D2 (ergocalciferol) supplementation, which the body will convert to D3 as needed.[60] Good plant sources are alfalfa, nettles, kelp, chickweed, many mushrooms and HealthForce Vitamineral™ Green, which contains plants high in non-toxic, vegan vitamin D. However, note that nothing other than actual sun can replace the sun for Vitamin D.

Essential fats

Essential fatty acids (EFAs) have many vital functions. They increase metabolic rate, improve metabolism, increase oxygen uptake, and increase energy production. EFAs and what the body makes from them are components of membranes that surround each cell. You will find more information on EFA's in chapter ten; don't miss it!

No boundary: ecology

We are interdependent with our environment, and the ecological costs of food production to raise livestock for meat and dairy are alarming. According to the United Nations Food and Agriculture Organization, the livestock sector generates more greenhouse gas emissions as measured in CO_2 equivalent – 18% – than transport. It is also a major source of land and water degradation. Says Henning Steinfeld, Chief of FAO's Livestock Information and Policy Branch and senior author of FAO report, *Livestock's Long Shadow – Environmental Issues and Options, "Livestock are one of the most significant contributors to today's most serious environmental problems. Urgent action is required to remedy the situation."* When emissions from land use and land use change are included, the livestock sector accounts for 9% of CO2 deriving from human-related activities, but produces a much larger share of even more harmful greenhouse gases. *It generates 65% of human-related nitrous oxide, which has 296 times the Global Warming Potential (GWP) of CO_2.* Most of this comes from manure.

Livestock production accounts for respectively 37% of all human-induced methane (23 times as warming as CO_2), which is largely produced by the digestive system of ruminants, and 64% of ammonia, which contributes significantly to acid rain. Livestock now use 30% of the earth's entire land surface, mostly permanent pasture but also including *33% of the global arable land used to producing feed for livestock*, the report notes. As forests are cleared to create new pastures, it is a major driver of deforestation, especially in Latin America, where, for example, some 70% of former forests in the Amazon have been turned over to grazing.

No boundary: animal awareness
"Animals are my friends... and I don't eat my friends." – George Bernard Shaw

As of the writing of this chapter, we are watching the Olympics unfold in Beijing, China. In a telling move so as not to offend visitors, the Beijing Catering Trade Association has forbidden all 112 specially designated Olympic hoteliers and res-taurateurs to provide dog meat dishes during the games, and "strongly advised" other establishments to put canine cuisine off the menu too.[61] According to the USDA's National Agriculture Statistics Survey (NASS) in the year 2000, Americans killed 9.7 billion animals for food, or approximately 26.5 million unnamed animals each day that as a society we would rather not admit have personalities, family ties, feelings, and individual natures quite similar to the dogs that Olympic officials in Beijing know we would be offended to see on a menu.

Three films are of utmost value if you are looking to shift away from meat-eating (or *kreophagy* as Howard Williams called it) and dairy consumption: *Earthlings* narrated by Joaquin Phoenix; *Meet (?) Your Meat* narrated by Alec Baldwin; *Fast Food Nation* based on the book by Eric Schlosser. Also make sure to pick up the books *Diet for a New America* and *The Food Revolution* by John Robbins, and view John Robbins' documentary *Diet for a New America*, based on the book. You will quickly understand how cruelly cows are treated before being killed for meat and "Indian leather." Every cow raised for dairy is eventually killed for meat after surviving a traumatic life as a dairy cow. In terms of animal cruelty, environmental degradation, and karma, vegetarian is just a stop on the tour through the stages of the dietary spectrum to cooked vegan and raw/live vegan. Albert Schweitzer said, *"Until he extends the circle of compassion to all living things, man will not himself find peace."* There it is – eating becomes an act of love and compassion for all living things.

The green colosseum: vegan athletes
"If care is taken to include a wide variety of foods, vegetarian diets can be nutritionally adequate to support athletic performance." – The US Olympic Committee on Vegetarian Diets

"Whether an individual is a recreational or world-class athlete, being a vegetarian does not diminish natural talent or athletic performance. As far back as the Ancient Games, Greek athletes trained on vegetarian diets and displayed amazing ability in competitive athletics." [62]

The Badwater Ultramarathon is a grueling 135-mile race in the desert of southern California, held during the hottest month of each year in temperatures up to 130 degrees Fahrenheit for some of the most extreme athletes in the world. It is billed as "the toughest footrace on earth." On July 12, 2005, in 24 hours, 36 minutes and eight seconds, vegan athlete Scott Jurek won the Badwater, shattering the course record by more than half an hour, and finishing a full two hours ahead of his closest competitor. Before the California race, *Jurek had never run more than 90 minutes on pavement.* Nor had he trained for the intense desert heat, except for arriving a week early to the Death Valley start area. Jurek returned to the Badwater in 2006 and beat everyone again.

In ancient Greece it was well known that Olympic athletes performed best when they ate plant-based diets, yet today the question still sits in many people's minds: can people perform as well athletically without animal-based protein? Most think not, yet when we look at the data we find that they not only perform as well, but vegan or vegetarian athletes perform *better* than their meat-eating opponents. According to T. Colin Campbell, PhD in his article Muscling Out The Meat Myth, *"...there's hardly another myth in nutrition so insidious yet so intractable as that which encourages us to believe that consuming lots of ... animal-based foods-makes for fitness, bigness, and strength of body."*[63] Dr Campbell explains that this myth is largely due to the discovery in the early 1900s that animal proteins prompt body growth more "efficiently" than plant protein, meaning that eating animal protein causes the human body to gain more body weight when compared to plant protein. We now know that this is not necessarily a positive outcome, and that the consumption of animal proteins is linked not only with the growth of muscle, but also the growth of cancer and other fatal disease.

Around the same time that other scientists were advocating the superiority of animal protein, Dr. Russell Chittenden, a professor of physiological chemistry at Yale University, was proving the opposite:

"He wondered whether consuming diets very much lower in high-protein foods (i.e., much lower intakes of animal-based foods) would bring about undue fatigue and loss of mental and physical fitness. What concerned Chittenden were the claims that a generous consumption of animal protein could really make for strength, endurance, and "manly" qualities, as some were saying. Initially, he organized an experiment to see if eating less protein and animal food would really make him and his colleagues weaker and less able to put in a good day's work. To the contrary, he found that their health, vigor, and overall fitness were considerably improved."[64]

Chittenden went on to experiment with groups of military men in training, men used to eating large amounts of meat, putting them first on one-third the amount of animal protein they were accustomed to, and then on a largely plant-based diet. The original test scores went from 3,000 to 6,000,(?) and with his second test group the athletes saw approximately a 35% improvement in their performance in just five months! The following is an impressive lineup of some plant-based athletes who are backing Chittenden's findings:

Bill Pearl (Mr. America, Mr. USA, and four times Mr. Universe)

Andreas Cahling (Mr. International)
Hercules Steve Reeves (Mr. America, Mr. World and Mr. Universe – and vegetarian at least part of the time during his competitive career)
Jack Lalane (TV personality and bodybuilder)
Monika Montsho (weightlifter, 1991 NW woman weightlifter of the year)
Cory Everson (bodybuilder, 6-time Ms. Olympia)
Carl Lewis (seven-time Olympic gold-medalist sprinter and at one time the world's fastest man)
Edwin Moses (Olympic Gold Medallist hurdler and world champion for more than a decade)
Dave Scott (triathlete, 6-time Ironman winner, the only one to ever win this more than twice.)
Martina Navratilova (tennis champion)
Billie Jean King (tennis champion)
Desmond Howard (football player, Heisman trophy winner)
Tony LaRussa (coach of Oakland Athletics)
B.J. Armstrong (US Basketball star)
Chris Campbell (1980 world champion wrestler)
Di Edwards (runner, Olympic semi-finalist)
Sally Eastall (marathon runner, UK No. 2)
Lucy Stephens (triathlete)

Do not doubt that vegans can be strong, vibrant, muscular, and athletic, winning in the Ironman, the Badwater Ultramarathon, and on occasion, your local wheatgrass drinking competition.

Vegan 3.0: the cuisine ahead
"Every man is the creature of the age in which he lives; very few are able to raise themselves above the ideas of the time." – Voltaire

Vegan 3.0 is built on the knowledge base of Vegan 1.0, and its dissemination in Vegan 2.0, by an organized, creative, engaged online globally-networked community. Vegan 3.0 is largely raw/live vegan, increasingly local, increasingly nutrient-dense, incorporating superfoods, higher in leafy greens and sprouts, and lower on the glycemic index. A healthy perspective at Vegan 3.0 can see the whole stages development of the Spectrum of Diet™, and an appreciation (and humor) exists for the importance of each stage along the way to raw/live vegan.

In the coming decade, Vegan 3.0 will see unprecedented numbers of vegetarians worldwide make the shift up the Spectrum to cooked vegan and raw/live Vegan, engendering a profound shift in awareness about the significance of the individual in effecting one's own, and global, concerns in a process of interdependent co-arising. Modern medicine, pharmaceutical companies, agriculturalists, institutions of learning, and government will follow…

The Spectrum of Diet™ is a pending trademark by David Rainoshek, MA

About the authors:

David Rainoshek, MA *in Vegan/Live Food Nutrition, is the co-creator of JuiceFeasting.com with his wife, Katrina Rainoshek. He is a Juice Feasting coach, author, lecturer, and has Juice fasted/Feasted for over 450 days, up to 92 days at a time. David served as Research Assistant to Dr. Gabriel Cousens for There is a Cure for Diabetes, and is now authoring several books for release in 2008, including:* **Juice Feasting: An Integral Hero's Guide, The Four Means to Get Your Greens,** *and finally, with Katrina, a series of children's books beginning with* **Julia and the Nut Mylk Tree.** *David and Katrina coach 92-Day Juice Feasts for clients and retreats worldwide including the yearly Global Juice Feast, a world-wide cleanse for 92 Days on www.GlobalJuiceFeast.com. David and Katrina teach about Juice Feasting and nutrition education to the world through their 92-Day Program on www.JuiceFeasting.com. David served as leading Research Assistant to Gabriel Cousens, M.D., as head juice-fasting coach, and taught the 10-week nutrition education classes to kitchen and garden apprentices at the Tree of Life Rejuvenation Center in Patagonia, Arizona in 2006–07. He has taught more than 100 raw food preparation classes to children and adults.*

David and Katrina are self-described as a Dietary Activists and proponents of Nutrient Density and Health Freedom for all. "Availability is not enough. For Live Food Nutrition to be the truly transformative and integral movement of our times, it must be made accessible to everyone." David and Katrina drive a Ford F-350 on Straight Vegetable Oil reclaimed from Asian restaurants, have covered over 70,000 miles to-date, and currently reside in British Columbia, Canada.

(Endnotes)

1   "Livestock's Long Shadow: Environmental Issues and Options." Food and Agriculture Organization of the United Nations, Rome 2007. Online: http://www.fao.org/docrep/010/a0701e/a0701e00.htm

2   Esselstyn CB Jr,, Ellis SG, Medendorp SV, et al. A strategy to arrest and reverse coronary artery disease: a 5-year longitudinal study of a single physician's practice. *J Fam Prac* 1995; 41:560-568. Online: http://www.HeartAttackProof.com

3   Gale, Catharine, et. al. "IQ in childhood and vegetarianism in adulthood: 1970 British cohort study." *BMJ*, doi: 10.1136/bmj.39030.675069.55, (Published 15 December 2006)

4   Appleby PN, Davey GK, Key TJ. Public Health Nutrition 2002;5:645-654.

5   Allen NE, et al. Br J Cancer 2000 Jul;83(1):95-7.

6   CAP. College of American Pathologists. Cholesterol Testing Information. http://www.cap.org/health_and_wellness/Cholesterol_CAP.html. Accessed February 7, 2003.

7   Key TJ, et al. 1999 Sep;70(3 Suppl):516S-524S.

8   Spencer EA, Appleby PN, Davey GK, Key TJ. Diet and body mass index in 38000 EPIC-Oxford meat-eaters, fish-eaters, vegetarians and vegans. Int J Obes Relat Metab Disord. 2003 Jun;27(6):728-34.

9   Cousens, Gabriel MD with Rainoshek, David. *There is a Cure for Diabetes.* North Atlantic, Berkeley: 2007.

10   Barnard, Neal MD. *Dr. Neal Barnard's Program for Reversing Diabetes.* Rodale, New York: 2007.

11   Sparks DL, Martin TA, Gross DR, et al. "Link between heart disease, cholesterol, and Alzheimer's Disease: a review." *Microscopy Res. Tech.* 50 (2000): 287-290.

12   Grant WB. "Dietary links to Alzheimer's Disease: 1999 Update." *J. Alzheimer's Dis* 1

(1999): 197-201.

13   Gillman MW, Cupples LA, Gagnon D, et al. "Protective effect of fruits and vegetables on development of stroke in men." *JAMA* 273 (1995):1113-1117.

14   Carroll KK, Braden LM, Bell JA, et al. "Fat and cancer." *Cancer* 58 (1986): 1818-1825.

15   Armstrong D, and Doll R. "Environmental factors and cancer incidence and mortality in different countries, with special reference to dietary practices." *Int J. Cancer* 15 (1975): 617-631.

16   Chan JM, and Giovannucci EL. "Dietary products, calcium, and vitamin D and risk of prostate cancer." *Epidemiol. Revs.* 23 (2001): 87-92.

17   Agranoff BW, and Goldberg D. "Diet and the geographical distribution of multiple sclerosis." *Lancet* 2(7888) (November 2, 1974): 1061-1066.

18   Abelow, BJ, Holford TR, and Insogna KL. "Cross-cultural association between dietary animal protein and hip fracture: a hypothesis." *Calcif. Tissue Int.* 50 (1992): 14-18.

19   Robertson WG, Peacock M, and Hodgkinson A. "Dietary changes and the incidence of urinary calculi in the UK between 1958 and 1976." *Chron. Dis.* 32 (1979): 469-476.

20   Robertson WG, Peacock M, Heyburn PJ, et al. "Should recurrent calcium oxalate stone formers become vegetarians?" *Brit. J. Urology* 51 (1979): 427-431.

21   Borger, C., et al., "Health Spending Projections Through 2015: Changes on the Horizon," *Health Affairs Web Exclusive* W61: 22 February 2006.

22   Anderson, Richard. *Cleanse and Purify Thyself: Book 1*

23   Mills, Milton. "The Comparative Anatomy of Eating." Online: www.vegsource.com/veg_faq/comparative.htm

24   Cousens, Gabriel with Rainoshek, David. *There is a Cure for Diabetes*. North Atlantic Books, Berkeley: 2008. Pg 44.

25   Cousens, Gabriel. *Conscious Eating*. North Atlantic Books, Berkeley: 2000. Pg 438.

26   Robbins, J. *Diet for a New America*. Tiburon, Calif.: H J Kramer, 1987, p. 333. Cited in "Infant Abnormalities Linked to PCB Contaminated Fish," *Vegetarian Times*, Nov. 1984, p. 8.

27   Robbins, ibid., p. 334. Cited in Jacobsen, S. "The effect of intrauterine PCB exposure on visual recognition memory." *Child Development*, 1985, Vol. 56.

28   Ellis, F R, and Montegriffo, V M E. "Veganism, clinical findings and investigations." *Am J Clin Nutr*, 1970, 23:249–255.

29   Berenson, G, Srinivasan, S, Bao, W, Newman, W P Tracy, R E, and Wattigney, W A. "Association between multiple cardiovascular risk factors and atherosclerosis to children and young adults. The Bogalusa Heart Study." *New Eng J Med*, 1998, 338:1650–1656.

30   Key, T J, Fraser, G E, Thorogood, M, et al. "Mortality in vegetarians and nonvegetarians: Detailed findings from a collaborative analysis of 5 prospective studies." *Am J Clin Nutri*, 1999, 70(Suppl.):516S–524S.

31   Bergan, J G, and Brown, P T. "Nutritional status of "new" vegetarians." *J Am Diet Assoc*, 1980, 76:151-155.

32   Appleby, P N, Thorogood, M, et al. "Low body mass index in non-meat eaters: The possible roles of animal fat, dietary fiber, and alcohol." *Int J Obes*, 1998, 22:454–460.

33   Dwyer, J T. "Health aspects of vegetarian diets." *Am J Clin Nutr*, 1988, 48:712–738.

34   Key, T J, and Davey, G. "Prevalence of obesity is low in people who do not eat meat." *BMJ*, 1996, 313:816–817.

35   Snowdon, D A, and Phillips, R L. "Does a vegetarian diet reduce the occurrence of diabetes?" *American Journal of Public Health*, 1985, 75:507–512.

36   Virtanen, S M, Laara, E, Hypponen, E, et al. "Cow's milk consumption, HLA-DQB1 genotype, and Type-1 diabetes." *Diabetes*, 2000, 49:912–917.

37   "Diet and Stress in Vascular Disease," Journal of the America Medical Association, June 3, 1961, p. 806.

38   Esselstyn, C B, Ellis, S G, Medendorp, S V, et al. "A strategy to arrest and reverse coronary artery disease: A 5-year longitudinal study of a single physician's practice." *J Fam Prac*, 1995, 41:560–568.

39   Esselstyn, C B. *Prevent and Reverse Heart Disease*. www.heartattackproof.com

40   *World Health Statistics Annual 1994–1998*. Online version: www.who.int/whosis. Statistical database food balance sheets, 1961–1999. Available online at www.fao.org. Food and Agriculture Organization of the United Nations. National Institutes of Health. Global cancer rates, cancer death rates among 50 countries, 1986-1999. Available online at www.nih.gov.

41   Fuhrman, J. *Eat to Live*. New York: Little, Brown, and Company, 2003, pp. 51–52.

42   *Cancer* 64 (3): 605-12, 1989

43   Chan, J M, and Giovannucci, E L. "Dairy products, calcium, and vitamin D and risk of pros-

tate cancer." *Epidemiol Revs*, 2001, 23:87–92.

44   Plant, J A. *The No-Dairy Breast Cancer Prevention Program.* New York: St. Martin's Press, 2001, p. 74.

45   Plant, J A. *The No-Dairy Breast Cancer Prevention Program.* New York: St. Martin's Press, 2001, p. 75. JA Plant reference: Kliewer, E V, and Smith, K R, "Breast cancer mortality among immigrants in Australia and Canada," *Journal of National Cancer Institute,* 1995, 87(15):1154–1161. See also Cancer Research Campaign, *Factsheet 6.2, Breast Cancer—UK,* 1996.

46   Barnard, Dr. Neal. *Breaking the Food Seduction.* St. Martin's Press, New York: 2003. Pg 68.

47   Lewinnek GE, Kelsey J, White AA III, et al. The significance and a comparative analysis of the epidemiology of hip fractures. Clin Ortho Rel Res 1980;152:35-43.*Clin Ortho Related Res,* 1980, 152:35.

48   Recker, R R, and Heaney, R P. "The effect of milk supplements on calcium metabolism, bone metabolism and calcium balance." *Am J Clin Nutr,* 1985, 41:254–263

49   CR Paterson, *Postgraduate Medical Journal*, 1978, Vol, 54, 244-248, http://pmj.bmj.com

50   Wolfe, David. *The Sunfood Diet Success System.* Maul Brothers, San Diego: 2006. Pg 335.

51   "American Gastroenterological Association Medical Position Statement: Guidelines for the Evaluation of Food Allergies," *Gastroenterology*, 2001, 120:1023–1025.

52   National Digestive Diseases Information Clearinghouse. "Lactose Intolerance," *National Institute of Diabetes and Digestive and Kidney Diseases,* March 2003.

53   Taylor, C. "Got Milk (Intolerance)? Digestive Malady Affects 30–50 Million," *The Clarion-Ledger,* 1 Aug. 2003.

54   "Cow's Milk Protein May Play Role in Mental Disorders," *Reuters Health,* 1 Apr. 1999.

55   Carrell, S. "Milk Causes Serious Illness for 7M Britons. Scientists Say Undetected Lactose Intolerance Is to Blame for Chronic Fatigue, Arthritis and Bowel Problems," *The Independent,* 22 June 2003.

56   Position of The American Dietetic Association: vegetarian diets. *J Am Diet Assoc.* June 2003 (Vol. 103, Issue 6, Pages 748-765)

57   Cousens, Gabriel. *Spiritual Nutrition.* North Atlantic Books, Berkeley: 2005. Pg 269.

58   Cousens, Gabriel. *Spiritual Nutrition.* North Atlantic Books, Berkeley: 2005. Pg 436.

59   Faloon, William. "Should the president declare a national emergency?" *Life Extension Magazine,* October 2007. Online: http://www.lef.org/magazine/mag2007/oct2007_awsi_01.htm

60   Roberts, Michelle. Boston University Medical Center, January 2, 2008. "Vitamin D2 is as effective as vitamin D3 in maintaining concentrations of 25-hydroxyvitamin D" Online: http://www.eurekalert.org/pub_releases/2008-01/bu-vdi010208.php

61   Coonan, Clifford. *The Irish Times,* August 9, 2008. "Beijing officials want dog meat off the menu during Olympics" Online: http://www.irishtimes.com/newspaper/frontpage/2008/0712/12157878 62830.html

62   Excerpted from "Vegetarian Diets" by the International Center for Sports Nutrition, *Olympic Coach Magazine,* Winter 1997. Online: www.olympic-usa.org

63   Campbell, T. Colin. "Muscling out the meat myth." Online: www.vsdc.org/meatmyth.html

64   http://www.vsdc.org/meatmyth.html

Vegan 2.0

2

Organics For Life

Cherie Soria

Once considered a niche market, with questionable economic benefits, organic farming is now the fastest-growing and most profitable sector of agriculture in the U.S. Demand for human and animal food, body care products, bedding, clothing, and even cleaning supplies produced without hormones, pesticides, or other chemicals, is exploding. Sales of organic food and beverages rose from less than $4 billion a year in 1997 to $13.8 billion in 2005 and continue to rise. This makes the organic industry one of the fastest-growing in the world -- and a market that even large corporations are now taking seriously.

The reasons for the high demand for organics vary as much as the consumers who purchase them. Chefs claim the superior flavor of organic food, while many people are becoming concerned with the rising rates of cancer and other diseases attributed to pesticides. Children are worried about the health of the planet, and scientists are concerned about bees and other wildlife dying off as a direct result of agricultural chemicals. The demand for organic products has now gone mainstream. Yet in spite of this growing interest, only a small percentage of all produce grown in the United States is organic. As a result, organically grown fruits and vegetables are often expensive and difficult to find. Still, despite the limited availability and extra expense, eating organic food has become a growing trend that has forced farmers and retailers to take notice.

Some of the many benefits of eating organic foods:

• Superior flavor (many top chefs use only organically grown foods)
• Reduced intake of chemicals and heavy metals
• Decreased exposure to known carcinogens
• Better working conditions for farmers and workers
• Greater variety of heirloom fruits and vegetables
• No genetically modified organisms (GMOs)
• Cleaner rivers and waterways
• Minimized topsoil erosion
• Preservation of ecologically vital insects and birds that are killed by chemical farming methods
• Support of sustainable food production, "fair trade" agriculture, and small family farms

A brief history of organic agriculture

There are many standards for organically grown food throughout the world. All of them require growing crops without the use of chemicals or synthetic fertilizers, pesticides, or other agricultural chemicals. Since the dawn of civilization and up until the mid-1940s, this method of food production was the norm. No distinction between "organic" and "conventional" agriculture existed, because organic *was* the conventional form of agriculture. In the early days of industrial farming, producing large amounts of food for a growing population was a priority. The possibility of using agricultural chemicals to increase crop production was quite appealing to many farmers. What began as a seemingly beneficial new method of producing more food became a widely accepted way to farm. Initially, increased crop yields were the main result that farmers observed, and the "agrochemical" industry was born. By the 1960s, farmers began to see unanticipated side effects, such as massive erosion of topsoil, disturbing loss of wildlife, including bees and other beneficial insects, and widespread fouling of rivers and streams. By the time these phenomena became apparent, most farmers were dependent on agrochemicals to maintain their new levels of production. Overextended with mortgages, loans, and liens, farmers found themselves trapped in a maze of toxic, unsustainable practices and unable to revert to lower-yielding "traditional" growing methods.

Over the next several decades, the side effects became increasingly ominous as agrochemicals penetrated the food chain. Of particular significance is the impact on human health. Farmers, farm workers, farm neighbors, and consumers began to experience birth defects, compromised immune systems, reproductive disorders, new types of cancers, and a host of other symptoms. Rachel Carson documented these maladies and many more in her landmark book, *Silent Spring*, which explored the far-reaching effects of industrial/chemical agriculture. Fortunately, there have always been farmers who remained loyal to traditional practices such as composting, mulching, encouraging the presence of beneficial insects, saving seeds, and other sustainable food-production strategies. When we support organic agriculture, we make a choice that benefits both us and our environment.

What does "Certified Organic" mean?

"Organic" refers to the way agricultural products are grown and processed. Organically produced foods must comply with strict regulations governing all aspects of production. Organic farming maintains and replenishes soil fertility without using toxic and persistent pesticides and fertilizers. "Certified Organic" means the item has been grown in accordance with strict uniform standards that are verified by independent organizations. Certification typically includes inspections of fields and processing facilities, detailed record keeping, and periodic testing of soil and water to ensure that growers and handlers are complying with the standards. Standards vary with geography, but buying certified organically grown produce (or growing your own using untreated organic seeds) is the safest way to ensure that you ingest the fewest toxic residues. A label indicating "100% Organic" ensures that only organic ingredients and organic processing methods are used, while a label that says "Organic" requires at least 95% organic ingredients combined with a limited number of strictly regulated non-organic ingredients. Finally, products labeled "Made with Organic" must contain at least 70% organic ingredients.

Why does organic food cost more, and is it worth the extra money?

Organically grown foods can be more costly than conventional foods, whose true costs are hidden. Organically grown foods are more labor- and management-intensive, and organic farming tends to be implemented on a smaller scale. Governments (funded by our taxes) subsidize conventional agriculture, whereas organic farmers receive little or no support for their efforts. The true short- and long-term costs of chemical/industrial agriculture are quite high relative to its benefits. And, the high price we now pay, in terms of health and environmental destruction, is only a fraction of what future generations will pay, in ways we can scarcely dare to imagine.

Are organic foods worth the money? An increasing percentage of the population now says "yes", and high on the list are the most vulnerable groups -- children and pregnant women -- but even organically grown dog food is gaining in popularity among concerned pet-lovers. Those who cannot afford to eat all organic can choose to buy fruits and vegetables that carry the lowest pesticide load. (See the Environmental Working Group's Shopper's Guide to Pesticides in Produce, reproduced below.) Organic living has become so popular that many people even choose their vacation destinations based on availability of organic produce, organic restaurant offerings, and eco-friendly lodging.

How will mainstream acceptance affect the organic food supply?

Along with increasing mainstream popularity comes increasing pressure to cut corners on organic standards, especially now that large corporations like Wal-Mart have jumped on the organic bandwagon. Low-cost organic food sounds like a good thing, but not at the expense of quality. Strictly enforced regulations are important for maintaining the integrity of organic food production. At present half of all U.S. farm products come from only 1% of our farms. Big business is squeezing out organic family farms, and that is bad news for all of us. The EPA says that agriculture is responsible for 70% of the world's river and stream pollution, due to chemicals, soil erosion, and animal waste run-off. Organic farming may be one of the last ways to keep both ecosystems and rural communities healthy and vital.

What are GMOs?
The term "GMO," or **genetically modified organism,** refers to organisms whose genetic material is altered in a way that does not occur by mating or natural recombination. Instead, the organism's genes are changed by "mutagenic" breeding. For example, a tomato may be cross-bred with a peanut, making it unsafe (and potentially life threatening) for people who are allergic to peanuts. But the greater danger is in introducing GMOs into our environment. Science cannot predict long-term effects, since these organisms -- and the "frankenfoods" they produce -- have not been around long enough for us to fully comprehend the fire we are playing with. One very real risk that some agricultural scientists fear is widespread crop failure as a result of some unforeseen genetic flaw. Given that all individual varieties of GMO seeds have identical genetic make-ups, if blight affected one type of GMO, it could wipe out an entire crop of that type of plant. GMOs are a threat to surrounding fields of non-GMO crops and pollen from GMO varieties of one species can easily cross-breed with non-GMO varieties of another, resulting in ever-increasing confusion among consumers over which foods are safe, as new varieties emerge.

What if Certified Organic produce is unavailable?
As mentioned above, in addition to buying organic produce (which is always GMO free), you can grow your own food using untreated organic seeds. Conventional seed crops are grown with the entire arsenal of pesticides, herbicides, insecticides, fungicides, and other deadly chemicals. Since seeds are not considered food for human consumption, seed farmers can apply these poisons right up until the day of harvest. Organic seed growers use environmentally friendly techniques that don't require toxic chemicals.

> If you cannot grow or buy organic fruits and vegetables, wash your produce well, using a mild biodegradable soap, and rinse it thoroughly. Peel vegetables that have been waxed or coated, as well as root vegetables that have been sprayed with chemicals or grown in fungicide-treated soil. Thin-skinned fruits and vegetables, such as strawberries and tomatoes, are less safe than those with thicker skins and are often less flavorful when not organic.

Another healthful step you can take is to choose produce that has been shown to carry the lowest concentration of pesticide residues. According to the not-for-profit Environmental Working Group (www.ewg.org), exposure to pesticides can be reduced by almost 90 percent by avoiding the most contaminated fruits and vegetables and eating the least contaminated instead. Eating the twelve most contaminated fruits and vegetables (peaches, apples, sweet bell peppers, celery, nectarines, strawberries, cherries, lettuce, imported grapes, pears, spinach, and potatoes) will expose a person to about 14 pesticides per day, on average. In contrast, eating the twelve least-contaminated foods (onions, avocados, sweet corn, pineapples, mangos, sweet peas, asparagus, kiwi, bananas, cabbage, broccoli, and eggplant) will expose a person to fewer than two pesticides per day.

The foods listed above are part of a larger ranking of 43 fruits and vegetables entitled "The Shopper's Guide to Pesticides in Produce" (reproduced below). Compiled by Environmental Working Group analysts, this list is based on the results of nearly 43,000 USDA* and FDA* tests for pesticides on produce, collected between 2000 and 2004. The full guide, and lots of other helpful information, are available online at www.FoodNews.org.

The Environmental Working Group's Shopper's Guide to Pesticides in Produce

RANK	FRUIT OR VEGGIE	SCORE
1 (worst)	Peaches	100 (highest pesticide load)
2	Apples	96
3	Sweet Bell Peppers	86
4	Celery	85
5	Nectarines	84
6	Strawberries	83
7	Cherries	75
8	Lettuce	69
9	Grapes - Imported	68
10	Pears	65
11	Spinach	60
12	Potatoes	58
13	Carrots	57
14	Green Beans	55
15	Hot Peppers	53
16	Cucumbers	52
17	Raspberries	47
18	Plums	46
19	Oranges	46
20	Grapes - Domestic	46
21	Cauliflower	39
22	Tangerine	38
23	Mushrooms	37
24	Cantaloupe	34
25	Lemon	31
26	Honeydew Melon	31
27	Grapefruit	31
28	Winter Squash	31
29	Tomatoes	30
30	Sweet Potatoes	30

31	Watermelon	25
32	Blueberries	24
33	Papaya	21
34	Eggplant	19
35	Broccoli	18
36	Cabbage	17
37	Bananas	16
38	Kiwi	14
39	Asparagus	11
40	Sweet Peas - Frozen	11
41	Mango	9
42	Pineapples	7
43	Sweet Corn - Frozen	2
44	Avocado	1
45 (best)	Onions	1 (lowest pesticide load)

Taking Advantage of Farmers' Markets

These days, only a fortunate few of us have the time to grow our own produce. The rest of us have to rely on someone else to grow our foods for us. One good source for fruits and vegetables is your local farmers' market. Not only is the produce reasonably priced, it is usually grown by people who love being farmers. Unlike big commercial farmers, most of the vendors at farmers' markets spend time in the fields tending their crops. Their energy goes into the food, and you can taste it! Foods purchased at farmers' markets are usually far fresher than the foods you find at grocery stores, since farmers often harvest their produce early in the morning and bring it to market the same day. For this reason, top chefs are often seen shopping at farmers' markets -- they know fresh, ripe produce is the most flavorful! Savvy shoppers arrive early in the morning to get the best quality and selection. On the other hand, if you're looking for bargain prices, shop just before the market closes or when you see vendors starting to pack up. Most farmers would rather sell their produce at a discount than haul it back home. Even after being out all day, most farmers' market produce is still fresher than grocery store fare.

When you shop at farmers' markets, be sure to talk to your vendors and inquire about their growing practices. Farmers who use organic (or better) methods but cannot afford the steep certification fees and the personnel to maintain the paperwork are legally prohibited from advertising their foods as organically grown, but if their practices are truly clean, it is important to support them with your dollars. Small family farms usually care deeply about the Earth and seek to uphold the laws that keep dangerous chemicals out of our food supply.

Often, when you ask whether a farmer's food is organically grown, they will tell you they do not spray. Spraying, however, is not the only issue. Chemical fertilizers are highly soluble and disrupt the carbon cycle and soil ecosystems, including microorganisms, nematodes, and worms, all of which are essential to good soil health. Organic growers use slow-release products such as compost, green manures, and colloidal rock phosphate ("rock dust"), all of which have positive effects on the soil's biological community and nutrient concentration. Organic fertilizers and natural nutrients like nitrogen are also much less likely to be leached out into the groundwater, making them safer for the environment. So ask vendors if they use chemical fertilizers. Most vendors are honest and will tell you the truth, but you have to ask -- and you have to know what questions to ask.

Be aware that not all vendors at farmers' markets are farmers, and many did not produce the foods they are selling. Many vendors buy blemished or misshapen produce from commercial food processors. Nothing is actually wrong with this produce, but it's not of the same high quality as freshly harvested premium produce from "backyard farmers". Other times, you may find produce to be too perfect and shiny, or out of season -- both are red flags that the vendor did not grow these foods. Most importantly, speak up for organics. If vendors say they use chemicals, let them know that you are committed to supporting sustainable agriculture and that you buy only organically grown produce.

If there are no farmers' markets in your area and you must rely on local grocery stores, get to know your produce manager. He or she can be your best resource for information about the freshest, most seasonal produce available. Ask how long they keep produce in their holding areas and which foods are shelved right away, "harvest fresh." Often, grocery store produce is stored in holding facilities for a period ranging from several days to several months. Many grocery stores now package their fruits and vegetables in plastic wrap to protect them and extend shelf life. Since nutrients and vitality begin diminishing at the moment of harvest, neither of these practices is optimal for the consumer. Fresher food is always better!

Using the seasons to your advantage
More and more people are recognizing the importance of buying food in season, when it is freshest, most flavorful and least expensive. If you have a dehydrator or a freezer, you can preserve foods at the height of their nutrient content by buying them in bulk and preserving them for use in the off-season. For example, you can purchase summer corn by the case, slice the kernels off the cobs, and then freeze them. Commercially frozen corn is always blanched first, which destroys many of the nutrients. Fresh fruits freeze well, and frozen fruit is great in smoothies. You can also dehydrate fruits and use them for snack foods, or rehydrate them for use in smoothies or as dessert sweeteners. Consult a seasonal produce calendar for your region, like the one available online at http://www.kqed.org/topics/home/cooking/whats-in-season.jsp, so you can plan your strategy for freezing and dehydrating.

Typically, produce purchased by the case is marked down 10% off the retail price. Don't be afraid to buy flats of berries or figs, even if you don't want to freeze or dehydrate them. It isn't difficult to eat a flat of berries; in fact, it's fun to eat all you want of your favorite foods -- and when they are in season, why not?

Vote with your dollars
Opting for organically grown food and other products is one of the most important

economic choices we can make on a daily basis to support our health and that of the planet. In so doing, we not only choose a higher-quality product, we also vote with our dollars, sending a powerful message to governments and food processors about the direction we want them to go.

About the Author:

*Cherie Soria is founder and director of Living Light Culinary Arts Institute and author of three books, including **Angel Foods: Healthy Recipes for Heavenly Bodies** and **Raw Food Revolution Diet: Feast, Lose Weight, Gain Energy, Feel Younger!** Cherie and her husband, Dan Ladermann, own and operate Living Light International, which consists of four green businesses: Living Light Culinary Arts Institute, Living Light Cuisine To Go, the Living Light Marketplace, and the eco-friendly Living Light Inn. The Living Light Center, an 8,000-square-foot state-of-the-art facility, is located on the picturesque Mendocino coast of northern California and is designed to provide the latest advances in raw organic culinary education. Living Light Cafe offers fresh, organic, mostly raw vegan cuisine, and uses only biodegradable packaging. Living Light Marketplace features books, juicers and other kitchenware, and products for conscious living. Living Light Inn, located a few short blocks away, provides Earth-friendly living at its finest, with organic mattresses and linens, whole-house water filtration, and nontoxic cleaning products. For more information about Cherie Soria and Living Light International, call 707-964-2420, or e-mail info@rawfoodchef.com or visit www. rawfoodchef.com.*

3

Enzymes

Viktoras Kulvinskas, MS

If You Eat Cooked Food, You Need Food Enzymes

Adequate cellular nutrition is dependent on a combination of factors: dietary choices, method of food preparation, degree of thorough chewing, as well as the body's functional efficiency in digesting and assimilating food. Eating food-based enzymes is a key to helping your body maximize your genetic potential, even if you sometimes choose less-than optimal lifestyle habits. Using plant-based enzymes increases the availability of nutrients to the billions of cells that are your physical body. Your choosing to "dine with enzymes" can mean the difference between a life of mediocre or marginal health, and the experience of high-level wellness and abundant energy.

What are enzymes?

The word "enzyme" comes from the Greek word *enzymas*, which means "to ferment" or "cause a change". Enzymes are the foundation for all cell regeneration. They play a key role in the transformation of undigested food into the nutrients that are absorbed on the cellular level. With proper nutrition, we have the energy to participate in the dance of living. An enzyme is a specialized protein structure that carries with it an energetic charge. Enzymes speed up chemical reactions that normally take place very slowly or not at all. It is the energy behind the protein structure that makes enzymes different from other protein-based substances. It is this energetic life principle, sometimes called *prana,* or *ch'i*, that animates all life forms. The father of modern enzyme therapy, Dr Edward Howell, once said that enzymes emit a *"kind of radiation"* that can be picked up on Kirlian photographs. Howell can be singled out from other researchers because he stressed that enzymes are not merely expendable, protein-based chemical catalysts that move along chemical reactions. He forcefully argued that enzymes are none other than **units of life-energy that use various protein molecules as their carriers.**

Enzymes are much more sensitive to destruction by heat or cold than vitamins and minerals. Food cooked over 118 degrees F for more than a half an hour will kill all naturally-occurring enzymes. In the event that dry heat is used, the critical temperature for enzyme destruction is about 150 F. Enzymes are the true workers in and out of our cells. As Dr. Richard Gerber MD states, "The enzymes catalyze specific reactions of chemicals either to create structure through molecular assemblies or to provide the electrochemical fire to run the cellular engines and ultimately keep the entire system working".

> There are thousands of different enzymes, so many that one cannot separate enzyme activity with the process of life itself. From moving a muscle to blinking an eye, no biological work can be accomplished independent of enzymes. Without enzymes, the body would be nothing but inorganic matter.

Types of enzymes
Enzymes can be grouped into three main categories. The first category consists of the **digestive enzymes,** which the digestive system collects, manufactures and secretes to break down food. Examples of digestive enzymes are protease, which digests protein; amylase, which digests starch; and lipase, which digests fat. Each enzyme almost always has only one specific function that it carries out. For example, the enzyme protease only digests protein. The enzyme amylase only digests starches.

The second type of enzymes is composed of **metabolic enzymes,** which are present in every cell, tissue, and organ and act as biochemical catalysts in the second-to-second functioning of living cells. The metabolic antioxidant enzyme superoxide dismutase (SOD), which is present in all cells, reduces free radical damage, and thus retards the aging process. Raw foods, especially sprouts and algae, are rich in SOD.

The third class of enzymes is made up of various **food enzymes,** which come from raw, uncooked foods. The process of enzymatic digestion begins when you masticate your food in your mouth. When you chew, you not only mix the enzyme ptyalin from your salivary glands into the food, but allow the food-based enzymes present in the food to be released onto itself. This occurs from the moment that you rupture the cell walls of the food with your teeth.

Most fresh, well-grown produce has at least enough enzymes to digest the specific amount of protein, starch or fat found in the food itself. As a general rule, the higher the caloric content of an uncooked food, the more enzymes Nature will have put into the food to handle the exact amount of nutrients present. Nature is so considerate and thoughtful, don't you think? So, foods high in protein will have a high amount of protease or protein-digesting enzyme. Examples are blue-green algae and sunflower seeds. Foods such as whole oats have a high amount of amylase or starch-digesting enzymes. Foods such as avocados and nuts have naturally-occurring lipase or fat-digesting enzymes. Nature is so balanced – I wish I could balance my checkbook as easily!

One of the myths still held by many health food consumers is that eating a raw vegetable salad alongside an otherwise cooked meal is sufficient to digest the cooked food portion of the meal. The reality of the situation is that since there is a direct correlation between the number of calories in a food and the amount of enzymes present, low-calorie salads have relatively few enzymes to help out in digesting any other food you may be eating. Unless the salad is composed of sprouts (which are naturally high in enzymes because they are young plants), you cannot count on raw salads to be of much help in digesting other foods.

Enzyme logic in dollars and sense
Let's play a little with the concept of enzymes by using our day-to-day experience of banking as a metaphor. Your body's enzymes can be likened to cash reserves in your own life-force bank account. Each time you eat enzyme-less food, you tax your system by making a withdrawal from this enzyme bank. Meal by meal you decrease your enzyme net worth, which can be equated with your life potential. Since at least half of all enzyme capital in the body is assigned to digesting foods, eating life-less cooked foods in effect puts a continual hold on 50% of your budget. Your individual budget limit is determined by your genetic inheritance.

If one's enzyme capital is frozen in this way, your ability to allocate funds to improve the quality of your life is then on hold to the tune of 50% of your net worth! You'll then have limited enzyme resources with which to make much-needed home improvements (cleansing and rebuilding organs and tissues) and protecting your enzyme life savings via a strong immune system. To complicate matters, your bills are coming due, and guess what, your account is low in funds! You're desperate, so you borrow (take stimulants such as coffee to keep going) because your credit rating (overall health) is bad due to years and years of withdrawals. You now wish that you had made more enzyme deposits in your life force bank account, so that you wouldn't be finding yourself in arrears, experiencing energy deficiencies. You get the point. Now that you know how health finances work, start investing in your future health by taking plant-based enzymes today, before life hands you a bill that you can't afford to pay! It could be the best investment, with a return of new youthful energy and freedom from some of the crises of middle age.

Enzymes throughout history
In the 1890s, the forerunners of the modern science of nutrition discovered

building-block substances in food. They named these building-blocks *proteins.* At the turn of the 20th century, a new word was coined to refer to a class of food-based, bio-active, organically bound chemical substances found to be essential for human health. These substances were called *vitamins.* And about a decade or so later, the importance of organic *minerals* in food was recognized to be equally essential to health.

More than 100 years after the birth of modern scientific nutrition, we find ourselves at an exciting juncture. A missing link in our understanding of the life-giving properties of food is being illuminated by the increasing acceptance of the critical role of food-based enzymes for health and longevity. **I predict that in the near future, the recognition of the impact of enzymes on health will have even more profound repercussions than many of the discoveries related to vitamins, minerals, and proteins have had.**

We can begin a discussion of nutrition as it relates to enzymes by talking about our first food: milk. Numerous medical studies and current public health statistics confirm what our prehistoric ancestors knew, that infants who were breast-fed on human mother's milk had fewer health problems than those infants who were raised on pasteurized cow's milk. Aside from the self-evident fact that human mother's milk is ideally suited for human infants and cow's milk is ideally suited for calves, **it is significant that the former is unheated and therefore enzyme-rich and the latter is heated and therefore enzyme-poor.**

More than 20 years ago, I discovered Dr. Howell's long out-of-print first book gathering dust in the basement of a medical library where I was doing health research. Published in 1939, this limited edition book was entitled, *The Status of Food Enzymes in Digestion and Metabolism.* With much effort I traced its author, who was in his 80s, and found him affiliated with an enzyme manufacturing company he himself had founded in the 1930s. Dr. Howell graciously gave me permission to reprint and update the book under the new title, *Food Enzymes for Health and Longevity.* About a decade later, Howell's classic was again republished in a simplified and popularized version by Avery Press and renamed *Enzyme Nutrition.* With this last release, the long-ignored discoveries of Dr. Howell spread to many health practitioners and seekers of health around the world.

Dr Howell's food enzyme concept

Dr. Edward Howell was the first nutritional scientist to develop a large experimental and theoretical body of work aimed at answering the complex and critically important question, "What are the connections between food or supplement-based enzyme intake, health, disease, and longevity?" Howell devoted his entire adult life to conducting numerous animal and human experiments in his attempt to strengthen the theory that food enzyme deficiencies promote disease and premature aging, whereas enzyme-rich diets promote good health and longevity. To this end, his book, *The Status of Food Enzymes in Digestion and Metabolism* cited more than 400 research papers, which in his day represented the cutting edge of science. Modern researchers have yet to comprehend fully the implications of that book. As Dr Howell once said, "To say that the body can easily digest and assimilate cooked foods may some day prove to be the most grievous oversight yet committed by science".

Dr. Howell theorized that on a largely cooked, low-enzyme diet, the digestive system borrows enzymes from the body's general metabolic enzyme pool to help digest enzymeless cooked food. Howell emphasized that the consequences of this adaptive measure were great, in that diverting enzymes from one system to another eventually weakened the functioning of these other systems and the body in general. For example, he argued that the immune system was compromised due to gradual enzyme deficiency and that this set the stage for numerous health problems such as allergies, cancer, and diabetes. If he were alive today, Howell would undoubtedly include AIDS on this list.

In treating his patients, Dr. Howell initially prescribed raw food diets but soon found this to be impractical because many patients lacked the willpower required to stay on such a regime. By 1932, however, he had already developed a plant-based enzyme supplement designed to replace the enzymes lost in a typical cooked food diet.

Dr Howell discovered that enzyme supplements from plant sources were uniquely effective. Below are just a few of some of Howell's basic concepts. (For a more complete discussion, please consult the book *Enzymes for Health and Longevity*).

- Food enzymes are essential nutrients.
- Being more fragile to the effects of heat than vitamins and minerals, food enzymes are destroyed by the high temperature of cooking.
- When food is chewed and swallowed in its raw natural state, enzymes immediately go to work in the upper cardiac portion of the stomach.
- Eating a low-enzyme, cooked food diet increases the size of the pancreas, a sign that this organ is being overworked. He further hypothesized that this condition is a precursor to various forms of dysfunction such as hypoglycemia, diabetes and metabolic imbalances.
- A deficiency of food enzymes in the diet gives rise to "digestive leukocytosis", (excess white cells in the digestive system and blood) which is not the case when raw, high enzyme foods are eaten.

More than 60 years ago, Dr. Edward Howell began to cultivate one special species of the many aspergillus plants that existed in the plant kingdom. He picked the "oryzae" strain because there were no harmful aflatoxins (a type of poison) associated with this plant. More importantly, however, this strain contained a rich store of the very same enzymes that the human body used to digest food.

For the first time in recorded history, Howell gave the powdered form of these little plants directly to human patients. He found that aspergillus oryzae was a key to treating a whole host of seemingly unrelated ailments. Because of the success of his clinical work, he dedicated his life to working out a theoretical and experimental platform to explain how these seeming miracles had been accomplished. The development of the "Food Enzyme Concept" in human nutrition was this great man's life's work.

This chapter would not have been written, nor perhaps would I be as alive and healthy as I am today, if it were not for the amazing properties of these "angel-hair-in-appearance" microscopic plants. I have eaten aspergillus plant digestive enzymes for more than 20 years. I have also experimented with other animal and vegetarian-based enzymes such as pancreatin, pepsin, papain and bromelaine. I have concluded that aspergillus enzymes are far superior to these other enzyme sources.

Recycling and specificity of enzymes

The editor of the *Scottish Medical Journal* (1966) wrote that *"probably nearly half of our daily production of protein in the body are enzymes"*. In a way, our bodies are like big enzyme factories. There is strong evidence that the body seeks to conserve its digestive enzymes. In the prestigious scientific journal *Science,* Liebow and Rothman (1975) describe an experiment in which it was found that pancreatic enzymes given by mouth can be absorbed intact from the gut, transported through the bloodstream and then be re-secreted into the duodenum by the pancreas. If only my home's heating system were as efficient!

There is an antagonistic relationship between the demands of the digestive system for a continual supply of enzymes and the need of the organs, glands and immune system for enzymes with which to do their work. The competition for enzyme resources can easily be relieved by the consumption of food-sourced enzymes. Dr. Guyton's authoritative *Textbook of Medical Physiology* (1986) states that the pancreas, stomach and possibly other organs secrete specific digestive enzymes according to the type and quantity of food present. The ingestion of plant enzymes may have a conserving effect on the body's enzyme potential, possibly aiding cell and organ regeneration by digesting the foods which normally would have required the body's own pancreatic enzymes.

Co-enzymes make super-enzymes

Organic minerals and vitamins are sometimes bound to enzymes that are integrated into the enzyme structure and are referred to as co-enzymes. According to Dr. Maynard Murray, MD, every naturally occurring organic mineral should be considered essential for optimal health. Minerals are essential for the working of enzymes, and enzymes are essential for the working of minerals. A few examples: If a certain enzyme is lacking an essential co-factor mineral such as zinc, then the enzyme cannot successfully activate vitamin A to do its work.

If a co-factor of vitamin C lacks the proline hydroxylase enzyme, this will lead to impaired collagen synthesis which will profoundly affect muscle recovery and wound healing. Co-enzymes give the enzymes the power to do their work. Medical researcher Dr. Hagivara MD concludes: *"Modern science has made it clear that all chemical changes within the cells of man are performed by the action of enzymes. It has been found that minerals have much to do with the activities of enzymes. In that sense, **minerals can be said to be enzymes for the enzymes.**"*

Enzymes are without a doubt the most important and most overlooked elements in nutrition today. A deficiency of merely one enzyme may cause the malfunctioning of an entire metabolic chain reaction in the body, thereby preventing some vital function from unfolding. If the food we eat is rich in enzymes, vitamins, and minerals, it will add to our lives. If it is deficient in any of these elements, this will take away from the total life force available to us. Vitamins, minerals, and hormones cannot work without the presence of enzymes.

Enzyme deficiency diseases
The length and quality of life is directly proportional to the amount of available enzymes in the body. The level of amylase in human saliva is approximately 30 times more abundant in the average 25-year-old than the average 81-year-old. In contrast, whales and dolphins, who live in the perfectly balanced aquatic environment and live entirely on raw foods have no difference in cell enzyme composition in young and old. (Murray MD, *Sea Energy Agriculture*)

If one were to analyze the bloodstreams of newborns and elderly persons, there would be little difference noted in the comparative blood levels of most vitamins and minerals in the infant and the old person. Amazingly, however, there are more than a 100 times more enzymes present in the bloodstream of a newborn than that of an elderly person! This, to me, is an incredible, startling fact! Given this, can we then not look at premature old age, or for that matter, the aging process itself, as a biological condition with a major characteristic being a pronounced enzyme deficiency?

Vibrant, healthy cells have high enzyme activity levels. Enzymes are the spark of life and are what makes living cells and tissues truly alive. It is a dubious strategy to expect energy and aliveness from life and then go about eating all that is dead and lifeless. Dr. Francis Pottenger's famous ten-year study showed just that. He fed one group of cats an enzyme-rich diet, and found these cats maintained their health and vigor throughout several generations. A second group of cats, who were fed a diet consisting of at least 80% cooked food, exhibited evidence of degenerative disease. Pottenger's data supported Howell's theories that raw food contains vital factors no longer present in cooked food.

The SAD (Standard American Diet) has a much higher percentage of cooked and processed foods than most other diets, hence it does not come as a surprise to see that more than 70% of Americans are suffering from some form of degenerative disease. The excess intake of cooked fats leads to the exhaustion of the body's ability to manufacture sufficient amounts of lipase, the enzyme responsible for digesting fat. This in turn can lead to obesity, adult onset diabetes, and cardiovascular disease. Eskimos on the other hand can eat up to a pound of lipase-rich raw blubber each and every day and not have any signs or symptoms of cardiovascular disease. However, when Eskimos began to cook their fats like Westerners, they began to suffer from the same degenerative diseases that Western cultures do.

Another medical researcher, Dr. Paul Kauchakoff, MD, experimented with the effects of cooked and raw foods on the bloodstreams of humans. Dr. Kauchakoff found that eating cooked foods caused an immediate increase in the leucocyte (white blood) cell count in the bloodstream, whereas the same food eaten raw did not change blood physiology. Before this important experiment, medical dictum taught that it was a normal physiological event for leucocytes to increase in the blood and migrate to the intestines as soon as food entered the mouth. The strongest hypothesis formulated to explain this phenomenon is that in the body's wisdom, white blood cells collect enzymes from the body's enzyme reserves and migrate to the digestive system to aid in the digestion of the cooked food. Every cooked meal can then be seen as a significant stress on the immune system, speeding the exhaustion of enzymes and ultimately shortening your life.

Enzymeless diet speeds ageing
Dr. James B. Sumner, Nobel Prize recipient and Professor of Biochemistry at Cornell University, wrote in his book *The Secret of Life – Enzymes* that the "getting old feeling" after 40 is due to reduced enzyme levels throughout the body. Young cells contain 100 times more enzymes than old cells. Old cells are filled with metabolic waste and toxins. In the textbook *Enzymes in Health and Disease,* co-edited by Dr. David Greenberg PhD, Chair of the Department of Biochemistry at the University of California School of Medicine at San Francisco, this editor suggests that for optimal health, longevity, and the reduction of many of the diseases of old age, the use of proteolytic (protein-digesting) enzymes should begin about the age of 40 and should optimally continue for the rest of the life-span.

In a similar vein, Dr. Max Wolf, MD, in his book *Enzyme Therapy,* strongly endorses the use of plant-based enzymes. Dr Wolf states: *"Indigestion due to greasy foods is common... Plant-based enzymes are helpful for weak digestions common in old age, or for digestive disturbances. Enzymes are helpful with large rich meals or hard-to-digest foods. Preparations fortified with plant lipase, prevent postprandial (after eating) discomfort or gallbladder attacks."*

Enzymes fight free radicals

Free radicals are not holdovers from the 1960s, but are highly reactive, electrically imbalanced molecules that damage other cells by trying to unite with them in a sort of sexual harassment on the cellular level. When this happens, the cell wall is ruptured and the contents of the cell spills out and begins a cascade of reactions that causes more free radicals to form. Free radical formation is not always pathological but is a natural event that occurs in the process of living. Eating poor foods and living an unhealthy lifestyle can increase free radical formation. However, our body manufactures special antioxidant enzymes (i.e., superoxide dismutase) to remove free radicals before they create cellular damage. In youth, our cells are able to produce sufficient amounts of the metabolic enzymes superoxide dismutase and catalase, which enable them to defend themselves by neutralizing free radicals. As we age we need to provide the cells with sufficient support, so that they can continue to maintain that balance.

Plant versus animal enzymes

Animal-based enzymes work very powerfully on food when the optimal acid-alkaline (pH) environment that these animal-based enzymes require is present. What animal enzyme manufacturers, and those that prescribe these products, do not tell you is that the optimal conditions that are necessary for animal-based enzymes to work optimally do not correspond to the actual *in vivo* (in the body) conditions of the human gastrointestinal tract. Outside of this narrow, optimal range, animal enzymes do not work as well as aspergillus plant-based enzymes.

Pepsin, which only digests protein, is taken from pig carcasses and works if – and only if – the acid environment stomach reaches a pH of 3 or less. This is not always the case, especially in humans who would need supplemental pepsin in the first place. *Pancreatin*, which is taken from cow carcasses, works best in the neutral or slightly alkaline environment of the duodenum at a pH of between 7.8 and 8.3. These conditions are also not always present.

In contrast, plant-based aspergillus oryzae enzymes function well in the wide pH range actually found in the human gastrointestinal tract. Aspergillus oryzae plant enzymes are active in the stomach during the first 30 to 60 minutes of the meal. When the acidity of the lower (pyloric) stomach climbs, the aspergillus enzymes are temporarily inactivated . As it passes into the alkaline environment of the duodenum, aspergillus becomes re-activated again.

Enzyme products help the "SAD" one

The National Digestive Disease Information Clearinghouse in Bethesda, Maryland published these 1993 statistics for the US, as follows: 116,609 digestive system cancer deaths; 20 million cases of gallstones; 66 million reports of "heartburn" each month; 20 million cases of irritable bowel syndrome; 191,311 total deaths due to digestive diseases; 22.3 million work-loss days due to chronic indigestion; 9 million work-loss days due to acute indigestion; 4.5

million hospitalizations due to indigestion; 13% of total hospitalizations due to digestive disorders; 5.8 million digestive system surgeries; and 7% of the total number of surgeries performed were digestive system related.

Indigestion brings in its malodorous trail a host of symptoms and discomforts such as heartburn, gas, bloatedness, nausea, burping, bad breath, body odors, headaches, abdominal pain, insomnia, nightmares, allergies, fatigue, constipation, diarrhea, irritable bowel syndrome, diverticulosis, cramps, spasms, skin problems, acne, pimples, food allergies, antacid dependency, post-meal mental fatigue, lack of concentration, memory loss, and nervousness. What are the harmful consequences of chronic indigestion? When food does not digest properly, starches go sour, proteins putrefy and fats turn rancid. Important nutrients become unavailable to the billions of cells that clamor for them. Excess acidity or alkalinity can set in, resulting in aches and pains and a loss of energy that is sometimes mistaken for psychological depression. The electro-voltage potential of your cells declines, leading to premature aging. To compensate for this generalized lack of energy some of us eat sugar or caffeine to "jump start" ourselves so we can "keep on going." If this negative cycle persists, we *will* keep on going—to an early grave.

Furthermore, chemical energy is stored in a molecule known as adenosine triphosphate (ATP). By way of enzymatic action, food is transformed into energy and then stored in the ATP molecules in our cells. The less efficient is our digestion, the less ATP energy will be created. Furthermore, when digestion is inefficient, fermenting and putrefying food has to be neutralized by our immune system, which requires ATP energy to do the cleansing.

The enzyme effect on allergies
Allergies are among the most common and costly of all health problems, afflicting an estimated 37 million people at a cost in excess of over 1.5 billion dollars a year. Nine percent of all patients seeking medical care at a physician's office do so for allergies. *(Asthma and other Allergic Diseases, NIAID, NIH Publ. No 79-387, 5/79)* Allergies can be caused by an innumerable variety of substances, including food, pollen, dust, molds, drugs, cosmetics, toiletries, fabrics, poison ivy, etc. These allergens can enter your body through your food, the air, your skin, and even via medical injections.

Food allergies evoke a wide variety of symptoms, including fatigue, nervous tension, headaches, dizziness, nasal congestion, runny nose, itching, rashes, abdominal cramping, nausea, vomiting, and diarrhea. Foods high on the allergy list are milk, wheat, corn, eggs, seafood, and chocolate. Many people are also allergic to berries, citrus, and tomatoes. It is possible to be allergic to any food, including whole natural foods. However, I have observed that many people who are allergic to unsoaked or cooked seeds, nuts, and grains are no longer allergic to them when they are sprouted or soaked, or they take food enzymes. Why does this positive change take place? The enzymes in these foods become enlivened with the sprouting process. The complex allergenic elements of these foods, i.e. the gluten found in wheat, become pre-digested and/or neutralized by the action of these enzymes.

Many foods contain these hard-to-digest elements. Dr. Howell cited experiments that showed that bacteria, yeast cells, large protein molecules, and fats can slip through the walls of the intestines and into the bloodstream. If this happens, the already stressed immune system will not be able to deal with these undigested food elements and foreign proteins floating around. He further demonstrated that protective enzymes in the bloodstream break down these substances and absorb or neutralize them. In this connection, it was also found that if enzyme levels were too low, allergies developed. When supplemental enzymes were administered and the measured enzyme level in the blood had significantly increased, the allergies disappeared. The allergic reaction itself is the body's way to remove the allergen from the system. If the allergic reaction is suppressed by medication, then the body is forced to store the allergen in the body. The long-term effect of suppression is the eventual development of degenerative disease.

Dr. Cory Resnick, in *Plant Enzyme Therapy*, discusses practical approaches in treatment of food allergies: *"By digesting dietary protein, plant enzymes administered orally at mealtime work to decrease the supply of antigenic macromolecules available to leak into the bloodstream. In addition, orally administered plant enzymes which have themselves been absorbed intact may help to 'digest' antigenic dietary proteins which they encounter in the bloodstream." (Pizzome et al, '92).*

Enzyme fasting and healing

When you fast or go on a liquid diet of raw fruit and vegetable juices, your digestive system no longer has to produce enzymes. According to what Dr. Howell refers to as the "law of adaptive secretion," the enzyme potential that is no longer directed into digesting food can now be utilized by the general metabolic pool. These enzymes are now free to repair and rejuvenate the tissues and organs that need attention in other parts of the body. Many a seriously ill person has surprised family, friends, and doctors by healing themselves of seemingly incurable diseases when they adopted a total life-enhancing regime that included a high enzyme diet including supplementary enzymes, sufficient rest, appropriate exercise, positive mental attitude, and a conducive social and physical environment.

For a person who is run-down and toxic, it is not impossible to adopt such a program at home, but for those who are sick, the supervision of a competent health professional is strongly advised. One can also travel to the health centers that specialize in educating and/or healing people who are dedicated to regaining their health. A few places in Europe include Josef Issel's Ringberg Clinic in West Germany, and Dr Essen's Vita Nova in Sweden. In the United States, Hippocrates Health Institute of West Palm Beach, Florida provides a beautiful residential setting where one can learn by doing.

Can children use plant enzymes?

Most children have strong digestive systems. However, the fact that they can digest less-than-optimal cooked foods does not automatically make these foods ideal for the future unfolding of their maximum health potential. Sure, kids will digest the foods served them and still be full of youthful energy, but the same health principles hold for children as they do for adults: namely, that the process of aging is accelerated when enzyme reserves are squandered by the burden of digesting excessive amounts of cooked food.

Plant enzymes and medication
If you are under medical care or taking oral medication of any kind, there are steps you should take to avoid any inactivation of an enzyme supplement by your medication. Sprinkle plant enzyme powder *on the food itself* instead of taking the capsules or powder directly into your body. Make sure, however, that the food has cooled down a bit or else the enzyme powder will be damaged by the high heat of your food. In this way, the predigestive action of the enzymes will work directly on the food and not have to come in contact with the drugs that may be in your stomach.

Despite the long-overdue surfacing of the truth about enzymes, don't be surprised if your family doctor still downplays the importance or even the existence of enzymes in foods. Traditionally, segments of the medical community take a conservative posture on many issues. In fact, the majority of doctors, dieticians and nutritionists do not fully appreciate the contribution of food enzymes to health maintenance and the prevention of disease. At the conclusion of this chapter you will probably know more about food enzymes than most physicians!

Do plant enzymes survive gut acids?
Less than one fifth of all medical schools in the United States teach even the elementary aspects of nutrition. Of those that do teach it, the true role of food enzymes is rarely if ever taught. According to the prevailing accepted dictum, enzymes found in foods are destroyed by the hydrochloric acid of the stomach and are of virtually no use in the digestive economy. However, Dr. Howell has shown that as soon as a particular food is masticated in the mouth, the enzymes begin to digest the food. This has been confirmed by Finnish Nobel Prize winner Artturi Virtanen.
When the food reaches the first part of the stomach, (upper cardiac stomach) the food enzymes are still actively working. It takes up to 50 minutes for the hydrochloric acid level to rise to the critical level where the acidity of the hydrochloric acid could inactivate the food enzymes in the food. Until this level is reached, food enzymes are still working. What is more, not all foods stimulate hydrochloric acid production appreciably. Foods like fruit, sprouts, grasses and many raw vegetables do not cause hydrochloric acid production to increase rapidly or in any great quantity. In this environment enzymes present in food have a longer time to do their work. According to Howell, even though saliva enzymes shut off in the presence of acid, food enzymes are not markedly disturbed.

After taking enzyme supplements, many people immediately feel a difference in the ease in which their food is digested. They also report an overall boost in their energy level. Others do not report any dramatic subjective improvement. The latter case is probably due to the relatively good health enjoyed already or the fact that the "bloom of youth" has not as yet faded. Whether you feel any immediate subjective improvements in your health as a result of taking enzymes is not as important as your understanding how enzymes do their work of enhancing digestion and assimilation, boosting the immune system and contributing to your body's total vitality.

In conclusion
Outside the human body, enzymes can produce dramatic effects very quickly. Enzymes are used in the process of making bread, wine, cheese, etc. Enzymes are used in laundry detergents, septic tanks, and in dissolving massive accidental oil spills. In these cases, there is no denying that enzymes do their work. Why then is there so much resistance to accepting that food enzymes do work in the human body?

In nature, all undomesticated animals eat an enzyme-rich diet. They live out their lives, largely free from degenerative diseases. The human animal is the only species that nourishes itself on a cooked, largely enzymeless diet. Our longevity and our well-being could be increased if we ate more whole foods with an emphasis on uncooked foods.

When food is cooked, there is a reduction in the bioavailability of protein, vitamins, and minerals so that your cells get much less nutrition. Unless you cook at 118 degrees Fahrenheit or below (as in sun-drying or dehydrating foods), you will completely destroy all of the enzymes present in the food.

Dr. Howell's powerful words say it all:

"There is no other mechanism in the body except enzyme action to protect the body from any hazard. It is ambiguous to say that "nature cures" when we must know that the only machinery in the body to do anything is enzyme action. Hormones do not work. Vitamins cannot do any work. Minerals were not made to do any work. Proteins cannot work. Nature does not work. Only enzymes are made for work."

Key references
Belfiore F, M.D. *Enzyme Regulation & Metabolic Diseases* Greenberg, D. Ph.D., *Enzymes in Health and Disease*
Innerfield, Irvin, M.D., *Enzymes in Clinical Medicine*
Holcenberg John S., *Enzymes as Drugs*
Howell, E., M.D., *Food Enzymes for Health & Longevity* Hogiwara, Y., M.D., *Green Barley Essence*

Kautchakoff, Paul, *"The Influence of Food Cooking on the Blood Formula of Man";* Proceedings: The First International Congress of Macrobiology, Paris

Martin, Gustav M.D., *Clinical Enzymolgy*

Rossi G. V.Ph.D., *'Diagnostic Use of Enzymes'*

Murray, Maynard, M.D., *Sea Energy Agriculture*

Ratcliff, *Enzymes, Medicine's Hope, Readers Digest* 6/61 Santillo, Humbart N.D., M.H. *Food Enzymes*

Sumner, J. B., *The Secrets of Life - Enzymes*

Wilkinson, J.H., *'The Digestive Enzymes'* & *'Aging*

Wilkensen, H., Ph.D., *Diagnostic Enzymology*

Wolf, Max, M.D., *Enzyme Therapy*

This chapter is extracted from the ebook "Don't Dine Without Enzymes"

About the Author:
"Viktoras is the father of the modern day living-foods diet that is gaining popular support in the medical community. We see in Viktoras one of the most eminent geniuses in the history of the wellness industry." David Allen, PhD, author, wellness pioneer, researcher.

Co-founder with Dr. Ann Wigmore of the world renowned Hippocrates Health Institute and developer of its wheatgrass and raw food program, Viktoras **Kulvinskas** *has received international acclaim as an author, lecturer, and health consultant. In addition to publishing five books on natural healing, he has contributed articles to many publications including "Vegetarian Times", "Vegetarian Voice", "Health Street Journal", and "Alternatives". His bestselling definitive work on achieving health through raw foods, wheatgrass, enzymes, and spiritual practice,* **Survival In The 21st Century** *is now in its 35th printing. He has spearheaded the global raw foods revolution for some 40 years now.*

He received his Master of Science degree in pure mathematics from the University of Connecticut. He was a computer consultant for Harvard University, the Massachusetts Institute of Technology, the Smithsonian Astrophysical Observatory, and the Apollo Project.

Viktoras has spoken at the United Nations on solving world hunger and health problems. His researches on blue green algae and enzymes have contributed to the widespread availability of these products. Viktoras continues his work today as the premier pioneer of the global raw foods healing movement.

www.viktoraslive.org

4

The Principle of 80% Raw

Brian Clement PhD, NMD, LNC

As most, when I first embraced the living food diet and relinquished conventional vegan fare, I was like a new convert, an evangelical. This, of course, represents insecurity, but at the time I thought that my new religion would frown upon me if I ever touched my lips with a morsel of cooked cuisine. For eight years, I maintained a 100% living/raw diet and gained deep insight and significant biological data on its enormous benefits. My gift was that, for part of this time, I was also working with clients and guests at the Hippocrates Health Institute. The vast majority of the people I assisted were catastrophically ill. What was continually amazing was how this unprocessed organic food could reignite life and vitality in weakened and depleted people. Although rare, I worked with athletes who were trying to gain the edge in their sport. I found the diet to be as effective for them as it was for those afflicted with cancer and other dreaded diseases.

In time, and with the experience of working with tens of thousands of people, both in Europe where I was directing and developing centers, as well as Hippocrates, then located in Boston, I realized that the proposition of consuming 100% raw food for the rest of one's life would be untenable for most people. Their bodies would flourish with a balanced living food meal plan, but social restrictions and lifetime habits of consuming certain cooked dishes placed road blocks in their ability to wholeheartedly adapt to the diet. The majority who attempted adherence most often over-consumed nuts, seeds, avocadoes and fruits. All of this concerned me, as it placed a spotlight on the harsh reality that this remarkable lifestyle is very difficult for the average person to follow. If we could just give each participant a lobotomy, washing away their memories and explain the exceptional benefits derived by eating this simple and pure food, I am sure that there would be no hardship in this noble pursuit!

Somewhere in my ninth year as a living food vegan, I was visiting my mother who offered me steamed organic broccoli. After I gave a thirty-minute lecture on the poisonous effect of consuming such unfathomable waste, it struck me that that was the way my mother was continuing to show her love. This was the turning point for me, and I left my devotee position to become, once again, a scientific professional. Within days, I enlisted a friend at Tufts University to work on immunological profiles concerning vegan food consumption with different percentages of raw intake. After a long day at work, he would often spend time into the wee hours analyzing this subject. I frequently joined him but was not of much help, as this was out of my area of expertise. Three months later, we came up with an interesting finding and put forth a dietary plan from which it was based.

Strengthening immune function
Those engaged in the conquest of disease were prime candidates to consume 100% living vegan food for a minimum period of two years. We found that it took approximately this amount of time to reengage and fully develop the immune system cells. At that point, 93% were able to add minimal clean organic cooked vegan foods without seeing a change in their immune system. Approximately 7% of the group required a longer period of superior adherence to the pure diet. The tipping point was when we included approximately 20% cooked fare. What became apparent was surprising, although understandable. When moving from the 20 to 25% intake, there was an average 17% drop in immune function. When moving up to approximately 30%, or 10% beyond the advisable limit, it appeared that one half of the immune function was compromised. This confirmed other studies that I had explored in the past. Leukocytosis is a seldom-acknowledged disease wherein white blood cells are engaged to attack and remove cooked foods. We also observed that the differentials eosinophils, basofils, neutrocytes, lymphocytes, etc. all were engaged in the battle to remove what the body obviously perceived as unwanted elements. Of course, the immune system developed over millennia to prevent microbes, mutagens, other life forms, and now, pollution, from creating disorders. In recent years, first in Europe, Asia, and now North America, much interest has been placed in seeing the structural differences that are caused by cooking certain foods. **Acrylomides** are the most notable, whereas dangerous carbohydrates such as french fries, chips, cereals, including organic cereals, etc. become masterful carcinogens (cancer causers). In the United States, California has actually legislated that such foods must have a warning on their label. All of this further confirms why the use of living/raw food at the Hippocrates Health Institute has been in great part effective in strengthening the immune system. Abstaining from cooked food is the first step in renewing physical health. The consumption of organic plant foods additionally offers phytonutrients that target and kill disease.

A viable food plan
Having established a biological blueprint of the effect that pure vegan food had on the immune system, we then formulated suggestions on how to design a via-

ble food plan. When first announcing this in the early 1980s, the acceptance from Hippocrates' participants was overwhelming. Their joy was palpable, since now they saw light at the end of the tunnel. For those who generally held good health, we advised that they should live on 100% raw for two years and at least attempt six months before broadening their food choices. On that bright May day in New England, living/raw food became viable for the general public and changed its status from an impossible dream. We also acknowledged that our eating patterns were, at times, born out of social and cultural rituals. Knowing that these patterns can harm health, we included positive food choices and encouraged the removal of damaging fare. Living food and its relevance depends upon its availability, acceptance, and benefit. When all three conditions are met, we believe that, in time, the world's population will once again regain a vibrant level of physical and mental health.

It has become apparent that small amounts of cooked food in healthy participants will empower them psychologically without physiologically causing harm. One of the ongoing concerns we face when people change to a living diet is sustaining healthy body weight. Although there is no difference between sprouted grain and cooked grain when it comes to developing body mass, we observe that peoples' perception of their ability to maintain weight is improved when they include cooked sprouted grains into the diet. The mind and its multitude of memories literally impact the function, shape, and size of the anatomy. Quantum biology has validated this when discussing the cell mind and its independence as well as its conformity. Take a scar into consideration. This is an injury that may have happened decades ago when the largest organ (the skin) has been perforated. Within days, the healthy body heals the tissue, yet there is often an imprint made from this injury. The cells remember this assault and literally re-create the shape, strengthening the very cells so that it is better protected from the next potential penetration. A bone that is broken will be stronger in the break than it was before the fracture, *and the mind, once experienced, will potentially not allow a problematic circumstance to once again occur.*

The body and its cells are now known to actually call out for familiar sources of sustenance. Anatomies that are overweight, with their many fat cells, actually call out for fat producing "foods". This furthers our understanding of addiction, whereas it is not only the mind and its patterns and the substance and its addictive qualities, additionally it is the body requesting those elements that keep it locked into the vicious cycle. On the other hand, a healthy body that is well fed, exercised, and without exceptional stress, will request the likeness of itself. At this point, unnatural cravings will slip away and a balanced, emotionally stable desire for food will establish itself. When one has experienced an all organic/bio living diet for a period of time, even the deepest emotional desires for harmful substances will wane. In recent history, we have used foods as a buffer from our emotional stress and mental confusion. There is a two-way action that occurs when making healthy nutritional choices over time. The first is a reestablishment of cellular and physiological health. The second is a reestablishment of food as a tool, not a narcotic. Together they ally in the battle against overeating, binge eating, under eating, and general disorder.

Establishing symbiosis

Your anatomy and your thoughts can get their arms around a future that permits a bit of alteration. We must consider a life on a living/raw diet as viable, healthy, and exciting. When releasing ourselves from the bonds of restrictive ideology, it frees us to establish symbiosis. It has been my observation in thousands of cases where people are living up to some "bigger than thou" concept, that they tend to try to gain balance from over consuming sugars (fruits, juices, honeys, syrups, etc.), fats (nuts, seeds, avocadoes, oils, including coconut, etc.), or large amounts of food. It is much better when one is either emotionally and spiritually balanced and able to eat 100% living food by choice, or emotionally and physically balanced and able to eat up to 20-25% cooked organic vegan food. I must once again remind you that all such suggestions are based on healthy individuals, not those conquering disease.

Here at the Hippocrates Health Institute on holidays (Christmas, Independence Day, Thanksgiving), we serve a small amount of familiar cooked vegan cuisine and we see the psychological impact this has on people. It often reminds them of happy times from their past and familiar surroundings that instill confidence. Years ago on a Christmas tour of homes, when I entered through the front door there was a fragrance of cloves and cinnamon permeating the atmosphere. Instantly I became a five-year-old boy walking into my grandmother's house on Christmas Day. She always had a big pot on the stove with these two aromatic exotics boiling away. This is aromatherapy at its very best. The same applies to foods. Unfortunately, the first girl I was in love with loved pies! Every time we were together, we would consume at least one. This is the downside of food memories, and too many of us suffer from its unforgiving grips. Emotional change must come before you are able to adapt a sane cohesive diet. Until you change your perception, your perception remains the same and often creates an unsteady future of food choices.

Twenty-five years ago, I was being interviewed on a national radio program. At that time, I was often using the term "complete health". Well into the interview, the host asked me what I meant by "complete health". I was stunned. Afterward, I listened to the program and I have been using this description ever since: At any time in your life you are able to fulfill your greatest dream with your physical capacity. Food must be looked at as a fuel, not as a friend, a social device, or a drug. When growing to the point where you have tamed your misconceptions and energized yourself with nourishment, your capacity emotionally and spiritually will once again fly high. Remember to constantly allow change and not to pigeonhole yourself into any corner. Those of us who spend our lives researching and finding new discoveries in nutrition may tomorrow offer you something that is not available today. On your own, you may discover something that is invaluable for all of us to know and employ. Together, we can bring our enthusiasm, knowledge, and wisdom to others so that the world will gain the same benefits that we receive.

About the Author:

Dr. Brian Clement, PhD., NMD., LNC, *has spearheaded the International progressive health movement for more than three decades. By conducting daily clinical research as the director of the renowned Hippocrates Health Institute, the world's foremost complementary residential health Mecca, he and his team have developed a state-of-the-art program for health maintenance and recovery. His Florida (U.S.A.) center has pioneered a program and established training in active aging and disease prevention. With hundreds of thousands of people participating in this program over the last half-century, volumes of data have been accrued, giving Clement a privileged insight into the lifestyle required to maintain youth, vitality, and stamina. Among Dr. Clement's many publications are **Living Foods for Optimum Health** and **Longevity** and **Lifeforce.** His latest book,* Longevity, *delivers cutting-edge knowledge coupled with a common sense practical approach that will raise your level of health and happiness. Dr. Clement is first and foremost a devoted husband and a caring father of four. In addition to daily counseling and research studies, Clement conducts conferences worldwide on attaining health and creating longevity, giving delegates a roadmap for redirecting, enriching and extending their lives.*

www.hippocratesinst.org

5

Deep Food: Accessing Nutrient Density From the Ground Up

David Rainoshek, MA and Katrina Rainoshek

This chapter is about true nutritional abundance. By looking deeply at our current food choices and their impact, we can far transcend the flashy, heavily advertised, excitotoxin-laden, nutrient poor, disease-causing "foods" that are ubiquitous in modern life. We can see the wisdom of accessing abundance at every level: nutritionally, emotionally, culturally, and spiritually, with food from – and as – fertile ground for a deeper, more authentic expression of our individual and collective potential.

There are over 50,000 edible plants on Earth, yet according to anthropologist Jared Diamond, author of *Guns, Germs, and Steel,* approximately 90% of the human diet consists of just 15 foods[1]:

1. *Corn* **2.** *Wheat* **3.** *Rice* **4.** *Coffee* **5.** *Soy* **6.** *Potato* **7.** *Cacao (chocolate)* **8.** *Barley* **9.** *Chicken (flesh and eggs)* **10.** *Dairy (from goat)* **11.** *Dairy (from cow)* **12.** *Meat (from cow)* **13.** *Coconut* **14.** *Orange* **15.** *Cassava root (also known as Manioc and Tapioca)*

Over the last 11,000 years, as socio-cultural evolution worldwide has progressed from foraging to horticultural to agricultural to industrial to technological, few of these 15 food staples have concomitantly evolved in our industrial-technological stages to qualify as *Deep Food*: nutrient-dense; disease preventing and reversing; and health-promoting mentally, emotionally, spiritually, culturally, economically, politically, and environmentally. In recent centuries our foodstuffs have grown increasingly *shallow*, having been subjected to the impersonal claims of western industrial agri*business*, shipping, preserving, irradiation, flavoring, packaging, and the substitution of colorful advertising for true substance.

In the 21st Century, we find ourselves more fortunate than our ancestors, in that nutrient-dense foods, superfoods, and nutritional supplements are more widely available than ever before. **How can we heal the damaging aspects of the modernization of agriculture and food done by industry and technology, while incorporating the multiple benefits afforded to us by better organic practices, nutritional understanding, food availability and variety?**

We will investigate:
- Deep Food, nutrient-density, and the significance of these designations
- Why we are seeing a simultaneous arising of the best and worst foods ever available
- What our best nutrient dense foods are
- The personal and cultural significance of these foods
- Why eating a plant-based diet cannot stand alone in one's personal quest to live deeply in excellent health at every level
- The three fundamental qualities to cultivate in yourself to courageously and successfully claim and encourage Deep Food and abundant living for yourself and the world

Deep Food/Integral
Deep Food, as we are coining the term here, is defined by four main criteria we are using from the Integral All-Quadrants All-Levels Approach (AQAL Approach or Map) of Ken Wilber.[2] (Bear with us for a moment if this concept seems too complex for the subject of food. We think you will see that food quite deservedly merits the application of the AQAL structure, and in doing so we can gain a whole new understanding of food, and an appreciation for what we are defining as Deep Food.)

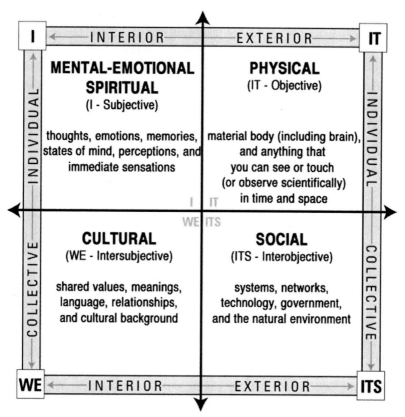

Figure 1: The AQAL Map Showing the Four Quadrants by Ken Wilber in *A Brief History of Everything*

This four quadrant AQAL model (see Figure 1) is extraordinarily useful because it represents the main perspectives or dimensions of every aspect of the manifest world: first person singular *mental, emotional, and spiritual* (I-Subjective), first person plural *cultural* (We-Intersubjective), third person singular (*physical* It-Objective) and plural (*social* Its-Interobjective). An Integral View, as opposed to a partial or reductionistic view, *takes all four of these quadrants into account.* As we will see, Deep Food signifies an Integral Approach to nutrition that needs to be understood and applied if we are to heal and transcend the pathologies of our industrial and technological stages of social development and their impact on food growth and consumption.

How can we tell if a food is shallow or deep? The most important factors (using the AQAL Map) in locating a food on the continuum from Shallow Food to Deep Food are:

PHYSICAL (IT-OBJECTIVE)	the soil and how it is farmed treatment or care of the food from harvest to table (packaged, preserved, flavored, frozen, cooked, fresh, raw, living)
SOCIAL (ITS-INTEROBJECTIVE)	the social – political – economic – ecological ramifications of the food
CULTURAL (WE-INTERSUBJECTIVE)	our relationship to the food, i.e. its cultural and mythological significance
MENTAL-EMOTIONAL-SPIRITUAL (I-SUBJECTIVE)	effect on the mental – emotional – spiritual states and development of an individual

Deep Food, in short, signifies a food or cuisine that drives the higher levels of development in any of the quadrants *without compromising development in any other quadrant*. This is very important. In modern times, reality has been so fragmented that our approaches to social, economic, political, scientific, and medical concerns have become *reductionist* or myopic. A simple example would be the mass production of foodstuffs via the mechanization of agriculture from farm to truck to fluorescent-lit grocery to table. From an economic standpoint of food costs, this lower-right quadrant (Economic "Its-Intersubjective") method of production may look great, but it seriously degrades the health of the individual, in body (the upper-right quadrant or Physical "Its-Subjective"), in mind (the upper left or Mental "I-Objective"), and it renders the food culturally bereft of deep significance (the lower left or Cultural "We-Interobjective"). Deep Food honors development in every quadrant, to the greatest extent possible, and once a person has the use of this term and its implications, authenticity and duplicity are easy to distinguish.

Deep Food/Physical: It-Objective/Nutrient Density

Ironically, Westernized cultures are simultaneously overfed and undernourished on low-nutrient, high-calorie foods ("empty" calories), creating the preconditions for diabetes, heart disease, hypoglycemia, hypertension, depression, chronic pain, cancers of all kinds, and the most obvious: *overweight/obesity*. A July 2008 Johns Hopkins University study published in *Obesity* projects that by 2030, 86% of Americans (the world's best case study for diet Westernization) will be overweight or obese, and according to study author Youfa Wang, MD, PhD, 24% of US children and 75% of adults will be overweight or obese by 2015.[34] What is going on here? We can start to answer this question by looking at the Social quadrant which includes political and economic realities of today's food supply.

Adam Drewnowski, an obesity researcher at the University of Washington sought answers, and investigated why economic status is the most reliable predictor of obesity in America. With a hypothetical dollar to spend, he purchased as many calories as he could, and discovered that he could buy the most calories per dollar in the *middle aisles of the supermarket*, among the towering canyons of processed food and soft drinks where a dollar could buy 1,200 calories of cookies or potato chips, but only 250 calories of carrots; 875 calories of soda but only 170 calories of orange juice.[5] Why is this?

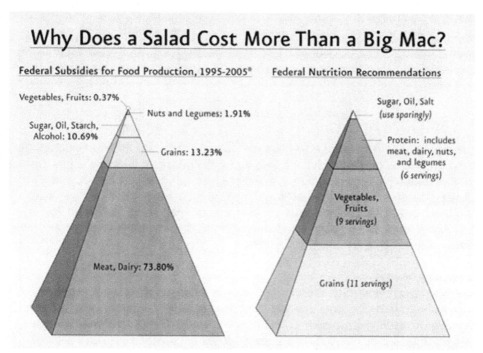

Why Does a Salad Cost More Than a Big Mac?

Figure 2: U.S. Federal Subsidies 1995-2005 vs. U.S. Federal Nutrition Guidelines (Physician's Committee for Responsible Medicine, August 2007)

Corporate interests are finding, whether by design or default, that cheap foods with long shelf lives, properly advertised, colored, flavored, conventionally grown and preserved (read: irradiated) can reap more profits at the store, and then down the road at the doctor's office, the pharmacy, and in the hospital - as opposed to fresh, unadulterated living, organic, disease-preventing, nutrient-dense foods grown and prepared with agricultural and culinary integrity. Government subsidies, seen in Figure 2, are not even remotely guided by the Federal Nutrition Recommendations, much less a plant-based diet. Our poor food environment is a fundamental symptom of how as a group we have settled for flashy, *shallow* foods, role models, television programming, politicians, lifestyles, emotional and spiritual experiences.

From The Ground Up
Despite the myths we have been told and sold, we are not Mars-bar eaters, Super Big Gulp drinkers, or Big Mac snackers, and do not suffer from a deficiency of these nutrient-poor junk foods. None of us is suffering from a deficiency of

Red Dye #40, Blue Lake #5, disodium inosinate, MSG, aspartame, or any of the other excitotoxins that have been deliberately placed in our foods to seduce and addict us for profit. For millions of years we have been physiologically, biochemically, and genetically designed to eat a diet of organic living plant foods. The overwhelming medical, sociological, and historical data corroborate this. Food is a fundamental way that we interface with our home the living planet and with our cultural ancestry (that existed predominantly *without heart disease, diabetes, and other diseases of overconsumption*). It is the most important and subtle way that we acknowledge an association or dissociation with who we truly are, and the stuff of which our greatest capacities are developed. When we are at a lack for the most basic nutritional elements, this affects every other level of our being profoundly as we ascend the Nest of Spirit (formerly known as The Great Chain of Being):

Matter (food)→Body→Mind→Soul→Spirit

Food is the ground on which the "higher" aspects of our being grow and mature. When matter is not cultivated and included with conscious care, individual and cultural pathologies are created – as we are now witnessing in full force in westernized cultures. As we discuss Deep Food from an Integral perspective, keep the basic progression of the Nest of Spirit in mind, as it is the Perennial Philosophy common to all the major world wisdom traditions – lending a far greater, globally unifying significance to Deep Foods.

Nutrients Matter

We will present data momentarily, but organic means food grown in nutrient-rich soil, without harmful agrochemicals, biological/genetic tampering, antibiological agents, or irradiation processes. Fresh-raw-live means that your food has not been compromised by cooking/processing before it came to you, and you are not going to insult your miracle food or your living body by heating and destroying the nutrients in what you eat.

> *When you cook food, according to the Max Planck Institute, you coagulate 50% of the food's protein. Other research shows that 70–90% of vitamins and minerals, and up to 100% of phytonutrients are destroyed when food is cooked.[6]*

Processing, cooking, pasteurization, and irradiation are all food handling methods that destroy the nutrient-dense qualities present in our foods when they are in their natural state. Because of these nutrient-destructive processes, we tend to eat more food in an effort to access a nutritional value equal to what we would have received from the uncooked food in its whole state. This additional eating is largely behind the Johns Hopkins projection of 75% overweight in the U.S. population by 2015. Nutrient dense foods have what is known as a high *satiety index*, meaning that your body is *satisfied* by the food sooner, and you experience this as an *aliesthetic taste change*, or the natural message to stop eating. In short, eating raw/living plant foods enables your body to get more (nutrient density) for less (calories eaten). For this reason the scientifically proven life extension method of CR (Calorie Restriction) happens naturally on a raw/live food diet. *See chapter 13 for more information on the healthy life practice of what we call Calorie Prudence.*

Nutrient-dense foods and cuisine have an abundance of bioavailable nutrition, including:

Protein (leafy greens are 20-30% protein)
Fat (including omega-3,[6], and 9 fatty acids)
Carbohydrate (living and raw carbohydrates are lower on the glycemic index than cooked carbohydrates)
Minerals (numerous sources suggest we need 92 mineral elements for optimal health)
Enzymes (only live, plant-based food sources contain living enzymes)
Phytonutrients-Vitamins-Antioxidants-Chlorophyll (plants contain hundreds or thousands of essential health-protecting/promoting phytonutrients, many of which are destroyed by heat)
Probiotics (healthy, beneficial *flora*)
Water (cooking and processing evaporates away valuable water from our food)

When most or all of these elements are in play, we have what Dr. Richard Anderson defines as a true food[7]; *"I propose that the true definition of a food is as follows: a substance that nourishes or fuels the body with life-giving forces (i.e. life-force, vitamins, minerals, enzymes, amino acids, etc.) without injury to its normal functions, thereby strengthening, energizing, and maintaining it. Food is not simply something one puts in the mouth, chews, and swallows. Food should not deplete or rob the body of its needed essence or harm it in any way. Dead or dying foods take an enormous toll on the body."*

Nutrient density is defined as a ratio of nutrient content (in grams) to the total energy content (in kilocalories or joules). Nutrient-dense food is opposite to energy-dense food (also called "empty calorie" food). According to the Dietary Guidelines for Americans 2005, nutrient-dense foods are those foods that provide the highest amounts of vitamins, minerals, enzymes, and phytonutrients per calorie.[8] For example, superfood algaes, vegetables, sea vegetables, and non-hybridized fruits are nutrient-dense. Processed, refined, pasteurized, irradiated food products containing added sugars, flavors, saturated fats, and alcohol are nutrient-poor. When you eat nutrient-poor foods, you must eat more food in an attempt (often futile) to get an equivalent amount of nutrition. Nutrient density can also be understood as the ratio of the nutrient composition of a given food to the nutrient requirements of the human body. Therefore, the most nutrient-dense food is one that delivers the most complete nutritional package in bioavailable form.

Our top nutrient-dense foods are: leafy greens; Blue-green algaes such as spirulina, chlorella, and Klamath Lake AFA; grasses; nuts and seeds; sea vegetables; green superfood powder concentrates; bee pollen granules; deep pigment phytonutrient-rich foods such as berries, pomegranates, etc. Dr Joel Fuhrman, author of *Eat to Live,* has created an excellent chart on the nutrient density calculations of various foods. Notice that leafy greens are the top foods listed!

Nutrient Density Chart

Sample Nutrient / Calorie Density Scores
Dr. Fuhrman's Aggregate Nutrient Density Index* (ANDI)
The higher the number the better the food

Food	Score	Food	Score
Kale	1000	Flaxseed	44
Collards	1000	Sesame seeds	41
Watercress	1000	Brown rice	41
Bok Choy	824	Salmon	39
Spinach (uncooked)	697	Avocado	37
Brussel sprouts	672	Pork loin	37
Swiss chard	670	Pumpkin seeds	36
Arugula	559	Skim milk	36
Radish	554	Pecans	34
Cabbage (cooked)	481	Potato	32
Bean sprouts	444	Grapes	31
Red pepper	420	Cod	31
Romaine lettuce	389	Banana	30
Broccoli	342	Walnuts	29
Cauliflower	295	Pistachio nuts	29
Green pepper	258	Chicken breast	27
Tomato sauce	247	Egg	27
Artichoke	244	Low-fat plain yogurt	26
Carrots	240	Shredded wheat	26
Asparagus	234	Whole wheat bread	25
Strawberries	212	Corn	25
Pomegranate juice	193	Almonds	24
Tomato	164	Feta cheese	21
Plums	157	Milk chocolate	21
Raspberries	145	Whole milk	20
Blueberries	130	Ground beef	20
Brazil nuts	117	Dates	19
Iceberg lettuce	110	Whole wheat pasta	19
Orange	109	White bread	18
Grapefruit	102	Peanut butter	18
Cantaloupe	100	White pasta	18
Tofu	86	Raisins	17
Sweet potato	84	Cashews	16
Apple	76	Apple juice	16
Peach	74	Swiss cheese	15
Green peas	70	Low fat fruit yogurt	14
Cherries	68	White rice	12
Kidney beans	56	Potato chips	11
Oatmeal	53	Saltines	11
Mango	51	Vanilla ice cream	7
Cucumber	50	Sugar cookies	5
Soybeans	48	Corn oil	3
Prunes	47	Olive oil	2
Sunflower seeds	46	Honey	1
Shrimp	45	Cola	.5

Figure 3: Aggregate Nutrient Density Index, from *Eat For Health* by Joel Fuhrman, M.D, DrFuhrman.com

The Magic Of Nutrient Density

In the context of a plant-source-only, raw/live, organic diet, it should be understood that we are not denying ourselves the fuel or nutrients we need. Nor are we in a cycle of deprivation. We are taking in a delicious, filling, natural, appropriate amount of calories that are nutrient-dense enough to activate an *aliesthetic taste change*. The aliesthetic change is experienced as when we feel pleasurably satisfied from eating. It is also known as the "stop eating" signal we get from our body. This taste change most commonly happens when eating raw and living nutrient-dense foods. Think about it: Who overeats a salad? Eating a processed, cooked diet laden with excitotoxins (such as MSG) provides the double insult of low nutrient density combined with the supersensory stimuli of artificial flavorings, driving body and mind to continue to ask for food long after our calorie needs would have been satisfied by a tasty nutrient-dense meal. You would think that by eating a lower-calorie diet that a feeling of restriction or deprivation would result, but when your body receives all the minerals, phytonutrients, vitamins, enzymes, protein, essential fats, complex carbohydrates, and water it requires through a plant-source-only meal, a feeling of deep satisfaction is experienced right down to the cellular level. We are satiated by these foods that are high on the satiety index. A completely new sense of abundance is realized as we begin to seek quality over quantity in our food. When we eat in such a way that everything we consume has purpose, we are living a life of true depth, which becomes indicative of the dynamic things we attract in every aspect of our life.

Health Begins In The Soil!

Societies and cultures throughout human history have risen and declined by this fundamental truth. In his groundbreaking work, *Collapse: How Societies Choose to Fail or Succeed*, Jared Diamond carefully examines the ecological reasons behind the collapse of societies throughout human history[9]. The methods by which we farm – for better or worse - significantly impact soil fertility, nutrition and human health, ecology, national energy policies, economics, culture, and national security. It has long been suspected that many of these [collapses] were at least partly triggered by ecological problems: people inadvertently destroying the environmental resources on which their societies depended. This suspicion of unintended ecological suicide – *ecocide* – has been confirmed by discoveries made in recent decades by archaeologists, climatologists, historians, paleontologists, and palynologists (pollen scientists).

Nowhere do we see the relationship of soil fertility, farming techniques, and the resulting health consequences of the food consumed more pronounced than in the United States. This is partly because there is so much data available to give us a picture of the results of this 70-year experiment. Each year since World War II, intensive agrochemical-based farming practices have produced agro-chemical-laden food of lower nutrient density at a significant cost. The US Department of Agriculture periodically publishes data on the nutritional content of food. Historically, since the 1940s, each publication of this data shows a decline in the average nutritional content of food. Wheat, for example, used to average a protein content of 19% in the 1940s, but today it averages about 12%. A prime example that this type of poor food production is not working is the very expensive US health crisis in nation of overfed, undernourished people. In 2009, the United States will spend $2.9 Trillion on health care,[10] yet ranks near the bottom in terms of overall health among industrialized nations. This is a crisis which we can trace back to conventional mechanized farming practices, the impact of the relative "strip mining" of the soil, agrochemicals in our diets (including in our newborns), and the nutrient-poor, genetically modified and irradiated foodstuffs produced and consumed since WWII.

Industrial Agriculture has accelerated soil erosion at an enormous pace. The United States loses two billion tons of topsoil a year to erosion, and according to the US Department of Agriculture the yearly cost is $40 billion—in lost productivity, silting of reservoirs, and pollution of waterways. In the last 40 years, nearly 1/3rd of the world's arable land has been lost to erosion and continues to be lost at a rate of more than 10 million hectares per year. Ninety percent of US cropland is losing soil above replacement rates. Loss is 17 times faster than formation, on average. At this rate, during the next 20 years, the potential yield of good land without fertilizer or irrigation is estimated to drop 20%.[11] We need to encourage sustainable organic agriculture to reverse this trend, and we as individuals have the power through a Deep Food approach. Health begins in the soil that feeds the food that feeds you!

Does Organic Matter?
In her research at Johns Hopkins University,[12] Dr. Virginia Worthington investigated the nutrient and toxic (heavy metal and nitrate) constituents of food in the U.S. She combined the research from all available studies that give numerical figures for organic content of specific nutrients and toxins in various foods, using 37 papers and 1,240 comparisons. For the five most frequently studied vegetables, lettuce, spinach, carrot, potato, and cabbage, she gives average percent differences for four nutrients. The figures are interesting: *"For example, vitamin C is 17% more abundant in organic lettuce (conventional 100%, organic 117%)."* In the case of spinach, average vitamin C content is 52% higher.

Mean percent additional mineral content in organic compared to conventional crops

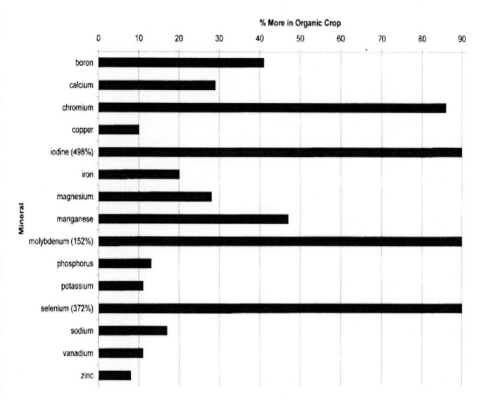

Figure 4: Mean percent additional mineral content in organic compared to conventional crops
Worthington, Virginia, MS, ScD, CNS, *The Journal of Alternative and Complementary Medicine*, 7(2): 161–73, 1991.

With well over a thousand individual comparisons, there were twelve nutrients with sufficient data for a statistical comparison: calcium, copper, iron, magnesium, manganese, phosphorus, potassium, sodium, zinc, beta-carotene, vitamin C, and nitrates. *"For each of the significant nutrients, the organic crops had a higher nutrient content in more than half of the comparisons. For the one toxic compound, nitrates, the organic crop had a lower content the majority of the time."*[13] For more on the importance of organic, please see chapter two by Cherie Soria.

Deep Food / Its-Interobjective/Political-Economic-Social-Ecological
"If people let government decide what foods they eat and what medicines they take, their bodies will soon be in as sorry a state as are the souls of those who live under tyranny." Thomas Jefferson (U.S. President)

Political. As you saw in Figure 2 earlier, "Why Does a Salad Cost More than a Big Mac?" government subsidies have little to do with protecting the public health, and are closer to keeping us at the feeding trough of the masses with corn, soy, wheat, and the animal products created by them. If you were one of the two billion people worldwide who saw the movie *The Matrix*, we can compare our present reality to the field of humans Neo is rescued from, all being fed liquid pink goo. We know it as corn syrup and hydrogenated vegetable oil, with corn starch, bleached white flour, food coloring and excitotoxins mixed in.

In 2005, the Consumers Union released *Out of Balance*, an eye-opening report on the state of political agency vs. the almost pornographic advertising/spending by U.S. food corporations.[14] It found that in 2004, the food, beverage, and restaurant industries' Super-Sized Mega Big Gulp Gordito advertising budget weighed in at US $11.26 billion, as compared to the mere Dixie Cup-sized $9.55 million[15] spent on communications for the federal and California *5 A Day* programs designed to encourage eating 5 or more servings of fruit and vegetables each day. Thus, the report said, *"Industry expenditures for food, beverage and fast food advertising are 1,178 times greater than the budgets for the California and federal 5 A Day campaigns."*

We could go on like this in a scathing, blood-boiling four-part book series discussing the US Farm Bill, US National Cattleman's Association, the US Food and Drug Administration, CODEX Alimentarius, the American Medical Association, Grocery Manufacturers Association, Big Pharma, and what Thomas Szasz calls our modern *pharmacracy*... (and you should check out the sources we have for you in this endnote).[16] So the questions arise, "Is there a political solution? What are we to do?" We will provide an opinion on this at the end of this section, but first let's look at some current economic, social, and ecological issues related to our food.

Economic. Shallow Foods have been created by a laser-pointed focus on economics, at the expense of every other quadrant: Mental-Emotional-Spiritual, Physical, and Cultural. Even realities in the Social quadrant such as Ecology are ignored, or used only to serve the economic goals of the Shallow Foods Economy. Shallow Foods are economically served by the following realities: low-cost mechanized conventional monocrop agriculture; cheap transportation (not for long with peak oil, however); and food processing to extend shelf life; irradiation, pasteurization, hydrogenation, homogenization, dehydration, freeze-drying, cooking, canning, freezing, added preservatives. In addition to these destructive practices which allow the Shallow Foods market to persist economically, industry is also leaving out, or taking out, many aspects of what makes for Deep Food and replacing them with pretty colors and food-scientist created flavors. One of our favorite images in Ram Dass' book *Be Here Now* says, *"Painted cakes do not satisfy hunger."* Quite right, and eating painted cakes is killing us.

Social. The Shallow Foods Economy reaps the unwanted dividends of high crime, violence, suicide, and depression, according to definitive research presented by Dr Russell Blaylock in his lecture, *Nutrition and Behavior*. Dr Blaylock presents an impressive array of studies on both juvenile and adult prisoners in the US system (highest per capita rate of prisoners in the world), which is further backed by Dr Gabriel Cousens research (*Conscious Eating - Food Effects on Body, Mind, and Spirit*) Dr. Cousens sites two pieces of telling research, which we will quote here in full:

When teenagers' diets were changed from their typical high white sugar, fast-food diet, a marked decrease in the teens' acting-out, violent behavior occurred. For example, Mrs. Barbara Reed, a probation officer in Cuyahoga Falls, Ohio, found that when she switched offenders from a diet of fast foods to a diet higher in fruits and vegetables, every one of the 252 teenagers in her case load stayed out of court as long as they maintained themselves on a healthy diet.

A two-year, scientifically precise study with 267 subjects by Steven Schoenthaler, Ph.D., published in the Journal of Biosocial Research, showed that while the average American eats approximately 125 pounds of white sugar per year, juvenile delinquents in custody averaged about 300 pounds per year. When this sugar intake was significantly reduced, junk food was reduced, and fruits and vegetables were increased, there was a 48% decrease in antisocial behavior of all types, including violent crimes, crimes against property, and runaways. This was true for all ages and races. This amazing result was achieved simply by changing the diet with no cost to the taxpayer.[17]

The US consumption of processed foods, concomitant high crime rate, and the results shown above should be all the evidence we need to walk swiftly and with purpose towards Deep Foods for our own social welfare.

Ecological. In the section, "Health begins in the soil!" we have already covered the deleterious effects of conventional agriculture, and the importance of adopting organic farming methods for human and ecological sustainability. One last point deserves highlighting, however, and that is the animal food industry as practiced in the US and other industrialized nations, and its effect on our natural environment. We discussed in chapter one the United Nations study, "Livestock's Long Shadow," which illustrates the massive greenhouse gas impact of the global cattle industry.

"It takes the equivalent of a gallon of gasoline to produce a pound of grain-fed beef in the United States. Some of the energy was used in the feedlot, or in transportation and cold storage, but most of it went to fertilizing the feed grain used to grow the modern steer or cow.... To provide the yearly average beef consumption of an American family of four requires over 260 gallons of fossil fuel." — *"Meat Equals War," web-site of Earth Save*

Raising animals for food involves a massive hoarding of resources. There is a tremendous loss in energy, materials, labor and caloric value. There is a tremendous amount of energy and grain that is required to feed the cows. The food required to feed 100 cows could potentially feed 2,000 people. The cows in the world consume two times the calories as the world human population. In the U.S. cows consume five times the amount of grain as humans. Better use of these resources could help solve the food crisis on the planet and prevent the death by starvation of 29,500 children per day (according to UN statistics) and approximately 40 million people who starve to death each year. Cattle farming, including dairy cows, causes losses of up to 85% of existing topsoil each year. In addition, the amount of water used in the dairy industry (and its by-products) is extremely high as compared to that required to feed a plant-based lifestyle, which can potentially save 1,500,000 gallons of water and 1 acre of trees each year when compared to a meat-based dietary approach. On average, one pound of beef protein takes up to 22 to 27 times more petroleum to get it to the table than a pound of plant protein.   Then there is the poo problem. According to the National Resources Defense Council, *"Giant livestock farms, which can house hundreds of thousands of pigs, chickens, or cows, produce vast amounts of waste. In fact, in the United States, these "factory farms" generate more than 130 times the amount of waste that people do. According to the U.S. Environmental Protection Agency, livestock waste has polluted more than 27,000 miles of rivers and contaminated groundwater in dozens of states."* At this point we can safely say, and we are speaking for the Earth here, "I am sick of all the sh#t!," and if you're not sure, a good read is *Your Call is Important to Us: The Truth About Bullshit* by Laura Penny.

Finally, an excellent primer by the Worldwatch Institute on the ecologically disastrous cattle industry called, "Meat: Now It's Not Personal," sums this section up perfectly: *As environmental science has advanced, it has become apparent that the human appetite for animal flesh is a driving force behind virtually every major category of environmental damage now threatening the human future—deforestation, erosion, fresh water scarcity, air and water pollution, climate change, biodiversity loss, social injustice, the destabilization of communities, and the spread of disease.*[18]

Deep Food / We-Intersubjective/Cultural And Mythological Significance
"One of the primary results - and needs - of industrialism is the separation of people and places and products from their histories. To the extent that we participate in the industrial economy, we do not know the histories of our families or of our habitats or of our meals." – Wendell Berry

Our processed, pre-packaged foods have little cultural or mythological density, further alienating us from our cultural heritage and ancestry. We find ourselves lost wanderers in a plastic-wrapped wasteland of Shallow Foods with no authentic orienting identities or significant mythologies, save those provided by the food industry: Ronald McDonald, the Trix Rabbit, Twinkie the Kid, songs about wieners – not the stuff of *enduring nations*. Western culture has been uprooted, having jettisoned – not included – the importance of being involved in our food as an agri*cultural* enterprise from farm to table. In school, we used to joke that out-of-touch kids thought food came from a supermarket. However we can, through a Deep Food awareness, reorient ourselves to an abundant variety of organic nutrient-dense plant foods, and re-learn the significance of real food in our lives with these cultural and mythological practices: Human Community; and Personal and Cultural Mythology.

Human Community. Experientially, contact with food and culture as a product of human (not industrial) agriculture and community is key. In the classic, *The Unsettling of America: Culture and Agriculture,* Wendell Berry conclusively demonstrates that today's agribusiness removes farming from its cultural context, and is destructive to the lives of farmers and to our culture as a whole. For Berry, food in all its stages *is* culture, mythology and religion. It is perhaps our most fundamental connection to the earth and the ongoing cycle of birth, death, and rebirth. The modern separation from the production and processing of food, mainly through the replacement of agri*culture* with competitive agri*science* and agri*business* – creates suffering not only in our physical health, but morally, culturally, and as communities of people. Berry writes, *"If a culture is to hope for any considerable longevity, then the relationships within it must, in recognition of their interdependence, be predominately cooperative rather than competitive. A people cannot live long at each other's expense or at the expense of their cultural birthright— just as an agriculture cannot live long at the expense of its soil or its work force, and just as in a natural system the competitions among species must be limited if all are to survive."*[19] This is a strong argument for the development of a cooperative localized food culture, and an essential component of Deep Food.

Personal and Cultural Mythology. In his film *Sukhavati: Place of Bliss*, mythologist Joseph Campbell explains that in the history of world mythologies the sun represents consciousness. *"The sun does not carry a shadow in itself. When the sun sets, the light sets with the sun. It is not the sun that is in darkness but we that are. So the sun represents the light and energy of life and consciousness not engaged in the field of time, but disengaged absolutely. In Buddhism the light is called the mother light, the light of consciousness and the undifferentiated light of consciousness."* Therefore, when you eat plants what you are doing mythologically and practically is *consuming consciousness*, because the plants are *sun foods*. The more we eat sun foods, the more light and consciousness permeates our being and radiates from our actions. Reality bears this out. Plant eaters have reduced rates of dementia and Alzheimer's, and consume more of the foods that maintain a sharp mind, including water, minerals, essential fats and amino acids. It is also a cuisine that protects our health, and that of the planet by encouraging sustainable agriculture, and ensuring that all on earth can be fed. My mentor and colleague Dr Gabriel Cousens often remarks that we could feed the world seven times over on a plant-based diet. From the authors' study and experience, health professionals using plant-based live food nutrition in helping their clients see an average 70-90% reduction in many prominent western diseases.

When we eat sun foods, we eat consciousness, which represents the father energy in mythology, yet we are also eating food from the earth representing the mother energy. In this way, since we truly are what we eat, and because these foods have such a profound ability to help us heal and prevent disease, we *become the mother, we become the father*, both through the food and in our growing up: standing on our own two feet and seeing to our own health instead of relying on so-called food manufacturers, doctors, governments, and the pharmaceutical industry to tantalize, sicken, coddle, and drain us dry. We become the authority and the guiding force for our own health reality, and with our newfound strength self-actualize our personal and collective true potential.

Finally, an excellent guide to the cultural mythology of food is *Nectar and Ambrosia: An Encyclopedia of Food in World Mythology* by Tamara Andrews. She writes, "*Food myths and food symbolism permeate ancient literary traditions. To people of times past, food was not mundane; it was magical. It was not only a means of sustenance but an affirmation of resurrection and renewal in the world... [Our ancestors] created food myths rich in symbolism, myths perhaps intended to keep accumulated knowledge alive from generation to generation... The ancients regarded agriculture not just as a scientific endeavor but as a religious art.*"[20]

Deep Food / Mental: I-Subjective / Nutrient Density As A Way Of Living

The food we eat is the most fundamental way that we acknowledge who we are (eaters of nutrient-dense plants), and our determination to have deep life experiences. When you eat *with purpose* the most nourishing food possible, free of toxicity and full of life and abundance, you will seek this in every aspect of your life experience. The most successful plant-based raw foodists we know practice what Integral Philosopher Ken Wilber calls "spiritual cross-training", in which consistent practices of self-development that are seemingly unrelated work synergistically to improve the performance of one another. In other words, you will be a better writer if you spend less time writing, and more time on meaningful exercise, spiritual practices, cultural activities, nutrition, and so on.

Through cross-training for our personal evolution, and not just hyper-focusing on cuisine, we recognize that shifting to a diet of nutrient-dense plant foods is not an act that exists in a vacuum *by itself*, but is part and parcel of a larger determination to acknowledge who you are at a fundamental level and to live your authenticity to the best of your ability. Those who are most successful at raw-live foods do it in the context of spiritual cross-training, and draw in with purpose the best persons, information, events, environments and experiences possible. This makes the challenge of moving up The Spectrum of Diet™ and into raw-live foods easier, as it is just one aspect of a greater life shift. While live foods may be your first shift towards the amazing life to which your deepest inclinations compel you, please view it – and make it – part of a larger world-centric act of love for yourself and all beings.

The Spectrum of Diet™ in Westernized Cultures

FAST FOOD	STANDARD AMERICAN	WHOLE FOODS	COOKED VEGETARIAN	COOKED VEGAN	RAW / LIVE VEGAN	JUICE FASTING TO JUICE FEASTING
EGOCENTRIC	SOCIOCENTRIC			WORLDCENTRIC		
SHALLOW FOODS / EXISTING <--> DEEP FOODS / LIVING						

Figure 5: The Spectrum of Diet™ in Westernized Cultures, David Rainoshek, M.A., www.JuiceFeasting.com

As we shift toward an organic, live-food diet, we also shift from low nutrient- to high nutrient density foods; from the creation of symptoms and disease to their transformation; dead food to vibrant, living food; maximum to minimum health care costs; below average to above average lifespan; millions dying of starvation to almost none; a *translative diet* of eating for comfort alone to a *transformative cuisine* of eating as a means and support for personal growth. Research and data from nations worldwide show that moving to a plant-sourced diet means the possible prevention and elimination of overweight/obesity, heart disease, diabetes, arthritis, hypertension, depression, and constipation, to name a few. Moving up the Spectrum of Diet™ is, in short, a transformation from a shallow narcissistic/egocentric existence of eating for oneself to an increasingly deep conscious worldcentric way of living as an act of love. This Spectrum, combined with the lens of the AQAL framework provides a very useful understanding of just how Deep our food and cuisine can be.

Deep Foods / Three Internal Essentials

There are three important qualities to develop when incorporating and encouraging Deep Food in a Shallow Food environment, which we will discuss vis-à-vis Zen instruction by Roshi Philip Kapleau in his classic, *The Three Pillars of Zen*. These essential qualities can be the foundation for *any* shift or growth, be it transcendental realization or a more earthly achievement, and they are: Faith, Doubt, and Determination.

Faith. First, one needs faith in live, plant-based, Deep Food nutrition, society, and culture; in the community of persons who will support them; and in one's own and others' ability to transform even the "incurable." This kind of faith comes naturally to some, and to many of us it is earned by a conscious decision to water this seed in ourselves by seeking out faith-building experiences, information and persons. Kapleau writes it is *"a faith that is firmly and deeply rooted, immovable, like an immense tree or boulder,"* that we must cultivate and maintain to eat at the level at which we want to achieve in our life.

Doubt. Second, you need to palpably feel what Zen masters call a "doubt-mass." This is a mass you feel in your gut about what conventional society tells you – and does not tell you – concerning agriculture, food and health. A strong doubt that your health and life is as good as it will ever get. Doubt that life gets more dull and painful and joyless as the years go on. *"It is a doubt as to why we and the world should appear so imperfect, so full of anxiety, strife, and suffering, when in fact our deep faith tells us exactly the opposite is true. It is a doubt which leaves us no rest. It is as though we knew perfectly well we were millionaires and yet inexplicably found ourselves in dire need without a penny in our pockets. Strong doubt, therefore, exists in proportion to strong faith."* – Roshi Philip Kapleau, *The Three Pillars of Zen*. Serious doubt about what you currently consider to be true must be developed which will drive you to keep moving up the Spectrum of Diet™. Most suffering is about getting stuck, or *dukkha* as the Eastern traditions call it. Doubt about the permanence of our current situation, no matter how terminal or permanent it may seem, can help to un-stick our wheels and create the thoughts and life practices that will foster transformation and healing.

Determination. Third, we are propelled by mature faith and doubt to a place of solid determination that we can – and will – get unstuck – *sukkha* - that we can find more beauty, peace, and abundance in the moments, days, and years ahead. A determination is in place to rise above the limitations, avarice, and sanctified misunderstandings that grease the machinations of the impersonal claims of postmodern society. We are determined to swim free of the momentum of mediocrity, and claim our inheritance of wisdom passed on to us by our ancestors who would surely have us jettison this path of individual and collective destruction we are now on and choose instead to consciously discover what the world is to be when: all are fed and we are not poisoning our air, soil and water. Perhaps then, too, individual religious dogma and mythos will be seen as a mere supporting structure for a mystical union of all traditions at the level of Spirit...

The progression on the inter-religiously acknowledged Nest of Spirit is from Matter to Body to Mind to Soul to Spirit, and each level includes and transcends the one before it like Russian dolls. If you want a transcendent experience – a *unio mystica*, with the Divine, or even if you just want to live happily at peace in your culture, nation, family, ecology, body and mind, then you will do exceedingly well to include the best foundation of Matter possible: a cuisine of Deep Food.

About the Authors:
David Rainoshek, MA in Vegan/Live Food Nutrition is the co-creator of JuiceFeasting.com with his wife, Katrina Rainoshek. He is a Juice Feasting coach, author, lecturer, and has Juice fasted/Feasted for over 450 days, up to 92 days at a time. David served as Research Assistant to Dr Gabriel Cousens for There is a Cure for Diabetes, and is now authoring several books for release in 2008, including: Juice Feasting: An Integral Hero's Guide, The Four Means to Get Your Greens and finally, with Katrina, a series of children's books beginning with Julia and the Nut Mylk Tree. David and Katrina coach 92-Day Juice Feasts for clients and retreats worldwide including the yearly Global Juice Feast, a world-wide cleanse for 92 Days on www.GlobalJuiceFeast.com. David and Katrina teach about Juice Feasting and nutrition education to the world through their 92-Day Program on www.JuiceFeasting.com. David served as leading Research Assistant to Gabriel Cousens, M.D., as head juice fasting coach, and taught the 10-week nutrition education classes to kitchen and garden apprentices at the Tree of Life Rejuvenation Center in Patagonia, Arizona in 2006-07. He has taught over 100 raw food preparation classes to children and adults.

David and Katrina are self-described as a Dietary Activists and proponents of Nutrient Density and Health Freedom for all. "Availability is not enough. For Live Food Nutrition to be the truly transformative and integral movement of our times, it must be made accessible to everyone." David and Katrina drive a Ford F-350 on Straight Vegetable Oil reclaimed from Asian restaurants, have covered over 70,000 miles to-date, and currently reside in British Columbia, Canada.

(Endnotes)
1   Diamond, Jared. *Guns, Germs, and Steel*. New York: W. W. Norton, 1997.
2   Ken Wilber is the founder of The Integral Institute (www.integralinstitute.org), and author of nearly 30 books, including *The Spectrum of Consciousness*, *A Theory of Everything*, and his magnum opus, *Sex, Ecology, and Spirituality*, which has been considered one of the four greatest books of the 20th Century, among Aurobindo's *Life Divine*, Heidegger's *Being and Time*, and Whitehead's *Process*

and Reality.

3   "Obesity Rates Continue to Climb in the United States." Johns Hopkins Bloomberg School of Public Health Public Health News Center, July 10, 2007. Online: http://www.jhsph.edu/publichealth-news/press_releases/2007/wang_adult_obesity.html

4   Youfa Wang, May A. Beydoun, Lan Liang, Benjamin Caballero and Shiriki K. Kumanyika. "Will All Americans Become Overweight or Obese? Estimating the Progression and Cost of the US Obesity Epidemic." *Obesity*, Advance online publication, July 24, 2008 DOI: doi:10.1038/oby.2008.351

5   Pollan, Michael. "You Are What You Grow." *New York Times*, April 22, 2007

6   Cousens, Gabriel. *Rainbow Green Live Food Cuisine*. North Atlantic Books, Berkeley: 2003.

7   Anderson, Richard. *Cleanse and Purify Thyself: Book 1*

8   "Dietary Guidelines for Americans 2005." U.S. Department of Health and Human Services. Online: http://www.health.gov/dietaryguidelines/dga2005

9   Diamond, Jared. *Guns, Germs, and Steel*. New York: W. W. Norton, 1997.

10   i,ii,iii Borger, C., et al., "Health Spending Projections Through 2015: Changes on the Horizon," *Health Affairs Web Exclusive* W61: 22 February 2006.

11   Kimbrell, Andrew. *The Fatal Harvest Reader*. Island Press, Chicago: 2002. Pg 68.

12   Worthington, Virginia, MS, ScD, CNS, *The Journal of Alternative and Complementary Medicine*, 7(2): 161-73, 1991. "This paper is an extension of work performed as part of doctoral dissertation at Johns Hopkins University, Baltimore, Maryland."

13   Online: http://www.nutrition4health.org/nohanews/NNSp02NutQualOrganicVsConv.htm *NOHA NEWS*, Vol. XXVII, No. 2, Spring 2002, pages 1-3.

14   *Advertising Age*, "50th Annual 100 Leading National Advertisers". June 27, 2005. Accessed August 5, 2005. Online: www.adage.com/images/random/lna2005.pdf

15   The 2004 communications budget for the federal 5 A Day program is $4.85 million and the 2004 communications budget for the California 5 A Day program is $4.7 million. This yields a combined total of $9.55 million.

16   Check out: *The China Study* by T. Colin Campbell, PhD; *Diet for a New America* and *The Food Revolution* by John Robbins; Mike Adams, The Health Ranger at www.NaturalNews.com; "Death by Medicine" by Gary Null; *When Healing Becomes a Crime* by Kenny Ausubel (or Google "Hoxsey"); *Food Fight* by Kelly D. Brownell; *Trust Us, We're Experts* by Sheldon Rampton and John Stauber; *Overdose: The Case Against the Drug* Companies by Jay S. Cohen; Pharmacracy: *Medicine and Politics in America* by Thomas Szasz; *The Secret History of the War on Cancer* by Devra Davis.

17   Cousens, Gabriel. *Conscious Eating*, North Atlantic Books, Berkeley: 2000. Pg 166.

18   "Is Meat Sustainable?" *The Worldwatch Institute*, July/August 2004. Online: www.worldwatch.org/system/files/EP174A.pdf. Also see "Meat and Seafood: The Most Costly Ingredients in the Global Diet" by Brian Halweil and Danielle Nierenberg, Worldwatch Institute. Online: www.worldwatch.org/files/pdf/SOW08_chapter_5.pdf

19   Berry, Wendell. "The Agricultural Crisis as a Crisis of Culture," *The Unsettling of America: Culture and Agriculture*. Sierra Club Books, San Francisco: 2004. Pg 47.

20   Andrews, Tamara. *Nectar and Ambrosia: An Encyclopedia of Food in World Mythology*. ABC-Clio, Santa Barbara.

6

God Sleeps In Stone: The Power of Minerals to Improve Health

David Wolfe

'God sleeps in stone,
Breathes in plants,
Dreams in animals,
And awakens in man.'
~Ancient Hindu Proverb

The ancient Hindus as well as many other ancient peoples understood the profoundly important substances hidden in stone. These magical substances, found in our rocks and then subsequently in the soil, which are then absorbed by our plants and ultimately wind up in us, are known as minerals.

Minerals are the atoms that make up solid, liquid, gaseous, and plasma matter. Some of the more popular minerals that we have all heard about include calcium, magnesium, potassium, sodium, sulfur, iron, zinc, gold, silver, copper, iodine, etc. It was the Greek Athenian philosopher, statesman, and orator Demosthenes who first formulated the atomic theory based on his observations of marble steps gradually wearing down after hundreds of years. From this observations he theorized that all solid objects were actually made up of very tiny particles he called atoms (and that we now call minerals). This theory developed into the discovery that these same minerals in stone are also found in us and in all other living things.

While most people have a general understanding that the body requires nutrients to function, most focus on the need for macronutrients such as protein, fat, and carbohydrates. Fewer individuals understand the role of micronutrients such as vitamins, amino acids, polysaccharides, and minerals. Even less realize that 95% of all bodily functions rely on minerals. Minerals orchestrate the delicate biochemistry of our bodies.

Demineralization among the human population (the absence of major dietary minerals such as calcium, magnesium, sulfur, iron, etc., and/or trace minerals such as zinc, selenium, manganese, copper, etc.) plus toxemia (the introduction of toxins) has now been confirmed to be intimately linked with poor health and disease. Therefore, in the present-day environment it is imperative that we limit our exposure to toxic materials and rebuild a properly mineralized body. The greater the amount of toxic matter introduced to our systems, the greater the need is for a healthy immune system to combat these life-depleting substances. Proper mineralization is key to creating a healthy immune system – so minerals can actually detoxify us.

Those new to eating our most natural food – raw plants and a raw plant-food based diet – often express concern over getting the proper amounts of vitamins (B vitamins in particular), but minerals are often overlooked. When consuming a raw plant-based diet, getting enough vitamins is rarely ever an issue. Vitamins abound in vegetables and superfoods (goji berries, cacao, maca, spirulina, chlorella, bee pollen, aloe vera, etc.) that are rich in vitamins A,B,C,E, and K. Many superfoods, vegetables, and fruits are excellent sources of vitamin C. Adequate amounts of B vitamins can be found in foods such as nuts, seeds, and in superfoods such as bee pollen, royal jelly, and spirulina. Even if the quality of the raw plants we are eating is not excellent, we can generally feel comfortable that we are consuming at least a reasonable amount of vitamins. Minerals, however, are entirely another story.

Nearly eighty years ago, American scientists recognized that as farming practices had changed, American soils had become grossly depleted of minerals. Mineral-depleted soils can only produce mineral-depleted food crops for humans and livestock. In an attempt to remedy the situation, the US Congress was informed of the problem. However, absolutely no action was ever taken. As a result of inaction and Faustian techniques of chemical agriculture, we are now three to four generations into a serious toxin overload and food-mineral-deficiency dietary crisis due to our intake of mineral-deficient plant and animal food (livestock). In following the principle of 'you are what you eat,' consuming mineral depleted foods does, without fail, produce a mineral-depleted population and contributes to the creation of obese individuals who cannot stop eating because they are incapable of getting the minerals that shut off appetite such as magnesium.

Thankfully, there have always been groups of radical organic farmers who have understood our needs, the needs of the plants, and ultimately the needs of our planet Earth. Certain 'tuned-in' farmers since prehistory have understood that the Earth itself has been using every technique at its disposal, including ocean water action, erosion, volcanic activity, earthquakes, continental drift, cataclysmic crustal movements, glaciation, the stone-dissolving actions of lichens, mosses, and forest floors, and more, to crush rocks into soils in order to create mineral geological varability so that all plants could grow to be healthier.

Numerous studies have now concluded that organically grown produce contains significantly higher amounts of minerals without the toxic effects of all the chemical reagents used in conventional farming methods. Plants grown organically without chemicals in reasonably good soils – or even better, using rock dusts and diluting ocean water (the ocean contains all minerals) in carbon-rich soils – thrive and develop healthy immune systems. These plants are naturally strong enough to resist the damage insects are able to inflict on weaker conventionally grown crops, negating the need for chemical pesticides. Once again, following the principle of 'you are what you eat,' when we consume mineral-rich plants with healthy immune systems, free of chemical toxins, we become mineral rich with healthy immune systems and decreased levels of toxicity.

The Effect Of Minerals On Enzymes
Much discussion has been given to the topic of enzymes in the last decade due to the increasing popularity of raw and living-food nutrition and the important role that enzymes play in our bodies. Enzymes can be considered the most unique aspect of living raw food. The enzymes we find in our food are catalysts allowing not only for the proper digestion of the food itself, but also for the proper metabolic functioning of each of our cells. In seeking optimal health, the amount of enzymes we have in our reserves directly correlates to our vitality.

Most people new to eating natural raw foods soon learn that the enzymes present in our food will be destroyed when our foods are heated over certain critical temperatures (between 120–170 degrees Fahrenheit). When food is cooked and does not have enzymes of its own, the body must pull from its enzyme reserves in order to aid in the digestive process. When our enzymes are being called on in this capacity, they are not able to perform their roles in metabolism.

Each cell in the body has 4,000+ different types of enzymes lying dormant and just waiting to be activated. To become active, both major and minor minerals are required in the process. Most people never fully activate all of their enzymes because they lack the minerals required to do so.

Our goal then becomes ensuring that every single cell has the minerals and nutrients required to activate the enzymes within it. When we are able to do this, we can increase the electromagnetic charge of our cells. Each cell can become like a super-charged enzyme factory. At the cellular level, this is the picture of health, with each cell resonating and capable of transmuting whatever nutrients are needed using catalytic enzymes at that moment.

The Role Of Minerals In Creating The Acid/Alkaline Balance
Most experts in the field of nutrition today accept that creating a proper balance of acidity to alkalinity within the body is fundamental to good health and vitality.

The body is constantly striving to stay in balance in multiple various ways. For example, our temperature is usually around 98.6 degrees and our blood pressure, heart rate variability, and breathing rate remain within certain parameters. Like these examples, our bodies are also striving to maintain a balance in our pH (per Hydrogen), which is the measurement of acidity to alkalinity.

Our ideal blood pH range is 7.35 to 7.4. Other tissues in the body may be slightly alkaline or acidic, and a good rule of thumb is to aim for an overall pH of 7.0. When the body is overly acidic, it will begin, in time to break down. Imagine the effect acid rain has on corroding the structure of a building. This is not unlike the corrosion that takes place within our bodies when we are in an overly acidic state. We can assist the body in achieving proper pH levels by the foods we choose to consume.

The body needs both acid-forming and alkaline-forming foods to maintain a proper balance. It is important to note that acid-forming foods in and of themselves are not bad. The problem that occurs for most people is that they consume a diet that is too high in foods that create acidity and not rich enough in foods that promote alkalinity. It's necessary to eat foods that complement each other for this purpose.

The major determining factor in whether a food will be acid-forming or alkaline-forming is the mineral content of the food. Foods rich in alkaline-forming minerals such as calcium, magnesium, silicon, iron, or the Ormus elements will create alkalinity in the body. Foods rich in acid-forming minerals such as phosphorous, chlorine, iodine, or nitrogen will create acidity in the body.

Minerals can be found in different parts of each plant. They gravitate toward and build up in various places within the plant such as the leaves, roots, stems, or seeds. As an example, we can see this principle clearly demonstrated when analyzing wheat. The husk of a mature wheat plant may contain anywhere from 67%–87% of the plant's silica, which is an alkaline-forming mineral. The seed of the wheat plant, however, contains no silica at all. Conversely, the seed of the wheat plant contains an abundance of phosphorous – far more than any other part of the plant. Phosphorous is an acid-forming mineral. As we begin to look at this concept – from my book *Eating For Beauty* – known as the mineral directive principle, we will begin to see that different minerals concentrate in different parts of the same plant or animal. For example, leaves, stems, flowers, and seed husks tend to contain alkaline-forming minerals. Roots and seeds tend to contain acid-forming minerals. In animal foods, the acidity is found in the muscles (meat) and the alkalinity is found in the bones; both muscle and bone must be eaten in order for a carnivore to maintain the acid-alkaline balance.

Acid-forming foods include nuts, seeds (including grains), and most sweet fruits and sweet vegetables, such as carrots and beets. Other foods fall into a more neutral range, meaning they do not promote either acidity or alkalinity. This range includes food such as seaweeds, cucumbers, tomatoes, bell peppers, green apples, wild berries, okra, and most types of melons. On the other end of the spectrum, we find that wild land-based foods, herbs, and vegetables are the best at creating alkalinity. Please note that the system here differs from acid-alkaline charts found in books on the subject including Dr. Young's *pH Miracle*, *Alkalize or Die*, and others. These books categorize potassium in food as an alkaline mineral, and I do not. This mistake causes these authors to miscategorize many foods (such as nuts and beans) as alkaline when they are not.

The easiest way to remember which foods are acid forming is the 'root, seed, muscle' rule. Sadly, this is how most individuals on Earth eat, creating acidic conditions for themselves without even recognizing it. Those without this knowledge tend to grab things like a burger and fries or a sandwich and chips as a usual meal. In this example, the bun or bread is the seed (grain), the chips or fries the roots, and the burger or lunch meat is the muscle. Even vegetarians can fall into this trap by eating dishes of beans and rice, which is nothing more than a bowl full of seeds. The traditional omnivore 'root, seed, muscle' diet or vegetarian 'root, seed' diet won't cut it for any long-term health or balance. Alkaline foods, superfoods, and herbs must be present.

Even with a natural raw and living-food diet, the idea is always to create a balance by choosing foods that complement each other. You may enjoy having a meal of dehydrated crackers made from nuts and seeds and topped with an avocado. These choices alone make this an acid-forming meal. However, by sprinkling some kelp flakes on top of the avocado and including a green leafy salad with this dish, you've now complemented the acid-forming foods with those that will promote alkalinity.

Using Wheatgrass To Quickly Mineralize The Body
An excellent way to quickly and economically flood the body with minerals is through the use of wheatgrass juice. Grasses including wheatgrass are one of the few known plants that have the ability to absorb all minerals present in the growing medium. Most often this medium is soil, but wheatgrass can also be grown using a hydroponic system.

One way to ensure optimal mineral content in the soil or hydroponic system used to grow wheatgrass is by adding ocean water. Ocean water is an excellent source for all minerals, both known and unknown. In this technique, ocean water is diluted then introduced to the growing medium, such as the soil. In this form, the wheatgrass will absorb all 90 minerals in the ocean water. A commonly used dilution ratio is 20 parts rain water to one part ocean water. However, 30:1, 40:1 or even 100:1 (for homeopathic usage) have been used effectively as well.

Creating Beauty Through Mineralization
Becoming more beautiful is another side effect of remineralizing our bodies to achieve radiant health. In particular, there are five minerals that lend to creating a more perfect physical appearance: magnesium, silicon, sulfur, zinc, and iron.

The Importance of Magnesium

Magnesium, one of the most important minerals for our body, is also one of the most deficient in the modern diet. In fact, it's been estimated that as much as 80% of our population is deficient in magnesium, followed closely by deficiencies in chromium, and iron. To get a sense of the healing properties of magnesium, consider these therapeutic effects: it calms our nerves, is helpful in relieving PMS symptoms, harmonizes mental and emotional imbalances, decreases irritability, improves sleep disorders, increases bone health, relaxes muscles, aids in digestion by acting as a laxative, soothes migraine headaches, eases cramps or spasms, helps blood-sugar imbalances, and is vital in the proper functioning of our heart muscle. Chlorophyll-rich green foods are high in magnesium.

The Alchemical Beauty Secrets of Silicon

Silicon can be found in our blood vessels, bones, cartilage, connective tissue, hair, ligaments, lungs, lymph nodes, muscles, nails, skin, teeth, tendons, and trachea. Growing and healing bones have been shown to contain high levels of silicon, and it also lends to strong teeth and healthy jaw formation. Silicon allows for flexibility and elasticity in our muscle tissues. The amount of silicon in the collagen of our skin directly relates to appearance as we age.

Through the process of biological transmutation, the body has the ability to transform silicon into calcium. Biological transmutation is the alchemical process performed by the body that allows one substance to be transmuted into another element. This theory violates Lavoissier's law and was first scientifically formulated by the late Nobel-prize nominee and French professor C.L. Kervran in his five books and five thousand pages of research notes, all of which have been summarized in an English book translation of his work known as *Biological Transmutations*. As a child, Kervran noticed that his family's hens would peck incessantly at specs of mica on the ground and wondered why they never pecked at grains of sand. Later he would notice his mother in the kitchen cutting open the chicken gizzards, which revealed small stones and sand, but never mica. He later discovered that mica, which is a form of potassium and silica, was being transmuted into calcium.

Foods rich in silicon include young bamboo shoots, bamboo sap, bell peppers, burdock root, cucumbers, hemp leaves, horsetail, marjoram, mature blades of grass, nettles, New Zealand spinach, nopal cactus, oats, radishes, romaine lettuce, tomatoes, and young tender green plants in the springtime.

Signs of silicon deficiency include poor skin quality, brittle nails and hair, dental cavities, weak bones, weak tendons and ligaments, atherosclerosis, and lung disorders.

The Alchemical Beauty Secrets of Sulfur

Sulfur is the foundational mineral of all beauty. It can be thought of as the world's best cosmetic. Adequate sulfur intake is greatly important in creating beautiful hair, nails, and skin. It has the ability to transform one's complexion, giving it a soft glow and flame-like tint. Sulfur can be key to clearing up even the worst cases of acne. The curliness of one's hair is dependent on the sulfur-to-sulfur bonds of the amino acid cystine. Sulfur is responsible for making our hair, nails, and skin shine with radiance.

Sulfur is also a powerful detoxifier that helps relieve pain and inflammation by flushing waste out of our cells. It can reduce lactic acid build up, helping to alleviate muscle leg and back cramps.

Good sources of sulfur-residue foods include aloe vera, noni, arugula, bee pollen, blue-green algae, hempseeds, broccoli, brussel sprouts, cabbage, durian, garlic, hemp seeds, horseradish, hot chilies/peppers, kale, onions, pumpkin seeds, radishes, spirulina, and watercress.

Symptoms of sulfur deficiency include acne, arthritis, brittle hair, brittle nails, gastrointestinal challenges, immune system dysfunction, lingering muscle injuries, memory loss, rashes, scar tissue, and slow wound healing. Symptoms of sulfur deficiency are often inaccurately labeled 'protein deficiency.'

The Alchemical Beauty Secrets of Zinc

Zinc works primarily through the role of enzymes. The activity of the antioxidant enzyme super oxide dismutase, which is a powerful anti-inflammatory, is dependent on zinc. Sexual development, the health of our reproductive systems, fertility, night vision, and the beautification of our skin also relies on having proper amounts of zinc.

Zinc is a key member of a group of enzymes that help the body maintain its collagen supply. This is essential for skin complexion. In order for enzymes to digest damaged collagen and rebuild new collagen, zinc must be present. In this same manner, it also helps heal burns. Zinc is also helpful in reducing outward signs of aging, the prevention of wrinkles and stretch marks, and even the repair of DNA due to exposure to x-rays and radiation.

Zinc is much more readily absorbed after you have detoxified heavy metals from your system with the regular use of MSM (methyl-sulfonyl methane), chlorella, cilantro, and zeolite compounds.

The best sources of zinc, all of which must be eaten raw, include seaweeds, cacao, ants, poppy seeds, pumpkin seeds, pecans, cashews, pine nuts, macadamia nuts, sunflower seeds, sesame seeds, coconuts, or in angstrom-sized zinc supplements.

Signs of deficiency include acne, loss of taste and smell, slow growth in children, alopecia, rashes, skin disorders, sterility, low sperm count, delayed wound healing, delayed bone maturation, decreased size of testicles, and poor eyesight.

If zinc is acquired from food, it is impossible to overdose. It is, however, important to note that zinc supplements may produce toxic symptoms if taken for a prolonged period at a dosage of over 150 mg daily. Signs and symptoms of a zinc overdose include a decrease of copper in blood, drowsiness, lethargy, lightheadedness, difficulty with writing, restlessness, and vomiting.

The Alchemical Beauty Secrets of Iron
Blood rich in iron produces a soft glowing tint of beauty that is visible just beneath the skin. Iron-rich blood is the source of magnetism (charisma). It is considered to be the most active element in the human system and therefore needs to be frequently renewed.

In terms of molecular structure, the hemoglobin in our blood is nearly identical to chlorophyll in plants. At the center of the hemoglobin molecule we find iron. At the center of the chlorophyll molecule we find magnesium. This tells us that the blood of the plant (chlorophyll) is similar to our blood.

Iron is important to the process of respiration. Two-thirds of the iron found in the body is in the blood. Iron-rich blood carries oxygen throughout the body. It generates magnetic blood current and an electro-magnetic induction current in the nerve spirals that pass through the walls of the arteries and the veins and help build and nourish tissues.

The best iron-rich foods are yacon root syrup, cacao products, spirulina, Jerusalem artichokes, onions, burdock root, cherries, blackberries, collards, young lettuces, nettles, parsley, shallots, spinach, young swiss chard, grasses, most dark green-leafy vegetables, most red-colored berries, and sea vegetables.

Symptoms of iron deficiency can include lightheadedness, weakness, fatigue, or intolerance to cold.

Ormus Minerals
As we've demonstrated thus far, minerals clearly have a profound and significant role in maintaining our health. Almost nothing can happen without their presence. So then, how would this discussion change if we were to introduce the concept that our knowledge of minerals, up to this point, has been incomplete? What if there has been a whole separate category of minerals that current mainstream science has not yet been able to identify? Subsequently, the possibility exists that we have become deficient in these as well. In one of the greatest scientific discoveries of our time, this category of previously unknown minerals known as Ormus was recently uncovered.

Ormus, sometimes referred to as ORMEs (Orbitally Rearranged Monoatomic Elements), monoatomic elements, or m-state minerals, is a separate and identifiable classification of atomic minerals known for their unique form. These minerals, however, do not find placement on the two dimensional Periodic Table of Elements. The unique form of Ormus minerals appear to be in a state that is closer to that of aether, vacuum, or pure energy than common minerals or atomic compounds. As it seems, because of the limitations of our current testing procedures, Mendeleyev's Periodic Table does not list Ormus minerals and is therefore incomplete.

Until now, the paradigm used for testing minerals has looked like a cut, slash, burn, poison, then analyze procedure. The major and trace minerals we've been aware of were identified by a procedure that effectively only analyzed them after they were 'killed.' Ormus minerals cannot be studied in this manner. They are identifiable and measurable because they exist as physical matter, but not by using the current paradigm for mineral analysis. When reasonably isolated and dried with silicon, Ormus elements are visible and have the appearance of a powdery substance. Our latest research is indicating that when an Ormus element is 100% isolated, it may be that it actually is a liquid at that temperature; more research will likely confirm this.

The Ormus minerals seem to be intimately woven into the fabric of all living things. Researcher David Radius Hudson brought to light this amazing discovery and indicates that as much as 5% of the dry matter of our nervous systems could be Ormus elements. They may be more abundant in biology than the trace minerals (zinc, copper, iodine, chromium, etc.). Ormus minerals have a natural attraction for the heavens and under controlled circumstances (removal of light, heat, oxygen, and other factors such as the conditions found in tree bark) will fall upwards or levitate. It is believed that this is what causes plants and animals to grow upwards against gravity.

Ormus elements are found deep within our earth, in lava, in soils, in salts, in ocean water, in springs, etc. They appear in our reality as infolded forms (seeds), which under certain types of stimulation will cause them to unfold (sprout) into different metals. Thus, we identify them by the metal they unfold into (e.g. Ormus copper, Ormus gold, etc.).

Ormus elements can be found in many forms including superfoods, superherbs, concentrated polysaccharide supplements, fresh water springs at the source, etc. Ormus minerals can also be consciously attracted into one's biology psychically and meditatively. The foods richest in Ormus minerals are aloe vera, bee pollen, honey, and others listed in my book *Amazing Grace*.

With advances in technology, I believe we will be able to prove that Ormus minerals concentrate in super foods such as spirulina, chlorella, maca, kelp, hemp, asparagus, ginseng, and berries such as acai, blueberries, raspberries, spikenard berries, schizandra, goose berries, etc.

Conclusion
The discovery of the critical importance of mineralization leads us to the insight that our health can be radically improved by eating and growing mineral-rich foods. Taking this one step farther, it becomes clearer that our state of consciousness is intimately related to our level of mineralization. Proper and abundant mineralization naturally creates states of prosperity consciousness.

Mineral deficiencies create states of scarcity consciousness.

We are now living in the most incredible time period ever. We now have access to the best foods, the best supplements, and the best information. Together, let's get mineralized, achieve our full potential, and Have The Best Day Ever!

About the Author:

David "Avocado" Wolfe is considered by his peers to be one of the world's leading authorities on nutrition. David is the author of **Amazing Grace, Naked Chocolate, Eating For Beauty, and The Sunfood Diet Success System**. David works, in conjunction with www.sunfood.com, to develop, market and distribute some of the world's most wonderful and exotic organic food items. David and www.sunfood.com (formerly Nature's First Law) were the first to bring raw and organic cacao beans/nibs (raw chocolate), goji berries, Incan berries, cacao butter, cacao powder, powdered encapsulated mangosteen, maca extract, and cold-pressed coconut oil into general distribution in North America.

Known for extraordinary quality control and ethical production, these products and many others developed by David and www.sunfood.com lead the field. David Wolfe has degrees in mechanical and environmental engineering, political science, is a juris doctor in law, and holds a Master's degree in living-food nutrition. He has studied at many institutions, including Oxford University. David still participates in higher education as a professor of nutrition for Dr. Gabriel Cousens' Master's degree program on live-food nutrition. David Wolfe is the middle son of two medical doctors, which provides him with a unique perspective in the health field. Since 1995, David Wolfe has given more than 1,000 health lectures and seminars in the United States, Canada, Europe, the South Pacific, Central America, and South America.

He hosts at least six health, fitness, and adventure retreats each year at various retreat centers around the world. David is the founder of the non-profit Fruit Tree Planting Foundation, whose goal is to plant 18 billion fruit trees on planet Earth.

David is also the founder of and leading contributor to the Internet's only Peak Performance and Nutrition online magazine: The Best Day Ever. As part of his action-packed schedule, David also coaches and feeds Hollywood producers and celebrities, as well as some of the world's leading businesspeople and entrepreneurs.

David is currently completing several new books, and he occasionally plays drums for the raw rock and roll group – The Healing Waters Band.

In 2004, David starred as "Avocado" in the reality television show Mad Mad House, airing on the Science Fiction Channel. In addition to having a passion for nutrition and music, David's favorite hobbies include hiking, yoga, literature, writing, alchemy, chemistry, wild adventures, hot springs soaking, planting fruit trees, spending time with loved ones, and having The Best Day Ever!

www.sunfood.com
www.thebestdayever.com
www.ftpf.org

7

High Water Content Foods and the Necessity for Proper Hydration

Dorit

"He that takes medicine and neglects diet, wastes the skills of the physician." (Chinese proverb)

In this chapter we shall look at the element of Water, specifically in foods that have a high-water content, and see how a lack of this element in one's diet can cause all sorts of imbalances, chronic illness, and disabilities, even after switching to a live foods diet. The human body can last weeks without food, but only days without water. The body is made up of 55–75% water, and mature adults are about 70% water. In a very healthy, well-hydrated person this can rise to 80%, whereas in the elderly and ill it can drop to about 60% and continues to drop as health is compromised.

Water is the basis of blood, digestive juices, urine and perspiration. The water content of the body breaks down along these lines:

80% of blood
73% of lean muscle (including brain tissue)
25% of fat
22% of bone

Water is needed in the body to maintain the health and integrity of every cell. It keeps the bloodstream liquid enough to flow through blood vessels, thus transporting nutrients and oxygen around the body and assisting in the elimination of toxins through urine and feces. Additionally, it regulates body temperature through perspiration and keeps mucous membranes moist – such as those of the lungs and mouth; it lubricates and cushions joints; reduces the risk of illness by keeping the body clear of harmful bacteria; aids digestion and works in moisturizing the skin as well as serving as a shock absorber inside the eyes, spinal cord, and in the amniotic sac surrounding the fetus in pregnancy.

The body is unable to store water for any length of time and needs fresh supplies every day due to losses from lungs and skin, accounting for 50% of water loss. Losses from urine and feces account for the rest of the total losses. The amount we need depends on our metabolism, the weather, the food we eat, and our activity levels. Heavy or obese people carry less body water than people of a healthy weight. This is because as fat content increases, lean tissue decreases, leading to an overall decline in total body water. Body water is higher in men than in women and falls in both with increase in age. Most mature adults lose about 2.5 liters (women) to 3 liters (men) per day, and the elderly lose about 2 liters per day. This water loss needs to be replaced through food and beverages. Except for a diet containing a large proportion of high water content foods, typically foods usually provide about one liter of fluid and the remainder must therefore be obtained from beverages.

Water in Chinese Five Element Theory is associated with the organs of the kidney and the urinary bladder as well as the back, the bones, and the endocrine system. The water element represents energetic reserves, the will to survive, courage, our ability to procreate, movement and flow, self actualization, will power, trust and faith. When the water element is out of balance, the mental and emotional ramifications are that a person will experience fear and a struggle for survival, a lack of reserves and deep fatigue, timidity, and a lack of trust in life and in other people. The physical symptoms include fatigue and exhaustion, all disorders of the urinary tract, infertility, hypertension, all endocrine disorders, lumbar syndromes, ankylosing spondylitis, and dental pathology.

One of the Traditional Chinese Medicine concepts of diet is that one should eat food which has the energy of that season in order to be in tune with that season. Thus, one should eat some cold foods and salty foods in the winter in order to partake of the energy of that season (and head off problems that can arise later). Salty (Water) foods are generally cooling (yin) and encourage energy to move in and down. The opposite might be applied here as well. In the summer (fire, hot) we require more cooling foods, most of which have a huge water content in them (eg. watermelons, cucumbers etc). Fortunately for us humans, the elements are not static; they are constantly moving and changing just as we are, so these are just guidelines rather than a formula on which to base your life and eating style on a daily basis. **The element of Water is abundant in live plant foods.**

What happens if you choose to eat mainly foods with a low water content?
Although the people at most risk of dehydration are the elderly and children, nowadays it has become a big issue for those traveling frequently on airplanes.

A traveler can lose approximately 1.5 liters of water during a three-hour flight, and with the new restrictions prohibiting carrying our own preferred source of water on planes, this has presented an enormous challenge for health-conscious travelers. This is exactly why I now take very juicy fruits on flights with me. Symptoms of dehydration include dark-colored urine, weakness, tiredness, confusion, and hallucinations. Eventually urination stops, the kidneys fail and, the body can't remove toxic waste products. In extreme cases, this may result in death.

The various causes of dehydration include:
Increased sweating due to hot weather/humidity, over-exercising, continuous fever, lack of proper drinking water, or not enough high water content foods in the diet. Other causes can be attributed to insufficient signaling mechanisms in the elderly or ill. Sometimes they do not feel thirsty even though may be dehydrated, or sometimes the need for hydration is misinterpreted as hunger for solid foods. Another cause can be due to increased output of urine as a result of a deficiency of pituitary or adrenal hormones, diabetes, kidney disease, or medications that increase the output of urine like diuretic drugs for the treatment of high blood pressure. Increased output of feces (diarrhea) or vomiting due to illness such as cholera, dysentery, or food poisoning can also lead to severe dehydration as can a long, protracted recovery period from burns.

If you are still consuming an animal protein-based diet, you will need to increase your intake of water-dense foods, because such a food choice requires more water for digestion and for removing nitrogen from the animal protein. This is also true if you are consuming a high fiber diet that is not mainly raw/uncooked. This is because fluids are important in preventing constipation, especially if wholemeal or whole grain foods are consumed in large amounts.

The kidneys as regulator
As stated before, the kidneys are one of the organs associated with the water element because they regulate the amount of water in the body. A special gland in the brain called the hypothalamus monitors water levels. If there is too little water in the body, the hypothalamus asks the nearby pituitary gland to communicate the need to conserve water to the kidneys. This is achieved by the secretion of a chemical called an anti-diuretic hormone. Once the kidneys receive this message, they reabsorb more water and concentrate the urine. At the same time, we are prompted to drink by the sensation of thirst, which is signaled by the brain. Alternatively, if there is too much water in the body, the hypothalamus instructs the kidneys – via the pituitary gland – to dilute the urine and release the excess.

Drinking too much water can also damage the body. If too much water is consumed, the kidneys cannot excrete enough fluid. Water intoxication can lead to headaches, blurred vision, cramps, and eventually convulsions. For water to reach toxic levels in the body, an individual would have to consume many liters a day. Water intoxication is most common in people with particular diseases or mental illnesses (for example, in some cases of schizophrenia), and in infants who are fed high quantities of fluid with low electrolyte levels (for example, infant formula that is too diluted).

Water content in food

Most foods, even those that look hard and dry, contain water. Usually, the higher the water content, the lower the kilojoule count. Most fruits and many vegetables are 90% water. The body can get about half or more of its water needs from food alone. (The digestion process also produces water as a by-product and can provide around 10% of the body's water requirements). The quickest, most balanced way to ensure a regular supply of this very necessary fluid is by the regular and consistent use of fresh raw fruits and vegetables.

The following fruits and vegetables contain a high water content:
Cucumbers – 97%
Tomatoes and Zucchini – 95%
Eggplant – 92%
Peaches – 87%

It is preferable to eat fruits and vegetables in season, and for variety add them in salads, raw soups, and juices freshly made to satisfy your body's thirst and desire for nutrients that have a high portion of fluids. For dessert eat fresh fruit. For breakfast, treat yourself to a large juicy watermelon or a glass of freshly squeezed tangerine juice made in a blender for fiber and micro-nutrients in addition to a large percentage of valuable fluids.

If you are eating some cooked foods, then use "dry" ingredients, which are also a good source of fluid. These are the foods that act like sponges as they cook, such as beans and some whole grains. For example, a cup of red kidney beans can be 77% water. That is more than 3/4 cup of liquid, while 1 cup of whole grain couscous will often contain 1/2 cup of water.

These high water content foods can also help those who are obese to lose more fat than those people who eat more calorie-dense foods. So if you eat the foods mentioned above you are actually taking in higher-nutrient foods and ensuring that your diet contains a large percentage of water based foods. The recommendation, therefore, if you are concerned about obesity, is to eat plenty of fresh, raw salads with sprouts, zucchini, celery, carrots and other vegetables that have a high water content. These foods will provide a portion double the size for the same calories as a salad made without the water dense vegetables. For example, a bowl of chili augmented with lots of raw vegetables in addition to the beans can expand the serving size of that dish while still maintaining a low calorie count.

Fresh sprouts, all kinds of lettuce, cucumber, celery, and tomato all contain a high degree of water and are very helpful for novices to a raw, living foods lifestyle, as they are very easy to grow and provide a very abundant harvest. I strongly suggest planting a garden of these gems from the plant kingdom so as to enjoy the bountiful harvest without stretching your budget.

You may be thinking: *"But I live by myself and this will all just go to waste, as I cannot possibly use all of these at once!"* A very easy and popular way to make sure that your diet contains a high portion of water-based foods while using up all of your harvest, and a great way to start a living foods diet for those who are new to this lifestyle, is simply to start juicing.

Juices

Juicing helps you absorb *all* the nutrients from the vegetables. This is important because most of us have impaired digestion as a result of making less-than-optimal food choices over many years. With juicing, you can add a wide variety of high-water-content vegetables that you may not normally eat as they are just too "new " or too "raw" for you or because, initially, you are unable to digest them well. In addition, if you grow some or most of your own vegetables and fruit, you can use up any excess this way.

Recommended high water content foods for juicing

If you are new to freshly made juices, I strongly suggest doing what I call mono-juicing. This means juicing only one of the following and drinking about 3-4 ounces of it first thing in the morning (feel free to dilute it in some water if you feel a need to do so) :

Celery – the best vegetable source of naturally-occurring sodium, and it is high in potassium. The high water content makes it ideal for vegetable juicing, or just eating.

Fennel (anise) – can be useful for indigestion and spasms of the digestive tract. It also helps expel phlegm from the lungs.

Cucumbers – very refreshing and rehydrating in the hot summer months.

Once you are used to drinking these by themselves, then you can start mixing them together.

To further increase your juicing repertoire and to guarantee that you get a lot of high-water-content foods in your diet, then add the following to your juicing regimen:

Green leaf lettuce, red leaf lettuce, romaine lettuce, butter lettuce, endive, escarole, spinach, Swiss chard, purslane
Zucchini -(this and other summer squash varieties contain vitamins A and C, potassium, and calcium),

Carrots and other root vegetables -(use beets sparingly, though, because of the high sugar content and its detoxifying properties)

Gradually add other green leafy vegetables to the mix with some lemon juice or apples mixed in.

Next you can start including more cruciferous vegetables such as:
Asparagus – contains rutin, which may protect small blood vessels from rupturing and also may protect against radiation

String beans – Green beans are touted as being diuretic and have been reported to help to treat diabetes

Cauliflower – including the base

Broccoli – has a reputation for its anti-cancer anti-viral and anti-oxidant properties

Red or green cabbage – this has a reputation of being great for healing ulcers if you drink it right away

Chinese cabbage – excellent source of folic acid

Bok choy – high in beta carotene and reported to aid with digestion

Kohlrabi – has been reported to help stabilize blood sugar and is therefore useful for those experiencing hypoglycemia and diabetes. It can also be effective against edema, candida, and viral conditions)

Radishes – reported to have antibacterial and anti-fungal properties) One of my favorites; I particularly like it mixed with tomatoes and cucumbers.

Lastly, begin to add the most bitter of the green leafy vegetables to your vegetable juices:

Kale – an excellent source of calcium, iron, vitamins A and C, and chloro-phyll. For those who are novices to eating raw foods and are hesitant to eat raw kale, juicing is an effective way to add this very important and under-utilized powerhouse of a vegetable

Collard greens – if you are putting this in a blender make sure it's a power-ful one! When purchasing collard greens, make sure that the leaves are still attached to the main stalk. If they are not, then be aware that the vegetable rapidly loses many of its valuable nutrients once the leaves are detached

Dandelion greens – use sparingly as this might detoxify the liver too quickly and has an extremely strong taste!! These greens have a reputation for being helpful in addressing AIDS and herpes. They may also be useful in treating jaundice, cirrhosis, edema due to high blood pressure, gout, ec-zema and acne, and preventing breast and lung tumors and premenstrual bloating.

Mustard greens – are known as an excellent anticancer vegetable and may also be beneficial for colds, arthritis, or depression. Add only a small amount unless you love the taste of mustard. Otherwise, it will overpower the juice or smoothie. You might wish to add lemon juice to this mixture as well.

Chicory – beneficial for digestion, the circulatory system, and the blood and has been reported to help diabetics regulate their blood sugar levels. In my own recipe book I use this and watercress a lot, as I not only love them but also find that they are very under-utilized in the "raw community".

Finally, to add some real zest and taste to your juices, start including some herbs such as **mint** (helpful with digestive disorders), **parsley** (useful as a digestive aid and to purify the blood and stimulate the bowels. It is also believed to be an anti-carcinogen), and **cilantro (coriander);** although tremendous caution ought to be exercised with the latter, as you might start releasing too many heavy metals in your system and not eliminate them quickly enough.

Nuts
Dried nuts are much higher in fat and protein because they have lost their water content. If you have ever eaten nuts fresh from the tree, you'll know not only how much tastier they are, but also how smooth they are when you are chewing them owing to a difference in their texture. This is because they have not yet lost all, or most of, their water content. If you do not have access to freshly picked nuts, then use dry nuts to make nut milk by soaking them and then blending them with fresh water before straining through a sieve or nut-milk bag.

Fruits
Of course, for an easy, scrumptious, and nutrient-dense high-water-content meal, fruit is king. The variety and differences in the fruit realm is enough to keep all your senses satiated in the shortest time possible. For those who are looking for ease, convenience, and satiation, nothing is more rewarding than a wide selection of fruits. When I first turned my life around and said *au revoir* to the world of cooked foods, I was astounded by how there was always something utterly delectable and enticing to look forward to each season. It took me back to my childhood, which was replete with lots of fruit of all kinds. My memory of my raw adult life is full of the first few years of wheatgrass juice, E3Live, various other green drinks, smoothies, avocados, cherimoyas, sapotes, jackfruit, heirloom tomatoes, and figs, which are still my absolute favorite fruits. I was in seventh heaven. No cooked food could compare to the aromas, textures, sights, and juices of these jewels of the earth. Today, I still indulge in these when my instinct takes me there, but they are no longer the mainstay of my diet. You will find that the longer you work your way into the magical kingdom of raw, the more your desire for certain

ate and the more your need for others increase. When you practice e proportion of high-water-content foods, then it becomes really easy ices in response to your physical needs or/and demands rather than omfort " foods or something to eat to distract you from any life expe- ...... you are adverse to welcoming.

About the Author

Dorit's love for Life and all the experiences of a severe illness that brought her close to the brink of dying propelled her into writing **CELEBRATING OUR RAW NATURE– A Guide for Transitioning to a Plant-Based, Living foods Diet** *and then its sequel,* **Celebrating our Raw Nature, Plant based Living Cuisine** *(the all-raw version with an accent on Seasonal Meals and recipes for children). In addition to numerous guest appearances on television shows, Dorit is presently working on a DVD series and hosts a talk show called* Recipes For Life *on www.iamhealthyradio.com . The name of this segment comes from the title of her third book (not yet in print),* **RECIPES FOR LIFE**, *and is also the title for the DVD series. Adding variety to her work as a Certified Living Foods Chef, Dorit was a workshop leader for a medically supervised Cleansing and Detoxification Retreat at the Fox Hollow Clinic and Spa in Kentucky. She was the innovator and founder of the Movement Therapy Department at Canyon Ranch in the Berkshires, and under her direction this department became the most financially profitable department of Canyon Ranch. She also teaches workshops at Whole Foods Markets across the USA and at Erewhon Natural Foods Market In Los Angeles. Through her company, Serenity Spaces, she runs a catering business. As part of her community work, Dorit created a Raw Lifestyle Network Group for those wiishing to add more live, nutrient-packed high-energy foods to their diet. The group meets the first Sunday of every month at raw-friendly establishments, and meetings are free of charge.* **Serenity Foods** *is her packaged-food line under the distributorship of Vegan Traders and is available in several prominent natural foods markets in Los Angeles, California. In 2004, Dorit shot a pilot for TV release called The UNcooking Show. She is presently touring the United States and Canada to promote the message of Conscious Eating and to bring high energy and healing foods into the forefront, and is the founder and organizer of* **The Green Lifestyle Film Festival**, *headquartered in Los Angeles, California. To learn more please visit her websites: http://serenityspaces.org http://www.greenlifestylefilmfestival.com Or ring 310-854-2078*

8

The Value of Raw Vegetable Juices

Rev. George Malkmus

When God created that first man and woman, Adam and Eve, He placed them in a garden and told them what was to be the fuel (food) they were to consume in order to sustain life:

> *And God said, "Behold, I have given you every herb-bearing seed (raw vegetable), which is upon the face of the earth, and every tree, in the which is the fruit of a tree yielding seed (raw fruit): to you it shall be for meat (food)". – Genesis 1:29*

Humankind was to forage for food, just like all God's other vegetarian animal creations. People were to walk through God's nature, pluck these raw fruits and vegetables, and consume them in their natural raw form, in order to obtain the nutrients necessary to fuel their physical bodies. Later, gardens and orchards were planted. It is interesting to note that, even after the Fall of Adam and Eve, people thrived on these raw fruits and vegetables, living to advanced years, for the next 1,700 years, without a single recorded instance of sickness. It was only after the Flood, which destroyed all plant life, that God allowed meat to be added to the diet *(Genesis 9:3)* – I believe for survival purposes; and when people started cooking food, sickness entered the human race.

My personal experience of illness

In 1976, after being told I had colon cancer, I searched for an alternative way of dealing with it, rather than accepting the traditional medical modalities of chemotherapy, radiation, and surgery my mother had accepted before me for the same condition. At the time of mom's death, I had felt that it was these medical treatments, and not the cancer, that ultimately caused her death.

In my search for an alternative route, I turned for help to an evangelist in Texas by the name of Lester Roloff. He had been trying for years to get Christians to improve their diets, as a means of improving their health, without much success. He encouraged me in my decision not to go the traditional medical route! Rather, he recommended I should do something as simple as change what I ate – from the Standard American Diet (SAD), a meat-based, sugar dessert, basically cooked food diet I had consumed for the previous 42 years of my life – to the raw fruit and vegetable diet God gave Adam and Eve in the garden *(Genesis 1:29)*. Evangelist Roloff also encouraged me to drink lots of vegetable juices.

Overnight I made the diet change. For the next year I did not put a single piece of cooked food into my body. I ate raw fruits and vegetables, and drank one to two quarts of raw vegetable juices a day. Almost immediately I started to get well, and by the end of that first year, not only had I seen my baseball-sized tumor disappear (without medical intervention), but also all my other physical problems!

By the end of that first year, however, on a totally raw vegan regime, I had lost too much weight, and so I added some cooked food back into my diet in an effort to gain some weight. While I continued to eat 85% raw, I introduced baked sweet potatoes, whole grains, steamed vegetables, whole grain pastas, beans, etc. These cooked veggies brought my weight up to a reasonable level, and I maintained that weight for the next 20 years. Then in the late 1990s, though still healthy and feeling great, I felt I was still too lean and needed to add some weight to my body. Not wanting to add more cooked food, I went in search of a way to gain weight without compromising my diet. That is when weight resistance exercises became a part of my daily exercise routine.

Ever since my cancer experience in 1976, stretching and aerobic exercises had been a part of my daily workout regimen, but not weight resistance exercises. Once I added these exercises to my daily work out, I started gaining weight. As a result, in the past eight years, I have added several inches to my biceps/triceps muscles, three inches to my calves, four inches to my chest, and gained twelve pounds of weight. My stomach muscles are now rock hard. I am now 74-years-old and am free of any known physical problem, capable of doing anything physically I could do as a teenager, and with a mind that is functioning better than it did as a teenager. My wife Rhonda and I power walk from two to eight miles daily, depending on our schedules.

Why juice?
When God created us He placed within us a digestive system so that we could process raw fruits and vegetables, seeds and nuts He provided in nature. This digestive system was designed by God to take the raw plant source foods found in nature and break them down into a form that would make them useable at the cellular level of our bodies as fuel. Listen to what H. E. Kirschner, MD, has to say

about this digestive process (*Live Food Juices*, pp 20 and 21*)*:
"Why not just eat the raw vegetables? As we have indicated in the previous chapter, for optimum health you need far more than you could possibly eat. The stomach just couldn't handle that much bulk. Then too, if modern research is correct, the power to break down the cellular structure of raw vegetables, and assimilate the precious elements they contain, even in the healthiest individual is only fractional--not more than 35%, and in the less healthy, down to 1%."

"In the form of juice, these same individuals assimilate up to 92% of these elements. The juice of the plant, like the blood of the body, contains all the elements that build and nourish. It is a well-known fact that all foods must become liquid before they can be assimilated."

Thus, by juicing, we do much of the work of the digestive system (removing the fiber) *before* we put the food into our bodies. By removing the fiber, which contains no nutritional value (fiber is only the carrier of the nutrients), we are putting only the part of the vegetable that contains the nutrients (the liquid part) into our bodies. By doing this, we eliminate the need for it going through the digestive process. With the fiber removed, the nutrients can go directly to cellular level in mere minutes, and this raises the percentage of nutrients reaching cellular level from less than 35% when we eat the whole food, to more than 90% when we drink the juice.

The Hallelujah diet
This is one of the *keys* to the results people experience on the Hallelujah Diet. It is one of the primary reasons that, within one year or less from the time a person makes the diet change that we teach here at Hallelujah Acres, over 90% of all physical, as well as psychological and emotional problems, are gone. The body has within it not only the ability to rebuild itself when given the proper building materials, but also the ability to heal itself of almost anything that ails it. This self-healing mechanism was placed there by God at creation, and has been passed down to each of us through genetic coding.

If we want to get well, or stay well, the very first thing we must do is stop putting toxic foods into our bodies. These would include all animal-source foods (both flesh and dairy, including all cheese), refined sugar, refined flour, salt, trans-fats, and caffeine. These are the substances that cause most of the physical problems being experienced today. Then we start putting into our bodies the raw building materials the Lord designed us to use as fuel, especially in the form of concentrated raw vegetable juices: and the miracle usually follows. Don't be concerned about not obtaining enough fiber on The Hallelujah Diet, as we still consume loads of fiber in the various vegetables, fruits, seeds, and nuts, we consume.

In the Garden of Eden, there were no juicers, but neither was there a need, because soil nutrients had not yet been depleted and man's physical body was not racked with physical breakdown. Thus the 35% nutrient content of foods was plenty adequate to supply all nutritional needs. But today, because of the low nutrient value of our foods and the extensive repair job needed by the average body, we need to get nutrients to cell level in greater quantities, and juicing accomplishes that.

It takes approximately one pound of raw vegetables to make an eight-ounce glass of vegetable juice. It is difficult, very time consuming and inefficient to eat a whole pound of raw vegetables; more than 65% of the nutrients are lost in digestive processing. By drinking an eight-ounce glass of raw vegetable juice, you are putting into your body the nutrients contained in a whole pound of raw veggies, and over 90% of those nutrients reach cellular level.

An eight-ounce glass of raw vegetable juice, mid-morning and mid- afternoon, gives the body incredible energy as well as taking away hunger. At the Gerson Hospital in Mexico they are healing terminal cancers using eight, 8-ounce glasses of carrot juice per day, four 8-ounce glasses of green juices from organically grown vegetables, along with a vegetarian diet. It was one to two quarts of raw vegetable juices per day in 1976 that restored my body to health, and vegetable juices have been a major part of my daily nutritional intake ever since. There is absolutely no substitute for freshly extracted vegetable juice.

Thoughts on juicing
If you live in the United States, it is important that the carrots be grown in California, because California carrots are grown in mineral-rich soils. It is the trace minerals that make carrots sweet. The most economical way to buy carrots is in 25-pound bags, which will fit in most refrigerators and if kept sealed will stay fresh for a month. Twenty-five pounds of carrots will produce approximately twenty-five 8-ounce glasses of juice. Rhonda and I juice 25-pounds of carrots weekly!

If you have a juicer already, try to add at least two glasses of fresh vegetable juice to your diet each day, (approximately 1/2 carrot and 1/2 greens). If you're considering purchasing a juicer, I recommend the Champion juicer, the Green Life juicer or the Norwalk Press juicer, especially if dealing with a serious physical problem. A spinning basket juicer is certainly better than nothing but is inferior to other types.

Blenders cannot produce vegetable juice – they only blend together the juice and fibers of the vegetable, leaving the fiber in the juice, thus defeating the very purpose of juicing, because the food must still go through the digestive process. Blenders may be used to make a blended vegetable salad, which increases nutrient value by three to four times over when you chew your raw vegetables. Nutrients are released from our foods only when the cell structure has been broken open by chewing or blending. Chewing your vegetables and sending the food through the digestive system provides the least amount of nourishment from the foods eaten. Blending the vegetables in a blender provides the second-greatest amount of nutrients at cellular level. But it is from the juices that we obtain the greatest nutrient value, and they become the most powerful source of nutrition known to mankind.

Many caution the drinking of straight carrot juice because of its high glycemic index numbers. We had our own staff PhD, Michael Donaldson, do some research and laboratory testing regarding this. His research revealed that a single slice of whole wheat bread or a baked potato gave a significantly higher glycemic reading than a 12-ounce glass of freshly-extracted carrot juice. However, we do suggest that for most people it would probably be best if they temper the sugar content of carrot juice with as much as a 50% dilution, using cucumber, celery, spinach, kale, or other vegetable juices.

At Hallelujah Acres we suggest that those who have no known physical problems and just want to maintain their excellent state of health consume two to three 8-ounce servings of vegetable juices daily, plus three servings of an organic barley juice powder. On a recovery diet, which would be someone dealing with a serious physical problem, we recommend at least six servings of vegetable juices daily, plus six servings of a powdered barley juice drink.

The drinking of fruit juices is discouraged. Eating your fruits and juicing your vegetables is a better way to go. There is too much natural sugar in concentrated fruit juices, and it can cause problems. I recommend that no more than 15% of the daily diet be composed of fruit, and if a person is dealing with yeast problems, high or low blood sugar problems, that they eliminate it altogether, as well as the drinking of carrot juice, until the problem is resolved.

Please do not assume from all this praise for the benefit of freshly extracted juice that there is any value to be gained from drinking store-bought frozen, canned, or bottled juice. There is not! Practically all natural nutrients as well as enzymes have been destroyed by heat, because everything in it that is alive – friendly bacteria as well as nutrients – has been killed to prevent spoilage during its long shelf life.

A pure vegan diet that is high in raw fruits and vegetables – and freshly extracted vegetable juices – will go a long way in providing the nutrition we need to build and regenerate and maintain our living cells, while also helping to efficiently eliminate waste from the body.

Concluding thoughts
I have found the ideal diet comprises approximately 85% raw and 15% cooked. Slight daily variations are unimportant. It is not the raw foods and juices them-selves that do the healing! What they do is provide us with the concentrated building materials the body needs in order to heal itself. Self-healing is built into all of us, and when we bring conditions conducive to healing about within the body, the body will almost always do what it was designed to do: heal itself.

The use of nutrients to enhance our God-given capability of self-healing has proven to be an extremely effective means of helping to prevent or heal a wide variety of ailments. Here at Hallelujah Acres, we have received literally tens of thousands of testimonies from folks who adopted The Hallelujah Diet, reporting recovery from more than 170 different physical problems.

Once we understand the theory and experience the reality of using nutrition to help our body maximize its own healing capabilities, we will see that this is the exact opposite approach of drugs. All drugs are chemicals that are foreign and toxic substances to the body and merely cover up the symptoms of ill health rather than provide self-healing and wellness. If we opt for promoting self-healing through nutrition, experience will show that drinking the freshly-extracted juice of raw vegetables is the most efficient way to obtaining this nutrition. Fresh vegetable juice should be a vital part of the diet of anyone who is serious about using natural foods to build an immune system capable of preventing or eliminating disease.

About the Author:

George Malkmus was born in Yonkers, NY, on February 12, 1934. He became a Christian at a Billy Graham Crusade Rally in 1957. After four years of schooling in preparation for the ministry, he pastored various churches. His church in Glens Falls, NY grew in six years from just his family to over 600 members by 1976, the year he learned he had colon cancer. After making the diet change in 1976, and obtaining complete healing of all physical problems, he tried to share his diet with others in the Christian community but was met with not only rejection, but also often hostility. In was not until 1991, when he shared his diet with Rhonda, a lady who was so stove up with arthritis she could hardly move, that positive things started to happen. Within one year of applying the diet change that had brought healing to George, Rhonda had been totally healed of her debilitating arthritis and had lost 85-pounds. George and Rhonda married in 1992, the same year they started Hallelujah Acres. George and Rhonda's previous spouses are both deceased. George and Rhonda have 4 children, 17 grandchildren, and 8 great-grandchildren. Hallelujah Acres started in a restaurant and Health Food store in Rogersville, Tennessee. The store was 11 feet in width and had 16 seats. Each Saturday morning a "How To Eliminate Sickness" seminar was held in that store, and gradually people started to listen, apply what was being taught, and get well. These people could not keep from sharing with others their healing experience, and word started to spread. Today, there are millions of followers worldwide. In 1994, George started training others to share this health message. To date, more than 7,000 people have been trained, and today there are trained Health Ministers located in every state in the United States, as well as in 44 foreign countries. Today, Hallelujah Acres is physically located on 20 acres of beautiful land in Shelby, North Carolina, and publishes a free 64-page, full-color magazine, read by some half-million persons bi-monthly. Rev. Malkmus also publishes a free weekly electronic Hallelujah Health tip, with a current circulation of 90,000. Hallelujah Acres has four Life Style Centers where people can go to spend a week or two learning and experiencing the complete Hallelujah Diet and Lifestyle program. The Hallelujah Acres Medical Clinic, located at the Oasis of Hope hospital in Tijuana, Mexico provides an aggressive natural approach to dealing with cancers and other chronic degenerative diseases. At the time of writing, Hallelujah Acres has a staff of 70 full-time employees and recently purchased 300 acres of new land on which they plan to build some 1,000 residences – condominiums, town houses, and single-family dwellings – for those who would like to live in a healthy Christian Community. Rev. Malkmus appears frequently on television. He has appeared live on the 700 Club, Trinity Broadcasting, CBS, NBC, ABC Nightline, The Food Network, and numerous times on Fox News. He also does almost weekly remote interviews on radio stations around the world. Books he has authored include: Why Christians Get Sick; God's Way to Ultimate Health; Message of Hope and Healing; and his most recent book, The Hallelujah Diet; along with numerous CDs and DVDs. His first book, Why Christians Get Sick, has passed the million copies in print mark.

You can visit his website at www.hacres.com, where you can also sign up for his free publications, or you can contact him by email at george@hacres.com

9

Chlorophyll Rich Green Foods

Victoria Boutenko
Jill Swyers
Michael Saiber and Tamera Campbell

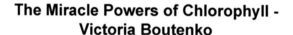

The Miracle Powers of Chlorophyll - Victoria Boutenko

Chlorophyll is as important as sunlight! No life is possible without sunshine, and no life is possible without chlorophyll. Many people enjoy the sun. We all feel better and look healthier when we expose ourselves to sunlight. In warm climates and weather, clothing is reduced to the very minimum as we immerse our bodies in the precious sunshine. However, not many people are aware that chlorophyll is liquefied sun energy. Consuming as much chlorophyll as possible is exactly like bathing our inner organs in sunshine. The chlorophyll molecule is remarkably similar to the heme molecule in human blood.[1]: it takes care of our bodies like a most caring and loving mother. It heals and cleanses all our organs and even destroys many of our internal enemies, such as pathogenic bacteria, fungus, cancer cells,[2] and many others.

To experience optimal health we need to have 80–85% of "good" bacteria in our intestines. Friendly bacteria manufacture many essential nutrients for our body, including vitamin K, B-vitamins, numerous helpful enzymes, and other vital substances. Such "good" or *aerobic bacteria* thrive in the presence of oxygen and require it for their continued growth and existence. That is why if we do not have enough oxygen in our cells, "bad" bacteria take over and begin to thrive, causing an extreme amount of infections and disease. These pathogenic bacteria are *anaerobic*, and cannot tolerate gaseous oxygen. Taking care of our intestinal flora is vitally important! "Good" bacteria can easily be destroyed with countless factors, like antibiotics, poor diet, overeating, stress, etc. In these cases we could have 80–90% of "bad" bacteria filling our bodies with toxic acidic waste. I believe that the dominance of anaerobic bacteria in our intestines is the prime cause of all disease.

Since ancient times, chlorophyll has served as a miraculous healer. Chlorophyll carries significant amounts of oxygen with it and thus plays a critical role in supporting the aerobic bacteria. Therefore, the more chlorophyll we consume, the better our intestinal flora and overall health will be. Considering that greens are a major source of chlorophyll, it is difficult to find a better way of consuming chlorophyll than drinking green smoothies.

Chlorophyll has been proven helpful in preventing and healing many forms of cancer[3] and arteriosclerosis.[4] Abundant scientific research shows that there are hardly any illnesses that could not be helped by chlorophyll. To describe all the remedial qualities of chlorophyll would be to fill a whole separate volume! The following list is just an example of the many healing properties of this amazing substance.

The many healing properties of chlorophyll include:
- Builds a high blood count
- Helps prevent cancer
- Provides iron to organs
- Makes body more alkaline
- Counteracts toxins eaten
- Improves anemic conditions
- Cleans and deodorizes bowel tissues
- Helps purify the liver
- Aids hepatitis improvement
- Regulates menstruation
- Aids hemophilia condition
- Improves milk production
- Helps sores heal faster
- Eliminates body odors
- Resists bacteria in wounds
- Cleans tooth & gum structure in pyorrhea
- Eliminates bad breath
- Relieves sore throat
- Makes an excellent oral surgery gargle
- Benefits inflamed tonsils
- Soothes ulcer tissues
- Soothes painful hemorrhoids

- Aids catarrhal discharges
- Revitalizes vascular system in the legs
- Improves varicose veins
- Reduces pain caused by inflammation
- Improves vision

Plants for survival

The most important goal of all life forms on our planet is a continuation of their life. What do we humans need to survive? Besides air and water, our primary need is food. We get our food from plants and animals. Where do plants get their food? They obtain their food from the soil and directly from the sun! Only plants "know" how to convert sunlight into carbohydrates. That's how they grow. From carbohydrates plants build new stems, roots, and bark, and most importantly, they build new leaves – because leaves can make more carbohydrates. This is why the mass of leaves is always superior in size in relation to the rest of the plant. Since the greens are always trying to increase absorption of chlorophyll, they continuously keep growing. Notice how quickly plants take over in our absence!

Plant life depends on sunshine, and human life depends on plants. Even when people eat animals, the nutrients derived from the meat are those that animal received earlier through consuming plants. That is why humans almost never eat carnivorous animals. Ancient Palestine teachings, Islam, and various other religions prohibit the eating of carnivorous animals such as lions, tigers, leopards, fox, eagles, pelicans, etc. My grandmother recalled that during the War, her hungry relatives tried eating the meat of carnivorous animals and birds and all became violently sick. At the same time, no living creatures, even carnivores, could survive without consuming some greens. We all notice how dogs and cats occasionally eat green grass.

With high oxygen content in chlorophyll and high mineral content in green plants, greens are the most alkalizing food that exists on our planet. By including green smoothies into our diet we can keep our bodies alkaline and healthy.

About the author:

*An adjunct professor at Southern Oregon University, **Victoria Boutenko** (of the well-known Boutenko family) is the author of **Green for Life, Raw Family** and **12 Steps to Raw Food**. The Boutenko family embarked on a diet of entirely raw foods in 1994, when they became seriously ill. This diet enabled them to heal all of their health problems. Now Victoria travels all over the world sharing her inspiring story and teaching classes on the raw-food diet. Based on the latest scientific research, Victoria Boutenko explains the numerous benefits of choosing a diet of fresh rather than cooked foods. Embracing the raw-food lifestyle is more than simply turning off the stove. Such a radical change in the way we eat affects all aspects of life. Victoria touches on the human relationship with nature, the value*

of supporting others, and the importance of living in harmony with people who don't share the same point of view on eating.
www.rawfamily.com

The healing power of wheatgrass - Jill Swyers

The "medicine of life"; "Nature's finest medicine": what is it, we hear, that could change our lives? This rich nutrient-dense chlorophyll-rich food is wheatgrass. The elixir of life! Wheatgrass is an excellent source of chlorophyll, which, as explained in the previous paragraphs, is a way of supplying the body with oxygen and in turn giving renewed energy. It cleanses, nourishes, rejuvenates and finally heals the body.

The benefits of wheatgrass
Wheatgrass is grown from a hard whole kernel wheat seed or wheatberry, as it is known in the US. It is used in a similar way as herbal medicines for its nutritional and therapeutic properties. This superfood purifies the blood, detoxifies the liver and cleanses the colon. It feeds and nourishes the body at the same time.

Additionally:

1. It is an energizer – chlorophyll wakes up and fuels the body! It is electrically charged, easily assimilated, and will aid the digestive tract.

2. It is a cleanser – wheatgrass removes unwanted toxins from the blood cells, organs, and tissues. It releases/removes excess fat, mineral, and protein deposits. It is able to kill unwanted bacteria and malignant cells in blood, lymph, and tissues.

3. It can strengthen the immune system and help alkalize the body, reducing the acidity. By balancing the pH, it will continue to build the blood and increase the oxygen capacity. It stimulates a healthy circulation, nourishes the cells, and increases red blood cells. It is also an anti-oxidant that prevents free radical formation.

4. As a healer, it stimulates and regenerates the liver. It can aid gastrointestinal problems, constipation, diarrhea, etc. it is possible to heal sores and wounds, improve blood sugar problems, and is effective in treating anemia, arthritis, diabetes, and many more conditions.

5. It can hydrate the body. Known for its anti-aging properties, it may be possible that it repairs DNA.

Superior qualities of wheatgrass juice

Wheatgrass is best consumed as freshly squeezed juice, and I will always stipu-late, "fresh is best". In saying that, it has to be easy for people to begin, so there are alternatives. Wheatgrass can come in many varieties and in dried forms, such as freeze-dried powder that is mixed with water to form a juice. Taste varies, according to the initial process and preparation, but to me, it is a medicine! The health-giving qualities speak for themselves:

*   Contains 70% chlorophyll – the life-force in wheatgrass
*   Rich source of vitamins A, C & E
*   Eight essential amino acids
*   Contains 92 of 102 trace minerals
*   Has a full spectrum of B vitamins including laetrile (B-17)
*   Contains calcium, iron, potassium, phosphorous, sulphur, sodium, cobalt, zinc, and magnesium
*   Known as a complete food, it has a balance of proteins, fats, and carbohy-drates

Wheatgrass can be grown from spelt, kamut, or barley grains. All methods of preparation are exceedingly beneficial, and it's all a matter of taste; but juicing is the most popular.

Wheatgrass as a protector

*   It can protect from low or high level radiation
*   Deodorizes the body
*   Protects from pollutants
*   Contains anti-bacterial compounds

I started taking control of my life many years ago, when I had suspected breast cancer, and other diseases, including being overweight. I have been drinking wheatgrass juice – 100ml/g / 2 oz. a day – for the past ten years and it has changed my life. Wheatgrass and green protein drinks are the secret to my life, and I introduce this secret into my teachings of the Hippocrates Healing Life-Change Program. A gradual process, this program is all about taking one step at a time.

Wheatgrass not only offers flavor and aroma like a fine wine or cocktail but also harnesses the sun's energy in chlorophyll and nutrients.
Wheatgrass, in short, is an energizing chlorophyll cocktail that:

*   Rebuilds the blood
*   Increases hemoglobin production
*   Heals wounds
*   Cleanses the colon
*   Is antibacterial
*   Alkalinizes the blood
*   Neutralizes toxins

- Cleanses the liver
- Stimulates enzyme activity
- Chelates out heavy metals

Nutritional components of wheatgrass juice

Wheatgrass has been recognized as a true superfood for more than two decades now. This particular analysis was performed by Irvine Analytical Laboratories, Inc. on 100 grams (2.8 oz) of wheatgrass:

Calories	21
Protein	1.25g
Carbohydrates	2g
Magnesium	24mg
Potassium	147mg
Zinc	0.33mg
Calcium	24.2mg
Sodium	10.3mg
Iron	0.61mg
Folic Acid / Folacin	29mcg
Vitamin A	427 IU
Vitamin B1 (Thiamine)	0.08mg
Vitamin B2 (Riboflavin)	0.13mg
Vitamin B3 (Niacinamide)	0.11mg
Vitamin B5 (Pantothenic HCl)	0.02mg
Vitamin B6 (Cyanocobalamin)	<1mcg
Vitamin C (Ascorbic Acid)	3.65mg
Vitamin E	15.2 IU
Biotin	10mcg
Chlorophyll	42.2mg
Choline	92.4mg

Add it to your wellness program and "raise a glass" of wheatgrass to your future good health. For further information on wheatgrass and algaes, please refer to Jameth Sheridan's chapter, 'Superfoods and Supplements'.

Resources:
Manual of the Hippocrates Health Institute (Florida)
Living Foods for Optimum Health by Dr. Brian Clement
Wheatgrass, Natures Finest Medicine by Steve Meyerowitz

About the author:
JILL SWYERS – LIVING FOODS FOR GREAT HEALTH & NUTRITION
Hippocrates Health Educator / Living Foods Consultant / Speaker / Practitioner /
Reiki Therapist / Naturopathic Nutrition / Trained Chef / Workshops / Retreats
"Healing & Enjoying the Hippocrates Lifestyle – One Step at a Time"

Since 1994, Jill Swyers has been teaching and guiding people on how to change their lifestyle – one step at a time, with nutrition. In 1998, Jill arrived at the Hippocrates Health Institute (Florida) as a guest, to do their 3-week program. Later that year, she went on to complete the 9-week Health Educator Program, becoming educated in Living Foods and Raw Foods, linking balance of the body with nutrition. As her main work is teaching the Hippocrates Lifestyle Program, with various different therapies, over the intervening years, Jill has returned annually to update her training, working as a volunteer. Since 1998, Jill has been traveling around the United Kingdom, Portugal, Ireland, and other countries, being invited to speak and bringing awareness to people, to help them reduce stress, gain energy, improve health as a preventative, and help to reverse dis-ease – "one step at a time." Jill continues on with constant learning, doing courses relating to healing, naturopathy, nutrition, health, herbs, healing massage, iridology, and integral hatha yoga teachers training, in order to understand how all therapies can be beneficial, and also to understand different subjects when working with different therapists. Having held various Hippocrates Lifestyle retreats at different centers in Portugal – cleansing and healing programs with a combination of Living and Raw Foods, including daily lectures and a variety of therapies / treatments linking to nutrition-based on the principles of energizing and revitalizing the body, mind, and spirit, Jill believes that a positive attitude and regaining one's health is the future.

Email: info@jillswyers.com
Website: www.jillswyers.com

Primordial, all-organic AFA – it's the wildness! - Tamera Campbell and Michael Saiber

Sea Vegetables And Freshwater Algae

There are tens of thousands of varieties of algae. Some are edible and health-giving, some are not. Two of the most popular edible algae are Spirulina and Chlorella which are hydroponically grown. Even though they are processed they are excellent foods that we recommend. There are also many wild-grown sea vegetables which are edible and nourishing.

"AFA has more bio-available chlorophyll than any other food. In biochemical research circles, the presence of chlorophyll in such high quantities is a clear indication of AFA's extraordinarily high life force. This inherent vitality helps keep the AFA's wide spectrum of nutrients at their absolute nutritional peak. For me, this partially explains the mystery of how AFA can have so many positive health benefits."
– Karl J. Abrams, Professor of Chemistry

At 8:45 pm, there's intense activity out on otherwise placid Klamath Lake. It's AFA harvest time! At 10:30 pm, David Robatcek gets a call from CEO Tamera Campbell, who is out on the lake helping the team to gather fresh AFA to be instantly batch-tested and frozen in vast banks of freezers to be later shipped to clients around the world. "David, we need the next shift to get out here in less than 30 minutes...." By 1:00 am, the day's harvest is complete. If, and only if, natural conditions are right, tomorrow will be another harvest day. As harvesters, we stand in humble relationship to nature. Our harvest is entirely dependent upon the creative intelligence of nature. Humans cannot determine, manipulate, or assist the outcome of this wild-grown crop. When the bloom is just right, we literally spring into action, night and day. We must move with clarity and speed, because we have only a small window of time each year to gather fresh AFA.

AFA stands for *Aphanizomenon flos-aquae*, an undomesticated aqua-botanical. As the rarest food found on earth, harvested only from Klamath Lake in Oregon, it is also the most nutrient-rich food known to humankind. It sets a standard for the entire "superfoods" category. Humans have indeed tried, but no one has ever been able to domesticate AFA. Going back over billions of years, nature remains to date the only gardener of the phylum and particularly of the species of AFA, a naturally occurring superfood without parallel. AFA, which has been fresh-frozen at the source to preserve innate potency, is available for daily use. Aside from having more bio-available chlorophyll than other foods, AFA is a pharmacopoeia unto itself. It is renowned for its multiple health benefits. AFA's combined elements work together harmoniously to tune both body and mind. That is why many call it an *adaptogen*. It remarkably tunes body and mind to a higher octave of health.

The love molecule
On the mental and emotional side, one extract from AFA contains a significant concentration of all-organic PEA (phenylethylamine), which increases focus and clarity. It is recommended for attention deficit disorder. Additionally, it lifts and brightens mood. In chocolate, PEA is known as the "love molecule". This extract from the AFA contains vastly more bio-available PEA than chocolate. PEA is a naturally occurring extract from AFA that promotes clear thinking and focus to provide optimal cognitive function.

Dr Gabriel Cousens, an alternative medicine MD with a background in psychiatry, writes: "*I've had people who've been depressed for years and years, and literally, within a few days after receiving [PEA from fresh-frozen AFA] or AFA their depression lifts. It is a specific food for attention deficit disorders and for depression*". PEA, found in wild-harvested AFA, contains the active ingredient that promotes mood balance and enhances focus with no side effects whatsoever. This is one reason we call AFA the "feel good food". Researchers at Rush University and the Center for Creative Development in Chicago conducted a study demonstrating PEA's anti-depressant effects: "*It has been proposed that PEA deficit may be the cause of a common form of depressive illness. PEA produces sustained relief of depression in a significant number of patients, including some unresponsive to standard treatments.*" Decreased urinary levels of PEA have been found in some depressed patients. PEA was found to be measurably and significantly lower in subjects with ADD. People using organic PEA from AFA report better attention at school and at work. It serves to balance mood and to increase concentration.

Runner's high, PEA and depression
A study by E. Ellen Billett, PhD, tells WebMD: *"What we are trying to say is now there is more chemical evidence for why runners' high occurs. We hope this information might give doctors more confidence in prescribing exercise for mild depression and as an adjunct to drug therapy."* The secret is PEA.. A Nottingham Trent University research team studied 20 healthy young men. The men had their PEA levels measured after one day of no exercise and after one day of moderate exercise. All but two of the men had increased PEA levels 24 hours after their exercise. Hector Sabelli, MD, PhD. is Director of the Chicago Center for Creative Development. He researched PEA while a professor at Chicago's Rush University. Dr Sabelli states that new findings fit exactly with all of his own experiments. *"What we have seen is that PEA metabolism is reduced in people who are depressed. If you give PEA to people with depression, about 60% show an immediate recovery -- very fast, a matter of half an hour."* Billett says that endorphins don't penetrate the brain as easily as does PEA. She thinks PEA may be the true basis for the good mood one gets from a workout; it is part of the reward of exercise.

Peak Performance
Fresh-frozen liquid AFA provides 64 pre-digested, 97% absorbable vitamins, minerals, and enzymes and has more biologically active chlorophyll than any known food. The presence and balance of these nutrient-dense factors is responsible for what Dr. Abrams calls *"the mystery of how AFA can have so many positive health benefits"*.

Dr. Fred Bisci, nationally renowned health lecturer and raw food advocate, recommends fresh-frozen liquid AFA for *"long-lasting energy boost"*. Olympians and professional athletes categorically state that AFA reduces fatigue and increases stamina. Ryk Neethling, an Olympic swimmer and World Record Holder states, *"Since eating fresh-frozen AFA, I've noticed an unmistakable boost in my energy. I have more stamina. Recovery time is dramatically shorter. AFA makes a big difference in my performance"*.

Stephen Molitor, an undefeated professional boxer using fresh-frozen AFA states, *"I don't feel weak or tired. I am amazed by my recuperation time between rounds. In one moment I am ready. It gives me focus like never before."* People going through a regular work day state they are able to function at more optimal levels altogether.

Anti-inflammatory benefits
Another extract from AFA provides anti-inflammatory properties. This is a soothing blue compound extracted from AFA. It is a special concentrate of the inflammation-reducing blue pigment naturally occurring in whole AFA. This extract has been clinically shown to reduce or eliminate pain and inflammation by selectively disabling COX-2 enzymes, connected to inflammation, and to support the "good" COX-1 enzymes, the ones that help us maintain normal joint, blood, kidney, and

digestive functions.

Effects on the immune system

AFA is the only food in the world known to support the natural and safe release of adult stem cells from the bone marrow. A study of AFA's effects on the immune system was conducted at McGill University in Canada. If was shown that consumption of a mere 1.5 grams of AFA resulted in rapid changes in immune cell trafficking. It was significantly demonstrated that AFA increases the immune surveillance without directly stimulating the immune system. Another extract derived entirely from AFA is stated to support the migration of stem cells to tissue in the body needing repair and is lab-proven to increase the number of circulating stem cells by up to 30% (about three to four million stem cells).

The AFA Combination

We have briefly touched upon some of the unique properties and extracts of AFA. Above all, it's truly the synergy of elements arranged by nature's own hand that is most responsible for AFA's ability to benefit both body and mind. AFA is a supportive food. It continually tunes the body to a more harmonious state of health. It helps bring the whole system into alignment and influences better food and healthy lifestyle choices. The most powerful and immediately usable form of AFA is the fresh-frozen liquid.

We are deeply moved to be caretakers of this primordial food, a gift from the wild to humanity, that continues to support the health and healing of many.

About the authors:

Tamera Campbell's areas of expertise are as varied as her numerous interests. Her dedication to the betterment of life for all inspired her 15 years as a dance instructor working with students ranging from the highly gifted to those with mental challenges, often volunteering her time and talents for the benefit of the community. Tamera is a 46-year-old mother of bright and beautiful E3Live™ babies as well as a frequent lecturer on detoxification and the body's elimination systems. In addition, she is the formulator of some of the top-selling green formulas on the market today, and her formulations are used by many world-famous doctors and healing clinics. She brings more than 20 years of experience in business management and operations to her current role of CEO and owner of Vision / E3Live™. These companies harvest and produce the revolutionary E3Live™, the world's first and only fresh-frozen Aphanizomenon flos-aquae (AFA). Vision/ E3Live™ is the world-wide leader of nutritional algae and an icon for 'greens' in the living foods community. Tamera has had the great fortune of working closely with Dr. Gabriel Cousens, Dr. Brian Clement of Hippocrates Health Institute, Dr. Fred Bisci, and many other highly respected and well-known healers who are living examples of the long-term benefits of the living foods lifestyle.

The discoverer and founder of E3Live™, and President of Vision / E3Live™, Michael Saiber was introduced to the raw living foods lifestyle more than 30 years ago after staying with Dr. Ann Wigmore. He is a true Renaissance man, having been a competitive swimmer, gymnast, and body builder, an art and

athletics teacher, and a highly successful businessman. His amazing background also includes helping and employing those he calls "special people" – people who live with challenges from congenital birth defects and disfigurements. His most important work has been as a lecturer on health and the impact of living foods in our diets – being credited with saving many lives due to his caring nature and expertise on the benefits of eating raw foods. Michael is the proud father of four children and a true example of a leader "walking his talk". At 67 years of age, he attributes his youthful appearance and boundless energy to this commitment to eating healthy foods.
www.e3live.com

(Endnotes)
1   Warburg, Otto. The Oxygen-Transferring Ferment of Respiration. Nobel Lecture, 1931. From Nobel Lectures, Physiology or Medicine 1922-1941, Amsterdam: Elsevier Publishing Company, 1965
2   Chlorophyllin Reduces Aflatoxin Indicators Among People At High Risk For Liver Cancer. Johns Hopkins University Bloomberg School of Public Health. Baltimore, MD. Proceedings of the National Academy of Sciences. November 27, 2001.
3   Chernomorsky, S. et al. Effect of Dietary Chlorophyll Derivatives on Mutagenesis and Tumor Cell Growth. Teratogenesis, Carcinogenesis, and Mutagenesis, *79* : 313-322, 1999.
4   Vlad M. et al. Effect of Cuprofilin on Experimental Atherosclerosis. Romania: Institute of Public Health and Medical Research, University of Medicine and Pharmacy, Cluj-Napoka, 1995

10

The Importance of Essential Fatty Acids

Rick Dina, DC

Essential fatty acids are involved in a wide variety of important physiological processes. These include the production of hemoglobin, oxygen transfer, energy production, recovery from fatigue, cell division, creating smooth and soft skin, creating stable heart rhythms, reducing platelet stickiness, regulating inflammatory processes, and hormone regulation. Fatty acids are a major part of our cell membranes, which surround and affect the functioning of every cell in our body. Fatty acid imbalances can create or contribute to unhealthy conditions, such as lack of proper nervous system development in infants and children, depression, cancer, diabetes, high blood pressure, and cardiovascular disease.

Of the many different fatty acids our bodies use for various functions, there are two fatty acids that we do not have the enzymatic capability to produce. They are known collectively as the two *essential fatty acids* (EFAs), since they must be obtained from our diet. The first, known as linoleic acid (LA), belongs to the omega-6 family of fatty acids, and the other, alpha-linolenic acid (ALA), is part of the omega-3 family of fats. Each family has six different fatty acid members. From LA, our body can make the other five omega-6 fats, and from ALA, our body can make the other five omega-3 fats. Fats other than those of the omega-6 and omega-3 families are created from other sources or processes, such as the breakdown products of carbohydrates or protein, or from other fats we consume.

LA, the omega-6 EFA, is the first member of the omega-6 family. It changes into gamma-linolenic acid, also known as GLA, the second member of the omega-6 family by a "desaturase" enzyme, one of the body's many metabolic enzymes.

. different enzyme changes GLA into DGLA, the third member of the omega-6 family. The next enzyme changes DGLA into arachidonic acid, or AA, the fourth member of the family. The fifth omega-6 fatty acid has little nutritional significance, and the sixth omega-6 fatty acid will be discussed later in this chapter.

In the omega-3 family, we begin with ALA, which is the omega-3 EFA. It undergoes three enzyme conversions to become EPA, the fourth member of the omega-3 family. EPA goes through two more enzyme transformations to become the sixth member, known as DHA. ALA, EPA, and DHA are the key players in the omega-3 family.

Depending upon which authority you are listening to, we need from 3 to 10 grams of linoleic acid per day, and about 2 to 5 grams of alpha-linolenic acid per day. Omega-6 fats are widely found in a large variety of foods, so getting enough of these is rarely ever a problem. Omega-3 fatty acids are much less abundant in typical modern Western diets. It is estimated, for example, that 90-95% of Americans are deficient in omega-3 fats, while having an overabundance of omega-6 fats. The rest of this chapter, therefore, will focus mainly on the omega-3 family of fatty acids.

Omega-3

The good news for those following a raw food diet is that the omega-3 essential fat, ALA, is found in virtually all fruits and vegetables. Although it has been challenging to get an exact figure, it is fair to say that 1000 calories of non-green vegetables and fruits contain approximately 1 gram of alpha-linolenic acid, which potentially meets half of your daily omega-3 needs. Sadly, there are very few people within the general population who consume such large quantities of fresh fruits and vegetables, which is why they are not usually considered a major source of EFAs. Fruits and vegetables also contain the omega-6 essential fat, LA, in about a 1:1 ratio with ALA.

Omega-6 (top) / Omega-3 (bottom) Conversion Chart

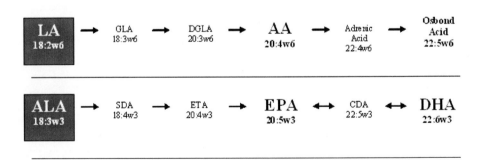

Leafy green vegetables supply about 10% of their calories from fat. 60–70% of this fat is alpha-linolenic acid. Interestingly, the plant uses ALA in the process of converting sunlight energy into carbohydrates, fats, and proteins. Approximately

150 - 300 calories of leafy greens (including broccoli) contain 1 gram of ALA, or half of your daily omega-3 needs. In other words, raw foodists who consume 1000 calories of non-green fruits and vegetables, and 150 - 300 calories of leafy greens have met their daily omega-3 requirements with only 1150 - 1300 calories. The consumption of this quantity of fruits, vegetables, and greens can easily be accomplished by following the recommendations for a healthy diet as provided by the International Living Foods Leaders Summit and which are described in this book. Leafy green vegetables also contain LA, but lesser amounts than ALA.

If this is not enough, then it is time to bring out the "heavy hitters" in the omega-3 plant world. The undisputed champion is flax seed. Flax, whether brown or golden, provides approximately 58% of its fat from ALA. One heaping tablespoon (US) of whole flax seed contains 2 grams of ALA, or an entire daily requirement. Hemp and Chia seeds are also excellent sources of omega-3 fats, with approximately two tbsp of either supplying 2 grams of ALA. Walnuts and soybeans contain ALA (omega-3), but they have about ten and seven times more LA (omega-6), respectively.

Knowing the ratio of omega-6 to omega-3 is very important. The optimal ratio of omega-6 to omega-3 is somewhere from 4:1 to 1:1. Some experts even suggest a ratio of 1:2, or half as much omega-6 as omega-3. A typical modern Western diet contains about 20 or more times more omega-6 fats than omega-3 fats, or a ratio of 20:1.

Why is the altered ratio such a problem? First of all, when consumed, the omega-6 essential fat LA gets converted into arachidonic acid, or AA, as described above. AA is the precursor for substances that initiate inflammation. The omega-3 fat EPA is the precursor for substances that control inflammation, so when we have a healthy ratio of omega-6 to omega-3, inflammation stays in check. When we have an excess of AA (omega-6) over EPA (omega-3), we tend toward an excess of inflammation, which not only contributes to obvious inflammatory conditions such as arthritis, but is also a major contributor to degenerative diseases such as heart disease, stroke, cancer, Alzheimer's, the complications of diabetes, etc.

AA is also found directly in domesticated land animals and dairy products. LA is found in abundance in processed foods, often including processed vegan foods. The oils commonly found in processed foods that contain the most LA include corn, cottonseed, soybean, sesame, sunflower, safflower, and peanut. Because the average modern person lives largely on animal products and processed foods and eats small amounts of fruits and vegetables, flax, hemp, chia, or cold water fish, we see then how we get such an overabundance of omega-6 fats in comparison to omega-3 fats. When we eat a large percentage of our calories from fruits and vegetables, especially leafy green vegetables, moderate amounts of nuts and seeds, and minimize or ideally completely avoid animal foods and processed plant foods, we tend automatically to get an optimum ratio of omega-6 to omega-3 fats, as well as a multitude of other nutritional benefits described throughout the rest of this book.

125

Another consequence of an excess of omega-6 fats over omega-3 fats is that even if you have enough of the omega-3 essential fatty acid alpha-linolenic acid, you may still end up with a deficiency of the other omega-3 fats made from it, such as DHA. In order to understand why this occurs, it is important to know that the very same enzymes that act upon the omega-6 family of fats also act upon the omega-3 family of fats. If we consume too many omega-6 fats, then the enzymes are so busy working on the omega 6 family that they are less available to work on the omega-3 family. This is known biochemically as "competitive inhibition." The idea is that both essential fatty acids are "competing" for the same enzymes to convert them into the other members of their respective families.

In a typical Western diet, there is "inhibition" of action upon the omega-3 fats, because the enzymes are too occupied with the excess of omega-6 fats. This is why some experts claim we need up to 5 or more grams of omega-3 fats per day, because they know that the typical person is eating too many omega-6 fats, and they want us to maintain the healthy ratio as described above. It is somewhat analogous to higher than necessary recommendations for calcium because nutritionists know the typical person will lose a lot of calcium from consuming an acid-forming diet. With an alkalizing diet, we don't need extra calcium to make up for the losses due to acidity. When we have a balanced ratio of omega-6 to omega-3 fats, there is generally no need for more than 2 grams of omega-3s per day.

DHA – the long chain omega-3

DHA is the longest chain omega-3 fatty acid, and is critically important for hormone regulation, optimal brain function, and for women who are pregnant or breast-feeding. Deficiency of this can contribute to diabetes, cancer, high blood pressure, depression, and learning impairment, as well as many common complications of pregnancy, such as pre-eclampsia, gestational diabetes, and post-partum depression. Cold water, fatty fish such as wild salmon, sardines, mackerel, trout, herring, and eel contain pre-formed EPA and DHA. When someone who eats a typical modern diet begins to include these cold water fish into their diets, there are often notable health improvements. They are now consuming the much needed omega-3 fats they were lacking before. This helps in areas such as lowering blood sugar, blood pressure, total and LDL cholesterol, reducing inflammation, and may even improve mood and brain function.

Unfortunately, fish also comes with some inherent problems. It contains cholesterol, saturated fat and its own arachidonic acid (AA), has no fiber, vitamin C or phytonutrients, is acid forming, and has varying degrees of environmental contamination, most notably mercury, dioxin, and PCBs. Even fish on the "safer" end of the spectrum are only supposed to be eaten a couple of times per week or month according to various authorities, such as the Environmental Protection Agency and the FDA of the United States. This is especially troubling for pregnant and lactating women, who are cautioned to eat even less fish than the general population, and none of certain species. DHA is one of the most important raw materials to create the brain, spinal cord, and peripheral nerves of the developing nervous systems of fetuses and infants, yet mercury is known to be very damaging to these structures, possibly even leading to birth defects.

How do vegans get their DHA?

The main question for vegans becomes how to secure a reliable source of DHA without consuming mercury and other environmental contaminants found in cold water fish. There have been many studies that have questioned the body's ability to convert ALA into DHA efficiently or effectively. I have examined many of these studies very carefully, and I would like to take this opportunity to take a look "beyond the headlines" that are often stated without a great deal of thought, consideration, or education behind them. We discussed how an excess of omega-6 fats inhibits the conversion of ALA into the longer chain omega-3 fats, such as DHA, by competitive inhibition. It is also well known that trans fats (from hydrogenated oils found in margarine and processed foods) and saturated fats (found in overabundance mostly in domesticated land animals and dairy products) interfere with the enzymes that convert the EFAs (LA and ALA) into their longer chain family members.

In one fairly representative study of pregnant women, commonly quoted in opposition to the idea that the body can effectively convert ALA into DHA, researchers gave ALA to participants in the experimental group in the form of margarine, with a 3.2 to 1 ratio of omega-6 to omega-3. The study did not discuss any other aspects of the women's diets, so we do not know the *overall* dietary ratio of omega-6 to omega-3 fats. This particular study was done in the Netherlands, however, so it is a fair assumption that the study participants were most likely consuming a typical Western diet, including more omega-6 fats than omega-3s, and an excess of saturated and trans fats. The control group received margarine with only omega-6 fats in it, and no omega-3.

Among other measurements, this study looked at blood levels of ALA, DHA, and AA, as well as another fatty acid known as osbond acid. Osbond acid is an omega-6 fat (the sixth fat in the omega-6 family) that is structurally nearly identical to DHA (the sixth fat in the omega-3 family), except that DHA has one extra double bond in the omega-3 position. Levels of osbond acid increase when there is not enough DHA, as osbond acid is functionally more similar to DHA than anything else the body can produce. In this way, it is seen by researchers as a "functional indicator" of DHA status. In other words, the poorer the DHA status, the higher the osbond acid level, and the better the DHA status, the lower the osbond acid level. This study noted an increase in osbond acid (not beneficial) in the blood of the women who consumed the omega-6 only margarine, while those who consumed the ALA (omega-3) fortified margarine did not see this increase (beneficial). In other words, the women who consumed ALA showed better functional DHA status than those who did not.

The title of this study was initially "Alpha linolenic acid supplementation in pregnancy has no effect on maternal cognition or DHA in maternal and infant plasma." Most health professionals only read the title and possibly the abstract (summary) of an article. They therefore often miss out on important information in the text of the article, such as the improvement in functional DHA status of women consuming ALA, despite having the odds heavily stacked against them by simultaneously consuming omega-6 trans fats in addition to their Western diets. Additionally, the

el in the cell membranes is what really counts and is a far better indicator
acid status than measuring only blood levels, as this study did.

studies have shown that we do effectively convert ALA into DHA, and that approximately 7% of ALA consumed ends up being converted to DHA. That would mean that 3 grams of ALA (found for example in the 1000 calories of non-green produce and 150 - 300 calories of greens mentioned earlier, which supplies 2 grams ALA, with one 1 additional gram of ALA added from either another 150-300 calories of greens, 1000 calories of fruits and vegetables, 1 tbsp hemp seeds, etc. or any combination of the above) would provide about 200 mg of DHA, which is an adequate daily intake based on the recommendations of most authorities.

In all fairness to the conversion studies, it must be noted that we have a population "at large" that consumes an average of 20+ times more omega-6 fats than omega-3 fats, along with unhealthy levels of trans and saturated fats. It is probably fair to say that the average person who fits this dietary profile indeed does experience inhibition of the enzymes that convert ALA to DHA.

Fortunately, there are ways of testing the fatty acid profile of our cell membranes. A few years back, we tested my wife, Dr. Karin Dina, who had been a mostly raw vegan for 15 years and was in her mid-thirties. At the time and for several years prior, her diet consisted of some fruit and lots of green vegetables, some nuts and seeds, with the consumption of flax seeds being extremely rare. She does not consume any processed food or isolated oil, and prior to this test had never taken any type of fatty acid or DHA supplement, or any algae product that might have provided an outside source of DHA.

All of her cell membrane omega-3 fats, including DHA, were within the normal reference range. So we can be quite sure that Dr. Karin does indeed convert ALA into DHA effectively. One case history does not prove everything, but if this healthy raw food vegan woman can convert ALA into DHA effectively, it is not too far of a stretch to speculate that others could do so as well. Research studies have shown that women produce DHA more efficiently than men and are even more efficient when pregnant and breastfeeding. This makes sense from a survival point of view, considering how important DHA is for the developing the nervous systems of fetuses and infants.

In the event that one does not have adequate cell membrane DHA levels, despite their best efforts, the good news is that there are vegan sources of DHA derived from algae. Algae is the original source of DHA for the fish who consume it (and on up the food chain) and thus contains DHA. As far as EPA is concerned, even the studies that question the conversion of ALA to DHA have always shown that plenty of EPA is made from ALA. Additionally, DHA can be converted to EPA. If one consumes adequate amounts of both ALA and DHA, it is extremely unlikely that EPA needs would not be met.

The bottom line is to minimize the excess of omega-6 fats, which comes primarily from processed food and domesticated land animals, and instead eat a diet based on fresh fruits and vegetables, including large quantities of leafy green vegetables. Flax, hemp or chia seeds can be consumed if there is concern about or need for additional ALA. These recommendations supply both optimal levels of ALA and allow for the conditions for the ALA to be converted into both EPA and DHA as needed. If necessary, there are specific algae-based foods or DHA supplements derived from algae that can be consumed, ensuring a reliable source of plant-based, pre-formed DHA without the health risks, ethical issues, and environmental planetary concerns associated with the consumption of fish.

About the Author:

Dr. Rick Dina, D.C. has been studying health and nutrition since 1986 and has been a raw food vegan since 1987. He worked at Hippocrates Health Institute in 1991 and then traveled the USA with the Juiceman company teaching the benefits of raw fruit and vegetable diets before entering chiropractic college in 1992. After earning his doctorate degree in 1997, he practiced at True North Health Education Center, a multi-disciplinary water fasting facility in Santa Rosa, CA, where he was involved in the care, supervision, and education of patients recovering from diabetes, high blood pressure, cardiovascular disease, autoimmune diseases, and other nutrition and lifestyle related health challenges.

In 2002, Dr. Rick taught a required course, "The Determinants of Health," at Bastyr University in Seattle, WA, the flagship 4-year naturopathic medical school granting doctorate degrees in naturopathic medicine. He and his wife, Dr. Karin Dina, D.C. teach raw food nutrition courses and lead retreats with organizations such as the Ann Wigmore Natural Health Institute™, as well as teach the acclaimed Science of Raw Food Nutrition™ series of classes at the Living Light Culinary Arts Institute™ in northern California.

For more information, please visit www.rawfoodeducation.com

11

The Key of Low
Sugar Consumption

Brian Clement, PhD, NMD, LNC

Three decades ago, when Hippocrates Health Institute resided in Boston, Massachusetts, banquets of fruit were common, and carrot and beet juice flowed like a river. In early spring, I received a call from a very important alumni, Edie May Huntsberg, who healed herself of cancer and wrote the famous book, *How I Conquered Cancer Naturally*. This publication sold a million copies, and Edie was the inspiration for more than half the people who attended the Institute. We were alarmed when she stated that her tumors were coming back in spite of medical checks showing her to be clear of cancer. Three months later, she put our minds at rest when she announced the tumors disappeared. This turned out to be a yearly event for the following two seasons. By the summer of the third year, she finally cracked the mystery of this odd phenomenon. Living in Southern California, many of her neighbors grew dates. They would often bring boxes to her, and like many, she would eat up to 3 lbs per day. When date season was over and the sugar supply waned, the tumors went into remission.

This was an unwelcome revelation to all of us working with the Hippocrates program. Personally, at that time my diet was well over 50% fruit and their juices. Not really wanting to face the music, I reluctantly established a group of nine alumni for a two-month study on the effects of fructose consumption. Five of the participants removed all fruit and fructose rich foods and juices, such as carrots and beets, from their diet; four were allowed to continue fructose consumption. In gathering weekly blood profiles, it rapidly became apparent that the immune system improved and the symptoms relaxed in the five who did not indulge in fructose. In the four who continued there was little to no improvement, and even

signs of decreased differentials (immune cells). We clearly established an understanding that our idea about fruit being natural, healthy, and healing was not quite
right. We made a swift concrete decision to remove fruit from all program participants who were in the conquest of cancer. We began to discuss this with sympa-
thetic local professors and scientists from such institutes as Harvard, Boston College, and Tufts University. Individually, they pointed out that in laboratory settings
they not only promoted the growth and development of cancer cells through the
use of sugar, but it equally spawns viruses, bacteria, molds, and yeast. Although
it was previously thought that sucrose was different than fructose, such was not
the case in human disease.

The sugar addiction

This monumental change was not joyfully received by those following the Hippocrates lifestyle. The foremost addiction that we all share is that of sugar. We fall
into one of two categories: current sugar addicts and recovering sugar addicts.
In retrospect, many of us surrendered our white sugar, honey, and maple syrup
and replaced it with fruit juice and copious amounts of sugar-rich choices. Those
effected acted like children with lollipops pulled from their mouths. Although intellectually I was completely committed to this change, emotionally it was as difficult
on me as the poor victims of our findings. I will never forget the first lecture tour
where I announced this significant change. If the audience had tomatoes, I am
sure my suit would have been stained. Some months after making this excruciat-
ing shift, I found myself flying to Los Angeles from the East coast. The passenger
next to me began small talk. To be polite, when asked, I told him I directed a
natural health center in Boston. He came alive and asked if it was Hippocrates,
where his aunt had healed herself. Surprised that he knew of Hippocrates, I
asked what he did. He said he was an agricultural expert specializing in fruit cul-
tivation. The next hour before we landed in Los Angeles, I had a crash course in
the history of fruit. I walked away with new powerful knowledge that provided me
with greater strength and commitment. Discovering that all fruits today, through
hybridization, contain from 28–34 times more sugar than their heirloom ancestors shone the light on fruit's dark side. For millennia, produce distributors have
understood that the sweeter the fruit, the greater the sales.

Shortly after we made the dynamic change to a greatly green and sprout diet, we
started to observe, clinically, diseases that were formerly difficult to defeat suc-
cumbing to the new cuisine. Statistically, our findings have established that many
cancers heal from two to seven times faster. Low- and high-blood sugar, which
took a long time, at best, to resolve, were now being turned by their sufferers in
record speed. Fungal and yeast problems were finally weakened and vulnerable
enemies, and viral and bacterial diseases that in the past seemed chronic now
seemed quite manageable. In the last 30 years, we have collected blood profiles
and medical records from tens of thousands of the Institute's participants. During
the 21-day session, four blood samples are taken. Upon returning home, these
participants are afforded life-long consultations. These consultations have harvested medical reports on numerous individuals over several years. From this,
we have created an understanding that a sugarless diet plays a profound role in
good health.

There is also an emotional component that surfaces when one either removes or greatly reduces the amount of fructose in the diet. Depression, attention deficit disorder, bipolar disorder, and schizophrenia sufferers all experience fewer swings and more stability when we replace sugar-rich foods with protein-rich greens. Over the last two decades, the allopathic field of diagnosis has provided even greater insight by the tool known as a PET scan. Diagnosing cancer has become far more simple and sophisticated by using this scan. During the procedure, patients have sugar injected into their blood stream. The cancer begins to gobble it up, and it shines like a star on the film. Great detail is evident when the cancer is moving (metastasis). You can actually view the route that it is taking. When quizzing the leading experts, they all agree that if we injected fructose, the same results would occur.

By their fruits...

For years, Hippocrates was the lone voice crying out about complications that sugar-rich foods often bring. Over the last decade, we have gained some powerful allies from both the scientific and living food communities. When the first Living Food Leadership meeting convened, I was pleasantly surprised to find out that the overwhelming majority of seasoned and experienced leaders had come to the same conclusion, both professionally and personally, that we had. There are now volumes written about sugar as a menace in all forms of disease. Progressive oncologists commonly tell their patients to remove all such "foods". In medical literature, sugar is now considered the most addictive substance.

There are those living food enthusiasts who claim that one cannot achieve enough caloric value (energy) from a green diet. They believe that fruit is the only viable way to gain such vitality. This is not valid, and, in fact, we have established that large amounts of fruit must be consumed consistently to gain an average amount of energy. Whereas sprouted grains, sprouted beans, sprouted nuts and seeds, and algae all provide energy and nutritional substance. Almost all fruit, including organic, is intentionally picked unripened. This makes produce far less perishable and viable for the distributors and shops that sell it. Although organic ripe fruit is alkalizing to the body, unripened fruit is acidic. Unripened fruit is like a baby that has been born prematurely and requires additional nutrients to become whole. When one consumes this acid-causing fare, it robs the tissue (bones, organs, etc.), of those missing nutrients weakening the anatomy of the partaker.

Between the exceptionally high unnatural sugar content and the acid-causing nutrient-robber effect, fruit should no longer be looked at as a mainstay. After decades of analysis, we established that when one has conquered their disease (cancer, virus, molds, yeast, fungus, spirochete, hypoglycemia, diabetes) they can consume up to 15% organic ripe fruit by weight of their total diet. What is interesting is that those of us who relinquished fruit do not have the same desire to consume it as readily as we once did. It is the lover you lost and were heartbroken by at first, but now you probably do not remember his or her name. There is a landslide movement away from fruit consumption in the legitimate field of natural health care. We cannot go overboard and condemn fruits in total, since they were originally the food of choice for humans. Before hybridization, the fruit was far more nourishing and absolutely less sugar-concentrated. The human anatomy was stronger and more functional and was able to use the fruit nutrients much better than modern man, with his weakened dysfunctional pancreas (sugar regulating organ). Seldom do we discover a fully functional pancreas.

Healthy children, on the other hand, are able to consume up to 40% of their diet as fruit, because they metabolize at a much faster level. We assume their organs are healthy and functional. Be sure you only use ripened varieties that are either collected by you or by a local source you fully trust. Dried fruit assaults teeth more than any other food, so be sure to floss your children's teeth and clean them immediately after consumption. Adults other than serious athletes should most likely avoid all forms of dried fruit. When engaging in extensive physical activity, one's metabolism mimics a child's and is able to break down and utilize the nutrients from the dried variety. Fruits, when eaten separate from other forms of food, can be a treat replacement. Due to social and ethnic norms, this is desirable. We would much rather see you eat a ripe organic fruit as a dessert than some absurd gourmet concoction with numerous conflicting ingredients.

Remember to be compassionate with yourself when removing this addictive fare from your diet. It is likely you will wander back to overindulgence. Forgive yourself and reestablish the strength that will keep you away from your cravings. When healing yourself, think of fruit as a sour medicine and avoid it with every drop of your energy. If you occasionally succumb to it, just remember it is far better than cake or ice cream. As a matter of fact, one of the things we teach our healthy guests to make is frozen banana ice cream. This has been a lifesaver, keeping people away from high-fat, high-white-sugar commercial brands. Occasional indulgences are not mortal sins; just do not make them permanent fixtures in your lifestyle. Those of you who still question all that you have just learned need to self evaluate why you have such a difficult time releasing this stimuli. Take baby steps and avoid all sources of sugar for a day, the next week two days, the following week three days. If you are honest with yourself, you will begin to feel greater strength, clearer thinking, and more overall stability.

Geography, availability and personal activity all play pivotal roles in the matter of how much fruit one can consume. Tropical fruit offers the most nutrition and the highest level of beneficial frequency. This is due to the abundance of Sun it captures during its ripening process. In the far north, where there are less solar rays available, the fruit's nutritional value largely comes via the soil and the deep root systems. Those living in the sunbelt would be better served to consume the tropical and subtropical varieties. Those residing in northern latitudes should gravitate toward hearty varieties. These ripened fruits actually fit the geography and the environmental influence necessary in accomplishing superior health. People exposing their bodies to daily sunlight receive many of the nutrients that are derived from fruit and thus desire and need less. Fully clothed individuals may want larger amounts of the local fruit, since they are not acquiring the necessary UV rays. Of course, green plants, including sprouts, harness the sunlight in a much stronger way than fruits, providing an excellent source of UV fulfillment.

With the barriers and boundaries that once stood now removed through global communication, we are fortunately exposed to exotic and new foods that have great value. Acai is one example. This fruit from a tall palm tree has very little sugar content, yet massive nutritional and antioxidant value. We have successfully been able to utilize small to moderate amounts of this fruit in its raw form even with those in the conquest of disease. Goji berries have a higher sugar content, but they are fully endowed with a wide variety of nutrients and antioxidants. Noni, a very low-sugar fruit in its raw form, enhances cellular communication that significantly raises overall health.

Bananas, dried fruit, and much citrus, melons, etc. are out of balance from hundreds of years of agricultural manipulation. These are examples of types of fruits to avoid. Most people do not realize that industry has the capacity to extract sugar crystals from fruit that mimic table sugar. Carbohydrates are the fuel for a healthy body. This does not mean that all carbohydrates are the same quality. Sprouted grains or beans dispense their vitality to the consumer over a two-and-half-hour period, whereas most fruits rush through the body spiking and plummeting energy. If you observe creatures who consume large amounts of fruit, such as chimpanzees, the food that they ingest has a major impact on their personalities. Sporadic behavior, rushing from a quiet contemplation to a crazed frenetic state, seems to be their rhythm. Gorillas, on the other hand, who in the wild consume sprouts (roots of green plants), appear stable and thoughtful. Their muscles are the strongest of any creature pound for pound. We should not misconstrue these statements. Monkeys or apes are not humans, although they are genetically similar to humans. What differentiates us is the human mind and the multifarious ways that we negotiate life. It is clear to those of us who have clinically observed diet that stability and strength come from a green plant-based cuisine versus a high water/sugar cuisine.

Changing lifestyle
Let us hope that you receive this information in the spirit in which it is offered. This is not in any way meant to be a criticism of those who are finding their way in the world of raw/living food consumption. As noted, I, as did most of my peers, personally experimented and overindulged in fruits and other dietary choices. At times, we were strong enough to emerge with clear thinking and analytical ambition. This often opened a new world in which we made greater discoveries for ourselves and those we guide. Each of you will also evolve in and with your lifestyle. This is quite natural and something I encourage. For those of you that are currently bringing about your own recovery, I support you in your utilization of our vast experience so that you can achieve your life's most important goal, conquering the disease. At this time, you do not have the liberty to experiment as healthier people may. Remember that when you have fulfilled your dream, your nutritional world will broaden and feel less restrictive. For those that are out of balance and continuing on the path of raw/living consumption but do not feel the inner physical and emotional strength that should reign, please adjust your food choices. Openly proceed acknowledging that human life is simultaneously powerful and fragile. Each of us is in the process of better understanding ourselves and others. Avail yourself to new findings and enhanced understandings. Allow those

guiding lights to lead you in the direction of self-fulfillment and passionate existence. It is our gift to acknowledge powerful vigor and humbling consciousness, as they both create the gracious life we all deserve.

About the Author:
Dr. Brian Clement, PhD, NMD, LNC, has spearheaded the International progressive health movement for more than three decades. By conducting daily clinical research as the director of the renowned Hippocrates Health Institute, the world's foremost complementary residential health Mecca, he and his team have developed a state-of-the-art program for health maintenance and recovery. His Florida (U.S.A.) center has pioneered a program and established training in active aging and disease prevention. With hundreds of thousands of people participating in this program over the last half-century, volumes of data have been accrued, giving Clement a privileged insight into the lifestyle required to maintain youth, vitality, and stamina. Among Dr. Clement's many publications are **Living Foods for Optimum Health** *and* **Longevity** *and* **Lifeforce**. *His latest book,* Longevity, *delivers cutting-edge knowledge coupled with a common sense practical approach that will raise your level of health and happiness.*

Dr. Clement is first and foremost a devoted husband and a caring father of four. In addition to daily counseling and research studies, Clement conducts conferences worldwide on attaining health and creating longevity, giving delegates a roadmap for redirecting, enriching and extending their lives.

www.hippocratesinst.org

12

The Body's Need for Adequate Salt

Jameth Sheridan, ND

Salt can help you heal, or it can take you down, depending on the type and amount.

Too much is, and the wrong type is extremely damaging to your health.

However, too little of the right type is just as bad. If you do not have enough of the correct type of salt, you will likely experience:

- Low energy
- Low blood pressure
- Blood sugar problems
- Cravings for the wrong type of salt
- Craving for animal flesh

At the 2007 International Living Foods Summit of raw food leaders, I brought up the issue of salt/sodium, because I felt and feel very strongly that many raw fooders were not getting enough of it. This may sound very strange, as mainstream health tells us to avoid salt. The issue of salt is a big one, and among the group there was lots of discussion, dissention, and debate about it. Ultimately, we all agreed to the statement that the optimum diet **contains adequate amounts of unprocessed salts, as needed.** The type and amount of salt are of critical importance.

My history with salt

When I got into health seriously in 1985, I was 100% salt-free for years. I was taught that all salt from all sources was evil, just like I was taught that all supplements and superfoods were evil. According to my gurus, refined, chemicalized, iodized table salt heated at 300–1200 degrees F, and unprocessed sources (like organically grown, whole food, unpasteurized miso with enzymes, probiotics, lifeforce, anti-radiation properties, and anti-cancer activity) were in the same category. My gurus included Natural Hygienists (old school raw foodists), some of whom where Chiropractors and Medical Doctors, and holistically oriented medical doctors. I was given both esoteric and very scientific, educated, and biomedically impressive-sounding reasons why salt was evil, based on their vast research, high intellect, and high degree of education. It all sounded good. Since my experience and knowledge of the body was limited at that time, I followed their program exactly and fervently. Although I followed a virtually salt free diet for years, sometimes I just craved it, and would eat it anyway. Later on, I became mostly a fruitarian, and my cravings for salt got stronger. Many other fruitarians also craved salt. Please note I am NOT a fruitarian now, and I do NOT recommend that anyone ever try to become one! I noticed that other raw fooders craved salt as well but avoided it for the same reasons I did: That is what our convincing gurus told us.

In 1990, I met my life partner, Kim, at the Natural Hygiene raw food convention. We would eat sea vegetables like Dulse and Kelp together. Being a well-trained, focused, and committed raw fooder, I diligently rinsed off every last bit of salt from the sea vegetables. However, I noticed that when she prepared the sea vegetables, she would not rinse the salt off very well at all. When I wasn't around, she would not rinse it at all. She was as hard-core as I was, so why was she not getting rid of this salt? She sensed something I did not yet, that we had been "throwing out the baby with the bathwater" when it came to salt. Eventually, I realized intellectually and experientially that she was right.

In one of the early '90s editions of the book we co-authored called *Uncooking with Jameth and Kim*, we recommended that people use Celtic Sea Salt. To my knowledge, this was the first time that the use of any type of salt was recommended in the raw food world. We were worried how this "against the grain" concept would be received.

Salt in nature

Salt occurs naturally in many foods to varying degrees. Fruits are extremely low or absent in them, vegetables generally are much higher. Celery is noted for its high, naturally occurring sodium content. Some may argue that all the salt we need should and does come from what occurs in natural foods. This is a strong argument, and it is not without merit. They may also point out that animals in nature do not eat salt. Also a good point. However, animals in the wild flock to naturally occurring salt licks. Some prey animals will even lick salt from the same salt licks as their predators, preferring to fulfill their salt cravings and risk possibly getting eaten. I am not talking about domesticated cats and dogs; I am talking about wild animals who have never had any processed foods in their life. Just because wild animals go to great lengths to add extra salt to their diets does not mean we need to, but it is something to consider.

What salt does
Salt/sodium is an absolutely essential mineral in the body. Without it, we would die. In fact, the body will do virtually anything to keep the proper balance of salt in the blood. The kidneys will work very hard to either eliminate excess salt or conserve the salt that the body has. The fact that our blood is salty and tastes salty is of extreme importance, and this will be discussed later on in this chapter.

Without going into a biology lesson that would only serve to confuse and you and try to arrogantly impress you (just like some of my previous gurus did) let's get down to some information you can *actually* use.

Salt and hydration
One of the functions of salt in the body is to hold onto water/fluids. If you have too much salt in your diet, you will hold onto too much fluid (fluid retention). In a way, you will have too much hydration, and your blood pressure may rise. Your kidneys will have to work harder to eliminate this excess sodium. On the flip side, if you do NOT have enough salt in your body, you will not be able to hold onto enough water/fluid. You will be DEhydrated and your blood pressure may get too low. Neither one is good.

You would think that if all you did was drink water, that you would be mega-hydrated. However, the opposite is true. When people water fast, meaning all that they put into their body is water, they become DEhydrated. I repeat. When all you put into your body is water, with nothing else added to it, you become poorly hydrated. What is the deal with that? The more water and no or low salt fluids you consume, the less salt your body has in it. With too much no/low salt fluids ingested, your body's sodium sinks to levels that are NOT physiologically optimum. You do NOT have enough sodium to hold onto the fluids in your body and you become DEhydrated. DEhydration is a significant cause of disease and toxicity, so much so that hydration is dealt with in an entire chapter elsewhere in this book. Also, with low-salt-induced low blood pressure, your circulation is impaired. Impaired circulation means impaired health. There is a way to avoid both toxicities and deficiencies in salt/sodium.

Salt does not equal salt
One of the problems with "salt" is that it is far too wide of a term. If a woman was mean to me once, should I conclude that all women are mean? If a black dog once bit me, should I conclude that all black dogs are bad? Absolutely not. That is another scenario of "all or nothing" or "throwing the baby out with the bathwater". Salt is not salt.

Table salt
Let's talk about regular table salt. *Regular salt is abysmal!* Whether it is mined from the earth or harvested from the ocean, its processing is immense. Regular table salt is the salt version of refined white sucrose sugar – *total garbage!* It is

heated from 300–1200 degrees Fahrenheit, bleached with something that we know can not be good, all other naturally occurring minerals are removed, and potassium iodide and aluminum silicate are added. What is left is a completely denatured, dead, processed, lifeless, bleached, toxic, isolated nutrient! This is similar to isolated vitamin C causing problems (see the Superfood and Supplements chapter), but naturally occurring vitamin C NOT causing problems. And the inorganic iodine that is added to table salt will literally KILL YOU if it is taken in enough quantity. Iodine in the form of whole seaweeds is non-toxic in any quantity. Refined table salt is a toxic isolated, purified, unnatural, drug-like substance with harmful effects on us due to what is left out and the chemicals that are added in.

"Sea salt"
Regular "Sea salt" is virtually the same as table salt, other than it may not be iodized. However, the same temperatures, processes, and chemicals are used to produce it. It is slightly less bad than table salt.

Unrefined sea salt
Unrefined sea salt is completely different than table salt or "sea salt". It is sun dried and 100% unrefined. No chemicals added, no oven drying. Whereas table salt and refined sea salts have 0% minerals, Unrefined sea salt naturally contains 8–16% minerals. Unrefined sea salt has approximately 84 elements contained in it. It is gray, rather than white, and slightly moist. Whereas regular table salt is akin to refined sugar, Unrefined sea salt is akin to whole fruit. Unrefined sea salt is an excellent choice for additional sodium. It may be listed under other names such as "sun dried sea salt". Just make sure it meets the criteria of unrefined sea salt. In the US, Celtic Sea Salt is an excellent brand of unrefined sea salt.

Sea vegetables
Sea vegetables are an awesome place get sodium from if you chose. They come with pure, unrefined sea salt on them. Sea vegetables are also a treasure house of other healing elements, so if you wash the salt off, don't worry, because the sea vegetable itself is so good (see superfood chapter for more info on sea veggies).

Miso
Miso is my sodium source of choice and, in my view, the #1 superfood condiment. Many wonder if miso is a raw food. Miso is teeming with life force, enzymes and active probiotics. You don't get more raw and alive than that. Miso undergoes a culturing process with probiotics that lasts months to years. The salt in miso has been metabolized by the probiotics, so it is really an organic sodium. Miso is so much more than salt. Miso has 35 times more of the cancer-suppressing isoflavone phytonutrient genistein than whole soybeans. This may explain, in part, why miso consumption is associated with lower risks for several cancers. Miso has also been shown to significantly enhance one's ability to withstand radiation and radioactivity (which we are all exposed to, to varying degrees). There are many types of miso, each with a different flavor. I recommend using a miso that is gluten-free (most are, but not barley miso).

Miso is made from soybeans or chickpeas, probiotics, and a grain (usually brown rice). However, miso is a pre-digested form and it is NOT associated with any of problems that soy is. And that is an entirely different issue. I will say here that the problems associated with soy stem NOT from people eating whole soy foods such as miso, tempeh (fermented whole soy), and to a lesser extent soy milk, and tofu, but rather from isolated soy extracts and RAW soybeans. Raw legumes are not good for you (they contain anti-nutrients to protect the sprout from being eaten when growing). After 20+ years into raw foods, I can tell you that they are best sprouted and steamed. Raw chickpea hummus is notorious for gas and gastrointestinal problems. If you have a problem with soy, NO PROBLEM; you can get soy-free chickpea miso and get all of the benefits of miso.

I consider unpasteurized miso to be the #1 superfood condiment. Pasteurized miso maintains many of the benefits, but unpasteurized miso is better. Miso is very salty, so it should not be consumed in the same quantities as spirulina or grasses, for example. However, too little sodium can be a huge problem, and consuming adequate amounts of healthy salt is essential to good health. Miso is also really good tasting! The bottom line is that miso rocks, hard!

Tamari and nama shoyu

Tamari is the world's first soy sauce. It lends an awesome, unique flavor to foods. It was the liquid by-product that rose to the top of miso cask (see miso section). For hundreds of years, this revered liquid was a rare commodity and reserved for special occasions. Eventually, master brewers figured out how to make tamari in greater quantities by culturing it independent of miso. This is how tamari is cultured today. Tamari, like miso, is cultured with its own probiotics and enzymes.

In Japan, where tamari comes from, it is automatically wheat-free. In other parts of the world, tamari sometimes has wheat in it. True tamari is 100% wheat and gluten free and is the best. Tamari is more flavorful than its cousin, nama shoyu, because of its greater content of amino acids. Nama shoyu is a (relatively) recent soy sauce. Nama shoyu is a modern, bastardized version of tamari. Breaking with thousands of years of Asian tradition (as far back as Asian records go), European wheat was added to nama shoyu (wheat was unknown until recently in Asia). During fermentation the wheat produces alcohol, which contributes to much of nama shoyu's flavor.

Nama shoyu (due to its wheat and gluten) has destroyed most prepared raw food cuisine for anyone with celiac, and has adversely affected people with wheat allergies.

Which one is better?
Tamari is superior to nama shoyu for several reasons:
• Tamari uses the time-tested, ancient methods of preparation
• Tamari (true) is wheat and gluten free
• Tamari is more flavorful, with a richer taste and more complex bouquet

Tamari is raw

There has been a gross misconception propagated in the raw foods community that tamari is cooked and nama shoyu is raw. This is NOT true. They are both cultured for up to years and then bottled. The confusion came with the names of the products. Nama shoyu was mistaken for "raw soy sauce" because the words for "raw" in Japanese sound like "namanamashii, "ki", and "mijuku". Tamari does not sound like "raw" in Japanese, thus it was falsely assumed that tamari was *not* raw. This is a case where a nutritionally inferior product (nama shoyu) has been used widely in the raw food community for the sole reason that it was thought to be 'raw', (and therefore *must* be better) even though tamari is clearly healthier. Please remember that health should be about health. Raw is one of the many critical aspects of health but, raw is not *always* better. Back to salt.

With all of its ancient traditions, better, more full-bodied flavor, wheat and gluten-free nature, and being every bit as raw as nama shoyu, there is no reason to NOT replace nama shoyu with wheat-free and gluten-free tamari. Tamari is just better on all counts.

Specific needs for salt

Salt and blood sugar: If you eat too much sugar, raw or not, you will crave more salt to balance your blood sugar. On the reverse, if you eat too much salt, you will crave sugar. To balance blood sugar, I add a pinch of a good, healthy source of salt, like Celtic Sea Salt, to my smoothies and any fruit recipe. Depending on various factors, I will add a little miso or tamari to my water and to my fruit or vegetable juices (especially if they have carrots in them).

Exercise and sweating: This is one of the conditions that I will add extra sodium to my water, juices, or food. Sweat contains lots of salt that needs to be replaced.

Adrenal glands and kidneys: Sufficient salt is required for proper adrenal and kidney functions. There are times of life and situations in life when you need more salt than others. If you do not recognize and address these, you will set up cravings for salt and salty foods. These cravings can include inherently salty (and inherently unhealthy) foods like animal flesh, or foods that have been intentionally salted like fried chips and other junk foods. If the need for a balanced amount of actual unrefined salt is addressed, these toxic cravings can be avoided.

What lack of salt did to me

I have been a vegan for 22 years as of this writing. About 4–5 years ago, I was doing a healing cleanse intensive. I was drinking large amounts of water, large amounts of juice, and was including a healthy amount of diuretic (causes passing of urine) plants like parsley. It was part of an experimental cleanse I was on. I did it for many months. Toward the end of this regimen, I started to crave "steak juice", you know, the salty blood that leaks out of the flesh when you cook it. What the F&%K, I thought to myself! I had been vegan for 17–18 years and had no cravings for meat, ever! What was going on? If I were a "regular" person, who was not committed to nutrition, ethics, and the environment, I would have thought that I "needed" red meat, and would of eaten it! However, I am proud to say that I was, and am, NOT a "regular" person.

who was not committed to nutrition, ethics, and the environment, I would have thought that I "needed" red meat, and would of eaten it! However, I am proud to say that I was, and am, NOT a "regular" person.

In addition to the "steak juice" cravings, I would literally salivate when I opened the fridge and saw the miso and tamari there. One time when I opened the fridge, my cravings were so long and strong and I was tired of salivating at the thought of tamari that I grabbed the bottle of tamari, and just started to drink it down straight! Right from the bottle like it was juice. What an immense relief it was! In my salt-deprived state, it INSTANTLY made me feel so much more energized and alive. And you know what it tasted like? The "steak juice" that I had craved. I never craved steak juice again. After a few rounds of drinking more tamari, and eating miso right out of container, I returned to greater energy, better mind-set, and greater health. I also added back these healthy salts (and Celtic/unrefined sea salt as well) in healthy quantities (I stopped drinking tamari straight).

What I did by limiting my salt so much was to set up cravings for anything that had it (tamari, miso, and blood). That's right, blood! Blood is very salty. Many people go on such low-sodium diets that they set up the same cravings, and many of them continue to, or go back to, hiring someone to kill an animal for them to eat the flesh and blood! I have seen this happen too many times due to the "throw the baby out with the bathwater" approach to salt/sodium.

Correct amount of salt for you!
Different factors such as genetics, blood pressure, blood sugar, how much you sweat, how much you exercise, outside temperature, humidity, how much sugar you eat, how much water and other low sodium fluids you drink, etc. will have an influence on how much salt you need. Salt is vital to good health. Sometimes you may require little or no extra, other times you may require lots extra. Too much of the wrong kind can cause you pain and suffering and contribute to disease. Too little of the right kind (see previous pages) can be just as bad. You can also have too much of the good salts. You are striving for balance. You do not have to be exact if you are using healthy sources. Do the best you can to consume the right amount of the right types of salt for you.

About the Author:
Jameth Sheridan, N.D. is a longtime Vegan, Raw Fooder, Herbalist, and hard-core holistic medicine researcher. He is an outspoken perfectionist on a deeply driven, on-going mission to uncover and spread truth, ethics, and full-spectrum health. He walks his talk and fully embraces as many aspects of a holistic lifestyle as he can, including non-toxic building. Dr. Sheridan is the single most recognized pioneer in bio-compatible nutritional superfoods. He brings a unique blend of scientific, yet vastly open-minded, deeply thorough approach, and an understanding of life force, whole foods, and mother nature to all that he does, with a deep reverence for all life. Dr. Sheridan researches, grows, and provides the highest quality superfoods under his own label, HealthForce Nutritionals, private labels, as well as makes custom formulas for other hard-core companies worldwide. Jameth is one of those unique people who is deeply

caring, compassionate, introspective, and humble, while at the same time he is not afraid to call upon his Warrior spirit to challenge the status quo or go against the grain, if, upon reflection, that is what he truly believes is right. He lives his life as a modern follower of codes of honor such as Bushido and Chivalry.

Dr. Sheridan's websites: www.HealthForce.com   www.RawFoodResearch.com

"The quality, therapeutic concentration, and affordability of a nutritional product can, and often does, mean the difference between lethargy and energy, sickness and health, and, quite literally, life and death. I don't want anyone to be tired, sick or dead because they could not obtain or afford the best possible product. If someone does not feel this same way, they should not be in the nutritional product business. I live and breathe this philosophy in both my personal and professional life and constantly strive to evolve HealthForce products and offer them at the best possible values. I would rather die than compromise these principles" – Jameth Sheridan, N.D.

13

Enlightened Eating with Calorie Prudence

David Rainoshek, MA and Katrina Rainoshek

> "We are living in a world today where lemonade is made from artificial flavors and furniture polish is made from real lemons." – Alfred E Newman

> "Did you ever stop to taste a carrot? Not just eat it, but taste it? You can't taste the beauty and energy of the earth in a Twinkie." - Astrid Alauda

In Westernized societies the disturbing Truth is that our food is lacking in Goodness – both in nutritional content and meal size – and our eating such food is resulting in the fading of Beauty. A July 2008 Johns Hopkins University study published in Obesity projects that by 2030, 86% of Americans (the world's best case study on the Westernization of diet) will be overweight or obese, and according to study author Youfa Wang, MD, PhD, 24% of U.S. children will be overweight or obese by 2015.[1][2] And it is no wonder: from 1970 to 2006, U.S. per capita daily calorie consumption has risen 19.9%, from 2,234 calories per person to 2,679 calories.[3]

Obesity carries with it a multitude of increased risk factors[4]: heart disease, depression, acid reflux, diabetes, dementia, arthritis, cancer, stroke, kidney disease, sexual dysfunction, and sleep disorders. With modern research data and its digital dissemination for all to read, the general debate is over on this one: Overweight is associated with numerous diseases, shortens life, creates direct and associated economic costs at $117 billion per year for 2001 in the U.S.,[5] with Johns Hopkins projections of U.S. $956.9 billion per year by 2030.[6] Mortality rates among the overweight and obese are telling: Ten-year analyses (1995–2005) reported in the New England Journal of Medicine of 527,265 persons aged 50–70 in the U.S. showed that being overweight increases the risk of death by 20 to 40 percent, and by two to three times (or more) in cases of obesity.[7]

Heavy burden – what to do?

We in the *over*fed, nutritionally *unde*nourished countries are headlong into a major global debate about what to do. You have three main views to consider: Business (and the political policies owned and dictated by business); modern medical advice (driven by Big Pharma, which profits from sickness); and most dear – our own internal experience that hears/listens to (read: is socialized by) the first two and that shops for and eats food, often confused and confounded by our bodies.

The shallow, consumer-culture answer promoted by everyone from McDonalds to the Grocery Manufacturers' Association is to *exercise more* – that way you can eat/buy as much as you want (please don't stop shopping) and still lose weight! Forbes Magazine reported that the number of US health club memberships has more than tripled since 1990. Americans over age 55 are the fastest-growing age group among gym members, up more than 266% since 1987 – more than twice the rate for US health club members as a whole.[8] Yet, we are more overweight than ever. So as a social policy, exercise alone is not working terribly well, even if it is a good idea.

Then we are advised by another sector of the consumer culture and many doctors – medical or otherwise – to *diet* (Dr. Atkins, Dr. Phil, The South Beach Diet, *Supercharged*, The Flat Belly Diet, Jenny Craig, Quick Weight Loss, Slim Fast, Diet Coke, etc.) An Amazon.com book search for "diet" yields 288,961 results as part of a US' $48 billion per year industry. On balance, studies show that 90–95% of us are unsuccessful on "diets" and return to our previous inglorious state of health, only to return later to the next diet craze when our heightened dissatisfaction with our current state synergizes profitably with the right marketing glitz.

Why diets don't work

Beyond misleading advertising, false claims, and the one-size-fits-all approach, here are some very simple reasons why these diets do not work for *you*:

SOS: The food of most diets, and the mentality with which you eat it, is not significantly different than what you were eating/experiencing before. This is known as a *translative approach* (as opposed to *transformative*): let's keep feeding you the same basic cuisine you are used to, with some interesting modifications (usually demonizing one of the macronutrients: fat, "carbs", or protein), and not expect you to shift your life in any significant way. Advocates/ purveyors of diets and their recipes use this similarity of taste experience to sell you on the ease of adopting their approach – what they don't tell you is that it is this very thing that makes falling off their plan back into familiar old territory so damned easy.

Caged bird: Dieting – semantically and internally as a practice-experience is limiting, causing lack, and deprivation – which temporarily feels good in an overabundance consumer culture, but that same culture bites you in the ass when the deprivation ceases to be an enjoyable, hopeful respite, *and what ubiquitously you are tempted with is anything but an apple...* and more like an apple-flavor extruded syrup vacuum-packed in a jello mold. The SOS aspect of diets and dieting further teases you – "fat-free" "low-carb" knock-offs of what you used to eat are a constant reminder to you that the authentic taste of former recipes is *just out of reach.*

Little room for development: Most diets stop early on the Spectrum of Diet™, or their center of gravity on the Spectrum is too low, leaving the dieter with nowhere else to go in the realm of dietary possibilities, missing out on the positive results that can be realized at the upper end of the Spectrum.

THE SPECTRUM OF DIET™

FAST FOOD	STANDARD AMERICAN	WHOLE FOODS	COOKED VEGETARIAN	COOKED VEGAN	RAW / LIVE VEGAN	JUICE FASTING TO JUICE FEASTING
EGOCENTRIC	SOCIOCENTRIC			WORLDCENTRIC		
SHALLOW FOODS / EXISTING <--------------------------------------> DEEP FOODS / LIVING						

Figure 5: The Spectrum of Diet™ in Westernized Cultures, David Rainoshek, M.A., www.JuiceFeasting.com

The whole truth? In addition, dietary approaches whose center of gravity are lower than Live Vegan on the Spectrum are partial truths at best, leaving out crucial, scientific realities accessed at the higher levels, which we will discuss in this chapter and throughout *Raw Food Works.* Mark Twain said, "Be careful in reading health books. You may die of a misprint." Well, it is probably not that bad, but this partiality does create knowledge gaps and pathologies at lower levels of the Spectrum. Followers of many diets are left frustrated and wanting, in terms of nutritional benefits and levels of healing, health, and longevity. In the light of lackluster results, the return to former ways of eating seems more inviting.

Short-term, limited focus: Most diets are focused on weight loss over health, results over complete science, and entertainment over long-lasting life practices that will stand the test of time. They are a sit-com, an amusement park, a temporary and passing show in an aspect of your life that is yearning for, and requires, deep authenticity.

To sum up, you are not in a new zone with "dieting" – a new internal geography vis-à-vis food, cuisine, and lifelong physical, mental, and emotional health has not been established. You are playing an old deck sold to you without all the same cards, and many of which are the Jokers. It is the SOS re-packaged (in many cases with fake ingredients), designed by a doctor or dietician (or talk-show host), often with a limited or fundamentally flawed understanding of the Spectrum of Diet™, focused on short-term weight loss (as opposed to longevity and life-transformation). So don't feel bad if you have failed at "dieting" in the past. Just like Thomas Edison and his 9,999 trials before finding the right filament for his lightbulb – you know what does not work, and that in itself is *extremely valuable information*. Let's put our past experiences in a useful context and get down to where it's really at.

Enter calorie restriction

When it comes to weight loss and health, exercise is good, but it doesn't work as a social policy to transform our health challenges (particularly when lacking sound nutritional guidance to go with it). "Dieting" and "fad diets" are (for most of us) short-lived, reaping temporary – then lost – gains, and with good reason. Diets on the lower parts of the Spectrum of Diet™ are also only partial in their level of acknowledgement of the whole of nutritional and physiological truths. We need an approach that takes into account the best aspects and jettisons that which is less than the best; encourages healing; reduces the preconditions for disease; is easily individualized based on numerous personal and environmental factors, and is desirable and enjoyable to maintain over a full lifetime.

Calorie Restriction, or CR as it known among modern professionals, is the clinical application and study of a millennia-old life-extension practice of Dietary Restriction (DR): reducing one's daily calorie consumption while maintaining a complete and healthy nutritional profile. CR has seen a significant amount of scientific research, articles, and books in recent years, with good reason. CR research is producing impressive results, including:

Proven benefits of CR

Extended life span	Lower blood pressure	Lower blood glucose
Lower circulating insulin levels	Reduced inflammation	Reduced body fat
Lower body temperature	Reduced free radical damage	Lower cholesterol
Strengthened immune system	Reduction of brain-destroying antibodies	Reduced heart disease
Reduced loss of brain cells	Improved muscle function	More efficient metabolism

In short, skilled practitioners of CR see a decrease in the underlying causes of many major Western diseases, decreased aging biomarkers, and a more youthful physiology. In this chapter we will investigate:

- The cultural history of Dietary Restriction and human longevity
- The science of Calorie Restriction, including a unifying hypothesis on the function of CR
- Calorie Prudence: the application of CR research as a Life Practice in the postmodern age
- Calorie Prudence and personal development

Let's be clear: this chapter will focus on the history of dietary restriction (predating clinical research), the science of Calorie Restriction, and the individual life-practice of Calorie Prudence in which a personal orientation of *prudence over restriction* is encouraged. With all the failed dieting and under-eating attempts in our Westernized food culture – many of which are coupled with mild to severe eating disorders among persons of every age and gender – being strict, feeling guilt and watering feelings of limitation and self-imposed deprivation won't cut it. Calorie Prudence will, with a nutrient-dense, plant-based raw/living cuisine, encourage a new way of thinking about and accessing the scientifically proven benefits of Calorie Restriction. It honors the cultural heritage of Dietary Restriction, and it does so in a spirit of abundance, joy, depth, and *completeness*.

Goodness – the cultural history of Dietary Restriction

> *"To lengthen thy life, lessen thy meals."*
> *– Benjamin Franklin (1706-1790)*

> *"Hunger is not the cause of death, for death approaches the man who has eaten."*
> *– Rig Veda X. 10.5*

> *"One-quarter of what you eat keeps you alive. The other three-quarters keeps your doctor alive."*
> *– Ancient Egyptian Hieroglyph*

Innate knowledge and successful practice of Dietary Restriction predates humanity itself, as evidenced by the fasting practice of animals in the wild. World-renowned fasting expert Dr. Herbert Shelton wrote about natural fasting occasions in "Fasting Among the Lower Animals,"[9] among them: during the mating season; after birth; when angry or excited; in captivity; when wounded; in disease; during food scarcity; in hibernation among animals, plants, birds, reptiles, and insects. Fasting in these cases is used for adjustment, adaptation, restoration and healing.

Humanity has been accessing the benefits of short- and long-term DR. in the forms of fasting, dietary moderation, seasonal eating, and food shortages for thousands of years. Dr. Gabriel Cousens writes in *Spiritual Nutrition*: *"Fasting... has its history in the spiritual practices of almost all religions. Socrates, Plato, and the Stoic and Neoplatanist philosophers such as Epicteus and Plotinus used fasting to purify the spirit in order to better perceive the Truth. Socrates and Plato practiced ten-day fasts. Pythagorus, the great mathematician, practiced forty-day fasts. Fasting is used in religions such as Judaism, Christianity, Hinduism, Islam, [Taoism], and Buddhism for a variety of different purposes – penitence, propitiation, a preparatory rite for initiations and marriage, mourning, to develop magical powers, purification, health, and spiritual development."*[10]

Scientific data backing DR. was not available until 1915–17, when Osborne and Mendel published their first observations on food restriction and prolonged lifespan in rats in the journal *Science*, followed 20 years later by the more well-known studies by Clive McKay at Cornell University. The positive human experience of various forms of dietary restriction is seen throughout the annals of human history. Accounts of resulting longevity or decreases in mortality rates range from the mythological to more scientifically defensible, and both serve our purposes here.

Mythology
Humanity has been accessing the benefits of short- and long-term DR. in the forms of fasting, dietary moderation, seasonal eating, and food shortages for thousands of years. Individual accounts of longevity and super-longevity have been part of the human story for thousands of years, beginning with the Old Testament account of Methuselah, who was said to have lived nearly a millennium. St. Paul the anchorite has been reported to have lived to be 113 years on only dates and drinking only water. The French Countess Desmond Catherine ate only fruit to the age of 145. Thomas Carn, born in London in 1588, lived to be 207, and a Mr. Jenkins, born in Yorkshire, England, lived [170 years] from 1500 to 1670; both ate no breakfast, had either raw milk or butter with honey and fruit for lunch (Carn may have had bread also), and either *had raw milk or fruit for supper. The French Countess Desmond Catherine, who lived to the age of 145, ate only fruit.*[11]

It might seem odd that a chapter on the benefits of CR would suggest that some of these accounts are *mythological*, but we are trying to establish broad acceptance and practice of Calorie Restriction as scientifically-proven in modern times, including ongoing research this year (2008). As we have seen in religious traditions worldwide, the eye of science has turned many aspects of religion on their heads, and this has radically shifted our views on what we take as literal truth, and what we view as inspirational mythological archetypes. Let's look at what the eye of science has to offer on some of these previous longevity claims.

Longevity claims and the eye of science
Consider the three examples of high-rates of centenarians in the social groups discussed by Dr. Roy Walford in his keynote speech at the 2nd Annual

Conference on Anti-Aging Medicine and Biomedical Technology for the Year 2010: the Vilcabamba of Peru, Azerbaidzhan in Russia, and The Hunza of Pakistan. These accounts have been referred to in many nutritional books in the last few decades of the 20th century, only subsequently to be proven false under further investigation by scientific researchers and academic review.[12] [13] [14] The comprehensive work, *Validation of Exceptional Longevity* collected and presented the work of 23 contributors from Europe and North America with the intention of developing rigorous scientific methods for validating the claims of exceptional human longevity, applying them to historical and contemporary data. We have all been fascinated with the *Guinness Book* records of long life – what the authors demonstrate is that even the most irrefutable cases are highly suspect, such as Pierre Joubert, who appeared in the *Guinness Book* as a 113-year-old man but actually died at age 65, whereas his namesake (his son) died 48 years later. After careful age verification, *the average lifespan of most of the alleged centenarians proved to be 88 years.*[15]

In addition, since the age of modern record-keeping, we have no credible accounts of anyone living longer than record-holder Jeanne Calment, having died in 1997 at the undisputed age of 122. In addition, we know:

- Only approximately seventy people in human history have been documented as reaching the age of 114.
- Only about twenty people reached the age of 115.
- Of the ten people regarded by the *Guinness Book* or significant scholars to have reached 116, three are subject to substantial doubt under academic review.
- Jeanne Calment is the only person with absolutely undisputed evidence to have lived to be more than 120.

Finally, in numbers you will see crunched in the next section on the science of CR, the longest-lived rats in groundbreaking CR research live to a human-equivalent of 105 to 135 years – the record holding mouse of Morris. H. Ross – and these results were achieved in a *controlled* laboratory environment. Thus, the verified, documented accounts of humans living *outside a laboratory* to ages of around 110–116 corresponds well to the equivalent range of longevity seen in calorie-restricted rats. I will leave the scientific validity of the aforementioned super-longevity claims for you to determine, but in the scheme of things, these previous longevity, super-longevity, and high centenarian accounts can serve as an important inspirational backdrop to the significant possibilities that we now have at our disposal with nutritional and health practices unavailable to previous generations.

Recent human evidence of CR and longevity
Right around the time that Osborne and Mendel were publishing their work on calorie restricted rats, the largest-ever study on human dietary restriction was underway in Europe involving three million people, care of food rations during World War I. Denmark was cut off from all food imports and, fearing food shortages, the Danish government appointed Dr. Mikkel Hindhede to coordinate

a rationing program, the results of which he later reported in the *Journal of the American Medical Association*.[16] Dr. Hindhede's plan was to shift the nation's grain from feeding cattle to feeding the three million people of Denmark. The dietary intake became predominantly vegetarian, lower in fat and calories, *resulting in a massive decrease in mortality rates by more than 34% from the average*. John Robbins in *Diet for a New America* cites a corroboration of this WWI Denmark study with WWII data from Norway during the German occupation, with similarly impressive results in reduced mortality:

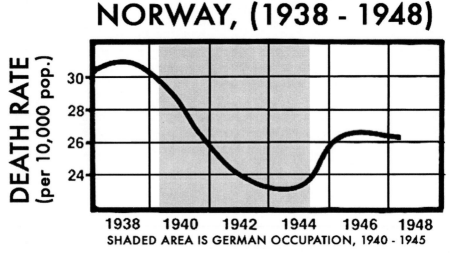

NORWAY, (1938 - 1948)

Figure 2: From the book Diet for a New America. Copyright © 1987 by John Robbins. Reprinted with permission of H J Kramer/New World Library, Novato, CA. www.newworldlibrary.com. Data derived from Mamros, H "The Relation of Nutrition to Health" Acta Medica Scandinavia, Supplement No. 246, 1950

More recently, good news out of the *Journals of Gerontology* in 2008 verified that the claimed prevalence of centenarians in Okinawa, Japan is reliable.[17] So we do have large human group evidence pointing to the possibility of increased longevity via better diet, reduced calories, or both. What does the historical record of scientific CR research have to say about increasing lifespan, and what kind of longevity window are we looking at?

Truth – the science of Calorie Restriction
Calorie Restriction is the *only* scientifically proven method for extending lifespan. Over the last 100 years, CR has consistently slowed aging, improved critical longevity biomarkers, and increased the lifespan of laboratory mice, rats, worms, flies, yeast, spiders, single-celled organisms, guppies, and rhesus monkeys, with results such as:

Life Form	Average Life Span	Calorie Restricted (CR) Life Span
Spiders	50–100 days	90–139 days
Single-celled organisms	7–14 days	13–25 days

| Guppy | 33–54 months | 46–59 months |
| Rat | 23–33 months | 33–54 months |

The roots of Calorie Restriction research go back to 1915–17 with Osborne and Mendel and their study of CR on rats.[18] They surmised that retardation of growth in youth by food restriction might slow down the maturation process and prolong the lifespan of rats. In his article in the journal *Science*, Osborne said, *"it appears as if the preliminary stunting period lengthened the total span of their life."* While early CR and growth stunting was a good first guess as to the function of CR in the body, it and numerous other hypothesis have been proven incorrect or partial. The unifying hypothesis on CR now widely agreed upon in the scientific community is known as *Hormesis*. In this section we will investigate key results in the history of CR research, identify the mechanisms at work, look at the latest human studies with CR, and wrap up with the Hormesis Hypothesis to explain the overall function of CR.

In animal studies, Calorie Restriction refers to several main types of nutritional adjustments to reduce caloric intake, including:

• Caloric restriction of up to 60% of that of the *ad libitum* fed (eating normally) control group
• Intermittent feeding (such as every other day)
• Reducing a major dietary component (e.g. fats)
• Increasing the non-digestible component of the diet with cellulose

As reported in peer-reviewed research, CR has led to incredible physiological results:

Extended life span	Lower blood pressure	Lower blood glucose
Lower circulating insulin levels	Reduced inflammation	Reduced body fat
Lower body temperature	Reduced free radical damage	Lower cholesterol
Strengthened immune system	Reduction of brain-destroying antibodies	Reduced heart disease
Reduced loss of brain cells	Improved muscle function	More efficient metabolism

These results boil down to a slowed aging process and greater chance of longevity. After Osborne and Mendel's findings, models for research on aging were popularized in the mid-1930s by noted nutritionist Clive McKay and his colleagues at Cornell University.[19] In the course of their research on cancer, McKay's team discovered that Calorie Restriction of up to 60% resulted in a doubling of their average lifespan. His longest-lived rats in each of his groups lived to be (in days) 1189, 1297, 1306, 1321, and 1421. Since McKay was primarily interested in cancer, these results were not followed up until the work of Morris H. Ross in the 1960s, also using rats.[20] Ross was mainly interested in the impact of CR on tumor incidence and the age of occurrence in his rats, and in the course of his research his longest-lived rats in each of his four CR groups died at 1287, 1322, 1480, and 1638 days. Let's pause for a moment and look at what these rat ages equate to in *human years*.

According to Anne Hanson, PhD, rats have a brief, accelerated childhood compared to humans, growing rapidly during infancy and reaching sexual maturity at about six weeks of age. Humans, however, develop slowly, not reaching puberty until about age 12–14 years. Rats become sexually mature at six weeks but reach social maturity several months later at about five to six months of age.[21] In adulthood, each rat month is roughly equivalent to 2.5 human years (Ruth, 1935).[22] Female rats enter menopause between months 15 and 18,[23] while humans enter menopause between 48 and 55 years. Based on this knowledge of rat and human development, we can use Dr. Hanson's chart below to calculate rat age to human age:

Rat's age in months	Rat's age in human years
1.5 months (puberty)	12.5 years (puberty)
6 months (social maturity)	18 years (social maturity)
12 months	30 years
18 months	45 years
24 months	60 years
30 months	75 years
36 months	90 years
42 months	105 years
45 months	113 years
48 months	120 years
51 months	128 years
54 months	135 years

Figure 3: Source: "How Old is a Rat in Human Years" by Anne Hanson, PhD (Animal Behavior, UC Davis). Online: http://www.ratbehavior.org/RatYears.htm

McKay's longest-lived rats in were living around 1300–1421 days (42.7 to 46.7 months), and Morris Ross's longest-lived rats on a more calorie-reduced diet were getting out to around 1400–1638 days (46 to 53.9 months), beating McKay's numbers pretty handily. In human years, that means McKay's *oldest* rats were living about 105 to 116 years, and Ross' *oldest* rats were living about 115 to 135 years. Remember, these were controlled laboratory conditions, so our documented, academically verified accounts of the longest-lived persons living to be upwards of 116 (and our anomaly, Jeanne Calment, dying at 122), give us a pretty good target as to the validity of previous claims and the upper limit for human longevity.

Getting closer: Rhesus monkeys
In 1987, the National Institute on Aging began a study of 30% CR in male and female rhesus macaques, aged 1–17 years.[24] To date, the mortality is lower in CR monkeys (15%) than the controls (24%). Notably, the CR group has a lower incidence of chronic diseases, including cancer, cardiovascular disease, diabetes, endometriosis, fibrosis, amyloidosis, ulcers, cataracts, and kidney failure. This is significant, as humans share a 93% common DNA sequence with rhesus monkeys.[25] More importantly, the reduction of these chronic diseases are associated with longevity biomarkers seen in human longevity studies, our next

stop on the CR Tour…

CR in humans: how do we know it works?

Humans live a *little longer* than mice, rats, worms, yeast, drosophila, and even rhesus monkeys, so without a large trial of CR with thousands of humans lasting the next 120 years, how do we know this even works? Enter the beauty of *biomarkers* – empirical measurements that predict survival rates, saving us decades of time in evaluating anti-aging interventions such as CR.

In CR research to date, the following biomarkers have been identified as most notable in animals on a calorie restricted diet:

- Body Temperature: Lower
- DHEAS: Slowed decline of this hormone (serum DHEAS levels decline in aging monkeys and humans. CR slows the rate of decline of DHEAS in CR monkeys)
- Hormones and Maturation: Longer growth/maturation period
- Blood Sugar: Lower
- Plasma Insulin: Lower
- Activity Level: Higher in later age

In a 2002 study[26] conducted by a National Institute on Aging (NIA) team led by G.S. Roth, researchers investigated data from the Baltimore Longitudinal Study of Aging in Male Humans (BLSA) begun in 1958. They considered three factors in relation to age and longevity: low body temperature, low plasma insulin, and higher DHEAS – all factors seen among longer-lived animals in CR studies. The researchers discovered/concluded:

- Significantly longer survival in men with lower body temperatures, lower plasma insulin, and higher DHEAS.
- The environmental or genetic factors that caused CR-like effects on body temperature, plasma insulin, and DHEAS in these men appear to be related to longevity.
- Data suggest that the same mechanisms that control aging in animals are at work in humans; thus modifying these mechanisms through CR may extend lifespan in humans.

The hormesis hypothesis of CR

In 2005, David Sinclair at Harvard University wrote, "Toward a Unified Theory of Caloric Restriction and Longevity Regulation"[27] in which he carefully reviewed the history of CR research to provide a context for a unified theory of CR. According to Sinclair, and corroborated by authors Paul McGlothin and Meredith Averill in their book *The CR Way*, the Hormesis Hypothesis has gained considerable support from a number of labs studying different aspects of CR and lifespan extension, and is now considered a unifying theory on the cutting edge.

Hormesis, put simply, is a beneficial stress. In the case of CR, you challenge your body with this beneficial stress. According to McGlothin and Averill, "With fewer calories available for energy production, your body shifts away from storing fat

155

to actually using fat and protein for energy. Soon your cells reproduce energy more efficiently and your stamina increases. Meanwhile, cell reproduction slows – giving the body time to protect against mutations and preserving cells that may be irreplaceable." This is one of the main reasons CR advocates and Vegan practitioners eat less dairy and see the same reduced cancer rates as societies that eat low/no dairy. Dairy raises the growth factor IGF-1, and as an adult, you don't want any more growth factors than absolutely required.[28] With CR and less fuel (calories), your body does not see any wisdom in accelerated cell replication! As McGlothin and Averill conclude, "The result: Your ability to protect against cancer increases; mutations that lead to cancer are likely to reduce; your body has more time to repair damaged cells and more rapidly kills cells that should be eliminated. In essence, CR greatly reduces the number of cells that are candidates to become cancer."[29]

INCREASED CELL PROLIFERATION/DIVISION MEANS SHORTER LIFESPAN AND HIGHER CHANCE FOR DISEASE

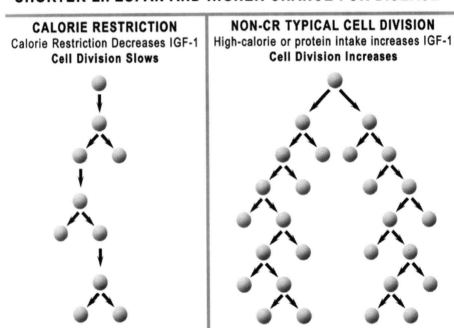

CALORIE RESTRICTION	NON-CR TYPICAL CELL DIVISION
Calorie Restriction Decreases IGF-1	High-calorie or protein intake increases IGF-1
Cell Division Slows	**Cell Division Increases**

Figure 4: Cell Proliferation, CR and Non-CR.

David Sinclair notes that hormesis is a radical departure from earlier hypothesis about CR, because hormesis is based on the premise that the results of CR are due to an *active* defense response of the organism in addition to passive mechanisms, as opposed to the purely passive mechanistic stance of earlier hypotheses that have now been disproved, or integrated into the Hormesis Hypothesis.

Thus, according to Sinclair, the Hormesis Hypothesis of CR is founded upon four main points:

Point 1: CR induces intracellular cell-autonomous signaling pathways that respond to biological stress and low nutrition.
Point 2: The pathways in Point 1 help defend cells and tissues against the causes of aging.
Point 3: The pathways in Point 1 regulate glucose, fat, and protein metabolism in a way that enhances the chance of survival during times of stress.
Point 4: The pathways in Point 1 are under the control of the endocrine system to ensure that the organism acts in a coordinated fashion.

Finally, Sinclair sums up the importance of this cutting-edge hypothesis and its relevance for all forms of animal CR studies vis-à-vis human longevity with CR: *"The contrast between this hypothesis and those that preceded it is stark. If this new theory is right, it means that the effect of CR is to provoke an active, functional response to stress, not simply to passively alter metabolism. It means that the response to CR is an ancient one that evolved to promote the survival of organisms during adversity. Being an ancient adaptive response, it also means that discoveries in simple organisms such as yeast, worms, and flies are likely to be more relevant to mammals than many had previously thought."*[30]

Calorie restriction in mid-life
Three critical pieces of research have thankfully proven that CR is effective when begun in our mid-to-later years. So if you were thinking it was too late for you or your loved one, think again. It is *never* too late to do something good.

Middle-aged mice: The first evidence of the efficacy of mid-life CR came in the 1970s from Drs Roy Walford and Richard Weindruch at UCLA Medical Center, who showed that even gradual restriction of caloric intake in middle-aged mice could extend average lifespan up to 60%."[31]

Drosophila: In research that could definitely claim the prize for Most Hilarious Title, the team of Mair, Goymer, Pletcher, and Partridge wrote, "Demography of Dietary Restriction and Death in Drosophila", hypothesizing that CR begun *at any stage of life* can reduce the mortality rate to that of animals on CR for their entire life. Two days after starting CR, and at various ages, fully-fed flies were no more likely to die than flies of the same age who had been doing CR their whole lives.

Stephen R Spindler Research: In 2001 Dr. Stephen Spindler, professor of biochemistry at the University of California-Riverside, underfed rats by 40%, and within a month they had a 400% increase in the expression of anti-aging genes, and a notable increase in the anti-inflammation, antioxidant, and anti-cancer genes. Spindler studied the expression of 11,000 genes in the livers of young normally-fed and calorie-restricted mice, and found that *60% of the age-related changes in gene expression with CR mice occurred within a few weeks after they started the CR diet.* In summary, Spindler's results, published in the *Proceedings of the National Academy of Sciences*, showed:

- No matter what age you are, you still get an anti-aging effect with calorie restriction
- Anti-aging effects can happen quickly on a low-calorie diet
- Caloric restriction of only four weeks in mice seems to partially restore the liver's ability for metabolizing drugs and for detoxification
- Caloric restriction seems to quickly decrease the amount of inflammation and stress even in older animals.[32]

Bottom line

I can hear a lot of young people rejoicing at the animal research showing that late-life CR practice is as effective as life-long CR practice. "So I can wait and start CR when I am in my 60s or 70s and chow on pizza until then?" Not exactly. We in Westernized nations are seeing aging/disease biomarkers among children, and increasing in severity as we age. Many Western diseases that kill us begin to surface in our 40s, 50s, and 60s. As a result, half of all Americans are on pharmaceuticals for just the things that are taken care of by CR: lower blood pressure, lower blood glucose, reduced inflammation (pain), lower cholesterol, etc. The wisdom is that health is what we consistently do, and beautiful, radiant health is an art best practiced in the present moment.

Beauty – the personal and artful practice of Calorie Prudence

We have now discussed the historical practice of Dietary Restriction and its scientific study as Calorie Restriction. Now let us look at the life practice of Calorie Prudence in your own experience, which is simple to appreciate in terms of the Spectrum of Diet™ (Figure 1).

For those of us in Westernized nations who have had access to the entire range of food, the Spectrum is actually a *stages progression* that involves mental, physical, and emotional changes and development as we move up the Spectrum toward raw/live vegan. As we shift toward an organic, live-food diet, we also shift from low-nutrient- to high-nutrient-density foods; from the creation of symptoms and disease to their transformation; dead food to vibrant, living food; and below-average to above-average lifespan.

Goals of CR

Some notable advocates who understand and apply the scope of CR research and practice are The Calorie Restriction Society, and Paul McGlothin and Meredith Averill of *The CR Way*. According to their current knowledge and practice, the stated goals of CR covering nutrition, diet, biochemistry, and personal practice are:

Food goals:

- Low, adequate calories
- Nutrient dense (high phytochemicals, vitamins, and minerals per calorie of food)
- High-fiber
- High Satiety Index (SI)
- Low Glycemic Index (GI) and low Glycemic Load (GL)

- Low-moderate protein intake levels
- Appropriate for the glycemically challenged, such as diabetics and pre-diabetics (one-third of U.S. population)
- Reduced cooking, emphasis on steaming/blanching

Body goals:
- Low blood glucose levels, including Fasting Blood Sugar (FBS) between 70–90
- Good glucose control (stable blood sugar)
- Low insulin levels
- Reduced inflammation
- Low growth factors such as IGF-1
- Hormesis
- Rejuvenation of brain cells
- Cancer protection

Personal practice goals:
- Meals eaten consciously, mindfully, and not in haste
- Awareness of when to stop eating, including the use of intuition
- Larger meal eaten earlier in the day
- Meals planned ahead of time
- Extended hours away from meals (dinner through breakfast)

When you read *The CR Way*, what you will find are fairly well-balanced, predominantly *cooked* vegan menus out there, with consciously chosen menu ingredients that truly take one a long, long way to meeting the goals listed above. Their suggestions for finishing your last meal early in the day, periodic fasting, and eating mindfully are excellent. In addition, they have nailed it on the personal practice goals one should have if wanting to achieve increased longevity on a plant-based CR diet. That being said, where the conventional CR approach is lacking is not in its understanding of the actual science of CR, but in the nutritional science culinary knowledge that goes with it, which is necessary to access the highest potential results of CR. We need a dietary approach that meets the science and goals of CR, while helping us to "dial down" caloric intake to appropriate/prudent levels *intuitively*. Cooked food – even cooked vegan food often involves realities that can contribute to overeating, such as:

Protein: denatured
Fats: destruction of omega-3 fats (read: rancid and *trans* fats)
Carbohydrates: increased glycemic index
Water: cooked out of food
Food Enzymes: partial or complete loss
Probiotics: partial or complete loss of biological activity
Excitotoxins: MSG, aspartame, artificial colors, conventional salt
Loss of phytonutrients
Creation of Advanced Glycation End Products (AGEs)

These potentially CR-negative qualities of cooked plant-based and animal-based foods have been extensively documented in *12 Steps to Raw Foods* by Victoria Boutenko; *Conscious Eating* and *There is a Cure for Diabetes* by Dr. Gabriel Cousens, MD; *Breaking the Food Seduction* by Neal Barnard, MD; *The Sunfood Diet Success* System by David Wolfe; and *Excitotoxins: The Taste that Kills* by Russell Blaylock, MD.

Calorie Prudence – Live

Why a raw/live food diet is so successful is that it turns on anti-aging and anti-inflammatory genes. This is because a live-food diet is a natural form of CR. When you cook your food, according to the Max Planck Institute, you coagulate 50% of your protein, 70–90% of your vitamins and minerals, and up to 100% of your phytonutrients. One of the phytonutrients, for example, called *resveratrol*, plays a very important role in activating the anti-aging genes. It is gaining growing recognition in fighting age-related diseases ranging from dementia to diabetes. At the raw-live stage of the Spectrum of Diet™, when properly accessed we actually eat up to 50% fewer calories compared to an eater at the fast food and SAD stages of the Spectrum, while maintaining a very high level of nutrition and health. The reason for this is that we are consuming *nutrient-dense foods*, not just calorie-dense foods. We are becoming nations of overfed, undernourished individuals.

When we say Calorie Prudence from a plant-source-only, live, organic diet, it should not be misunderstood that we are denying ourselves the fuel we need. Nor are we in a cycle of deprivation. Calorie Prudence will be best accepted and practiced long-term in a balanced way with a proper mental, emotional, and spiritual orientation. CR and fasting advocates are quick (and correct) to note that CR done appropriately is not a regimen of self-destructiveness or denial, as seen in anorexia or other unhealthy examples of under-eating in which a *dissociation* with the body is in play. That being said, we must look even beyond the most obvious of eating disorders in postmodern culture to the largely unperceived dissociation with the body, as evidenced by our center of gravity still falling squarely on the Fast Food and SAD stages of the Spectrum. Moving up the Spectrum of Diet™ is a sound way to resolve our dissociation and reclaim our connection with our bodies.

More calorie counting?

We are talking about long-term Calorie Prudence here, so one way you will be able to tell if you are calorie prudent is your weight. The easiest way to calculate your target weight range is to give yourself 100 pounds for the first five feet of height, and five pounds for each additional inch over five feet. For example a person 5'7" has a target range of around 135 lbs.

The window you want to stay in to know you are being Calorie Prudent long-term is at your target weight and down 3–5% from it. In our example of someone 5'7", the long-term CP weight range is going to be 128.25 to 135 lbs. The reason I am giving you this measure as opposed to calorie-counting is that we can (and probably have on former "diets") drive ourselves nuts counting calories to achieve a result. The benefits of Raw/Live and Calorie Prudence should ultimately be a result of eating and living well, and with the huge community of creative and knowledgeable people and available resources in Vegan 2.0 and Vegan 3.0 (see chapter 1, "Vegan 2.0: Everyone@Plant-Based") that we now have access to, this is too much fun to pass up. That being said, there are some other things that can help you move towards your target weight range, and help you maintain your health and weight:

Eating a low-glycemic index, plant-based Raw/Live Diet, with 10–30% total fat calorie intake max. For eating lower on the glycemic index, check out Dr. Gabriel Cousens' food phases chart in *Rainbow Green Live Food Cuisine*, the work of Brian Clement of Hippocrates Health Institute, and *The Four Means to Get Your Greens* approach by David Rainoshek, MA, which includes Victoria Boutenko's green smoothies as discussed in her book, *Green for Life*. When it comes to percentage of calories from fat, you have two main issues here: One, we tend to eat an excessive amount of fat *no matter what stage on the Spectrum we are at*. Two, there is an ongoing discussion in Live/Raw community, including professional advocates, on what an appropriate amount of fat is. The general window in the debate ranges from 10–30% total calories from fat. In short, move towards 10–20% total calories from fat, and choose your fat sources well. This is not the chapter to find complete guidance on this one: read the rest of the book!

Final words: development
I hope that the hard-core realities of human longevity, and the possibilities of excellent health and more years to live with Calorie Prudence and Raw/Live Foods, can act as a clarion call for us to get off of our duff. Mythologist Joseph Campbell wrote in *The Hero With a Thousand Faces*, *"The modern hero, the modern individual who dares to heed the call and seek the mansion of that presence with whom it is our whole destiny to be atoned, cannot – indeed must not – wait for his community to cast off its slough of pride, fear, rationalized avarice, and sanctified misunderstanding. 'Live,' Nietzsche says, 'as though the day were here.'* **It is not society that is to guide and save the creative hero, but precisely the reverse."**

About the Author:
David Rainoshek, MA *in Vegan/Live Food Nutrition is the co-creator of JuiceFeasting.com with his wife,* ***Katrina Rainoshek.*** *He is a Juice Feasting coach, author, lecturer, and has Juice fasted/Feasted for over 450 days, up to 92 days at a time. David served as Research Assistant to Dr Gabriel Cousens for There is a Cure for Diabetes, and is now authoring several books for release in 2008, including:* ***Juice Feasting: An Integral Hero's Guide, The Four Means to Get Your Greens*** *and finally, with Katrina, a series of children's books beginning with* ***Julia and the Nut Mylk Tree.*** *David and Katrina coach 92-Day Juice Feasts for clients and retreats worldwide including the yearly Global Juice Feast, a world-wide cleanse for 92 Days on www.GlobalJuiceFeast.com. David and Katrina teach about Juice Feasting and nutrition education to the world through their 92-Day Program on www.JuiceFeasting.com. David served as leading Research Assistant to Gabriel Cousens, M.D., as head juice fasting coach, and taught the*

10-week nutrition education classes to kitchen and garden apprentices at the Tree of Life Rejuvenation Center in Patagonia, Arizona in 2006-07. He has taught over 100 raw food preparation classes to children and adults.

David and Katrina are self-described as a Dietary Activists and proponents of Nutrient Density and Health Freedom for all. "Availability is not enough. For Live Food Nutrition to be the truly transformative and integral movement of our times, it must be made accessible to everyone." David and Katrina drive a Ford F-350 on Straight Vegetable Oil reclaimed from Asian restaurants, have covered over 70,000 miles to-date, and currently reside in British Columbia, Canada.

RESOURCES

Spiritual Nutrition by Dr. Gabriel Cousens, MD. Chapter 22, "Undereat!"
Rainbow Green Live-Food Cuisine by Dr. Gabriel Cousens, MD. Chapter 5, "Health Secrets of Live Foods"
The CR Way by Paul McGlothin and Meredith Averill, www.livingthecrway.com
The Longevity Diet by Brian M. Delaney and Lisa Walford
The Anti-Aging Plan by Roy Walford, MD and Lisa Walford
The Calorie Restriction Society, www.CalorieRestriction.org

(Endnotes)
1   "Obesity Rates Continue to Climb in the United States." Johns Hopkins Bloomberg School of Public Health Public Health News Center, July 10, 2007. Online: http://www.jhsph.edu/publichealthnews/press_releases/2007/wang_adult_obesity.html
2   Youfa Wang, May A. Beydoun, Lan Liang, Benjamin Caballero and Shiriki K. Kumanyika. "Will All Americans Become Overweight or Obese? Estimating the Progression and Cost of the US Obesity Epidemic." *Obesity*, Advance online publication, July 24, 2008 DOI: doi:10.1038/oby.2008.351
3   United States Department of Agriculture (USDA) Economic Research Service. "Loss-Adjusted Food Availability." Online: http://www.ers.usda.gov/Data/FoodConsumption/FoodGuideDoc.htm
4   Haslam DW, James WP (2005). "Obesity". Lancet 366 (9492): 1197–209.
5   Wolf AM, Manson JE, Colditz GA. The Economic Impact of Overweight, Obesity and Weight Loss. In: Eckel R, ed. Obesity: Mechanisms and Clinical Management. Lippincott, Williams and Wilkins; 2002.
6   Youfa Wang, May A. Beydoun, Lan Liang, Benjamin Caballero and Shiriki K. Kumanyika. "Will All Americans Become Overweight or Obese? Estimating the Progression and Cost of the US Obesity Epidemic." *Obesity*, Advance online publication, July 24, 2008 DOI: doi:10.1038/oby.2008.351
7   Adams KF, Schatzkin A, Harris TB, et al. "Overweight, obesity, and mortality in a large prospective cohort of persons 50 to 71 years old." N Engl J Med. 2006 Aug 24;355(8):758-60.
8   International Health, Racquet & Sportsclub Association (IHRSA). Online: www.ihrsa.org
9   Shelton, Herbert. *The Hygenic System, Volume III: Fasting and Sunbathing*, "Chapter 2: Fasting Among the Lower Animals." San Antonio: 1950.
10   Cousens, Gabriel. *Spiritual Nutrition*. North Atlantic Books, Berkeley: 2005. Pg 337-38.
11   Cousens, Gabriel MD. *Spiritual Nutrition*. North Atlantic Books, Berkeley: 2005. Pg 330.
12   Leonard Hayflick, *How and Why we Age*. Ballantine Books, New York: 1994. Pg 196-203
13   James F. Fries and Lawrence M. Crapo. *Vitality and Aging: Implications of the Rectangular Curve*. W. H. Freeman and Company, San Francisco: 1981. Pg 11-23.
14   Alex Comfort, *The Biology of Senescence*, 3rd Ed. Elsevier North Holland, Inc., New York: 1979. Pg 81-86
15   Jeune, Bernard and Vaupel, James W. *Validation of Exceptional Longevity*. Odense University Press, Odense: 1999.
16   Hindhede, M. "The Effect of Food Restrictions During War on Mortality in Copenhagen." *Journal of the American Medical Association*, 74 (6):381, 1920.

17	D. Craig Willcox, Bradley J. Willcox, Qimei He, Nien-chiang Wang and Makoto Suzuki. "They Really Are That Old: A Validation Study of Centenarian Prevalence in Okinawa" *The Journals of Gerontology Series A: Biological Sciences and Medical Sciences* 63:338-349 (2008)

18	Osborne TB, Mendel LB, Ferry EL. The effect of retardation of growth upon the breeding period and duration of life in rats. *Science*. 1917;45:294-295.

19	McKay, CM, Crowell MF, and Maynard LA. (1935). "The effect of retarded growth upon the length of life and upon the ultimate body size." *J Nutr. 10*, 63-79.

20	Ross MH. (1961). "Length of life and nutrition in the rat." *J. Nutr. 75*, 197-210.

21	Adams, N. and R. Boice. 1983. "A longitudinal study of dominance in an outdoor colony of domestic rats." *J. Comp. Psychol.* 97(1): 24-33.

22	Ruth, E. B. 1935. Metamorphosis of the pubic symphysis. I. The white rat (Mus norvegicus albinus). *Anat. Rec.* 64: 1-7.

23	Durbin, P. W., M. H. Williams, N. Jeung, J. S. Arnold. 1966. "Development of spontaneous mammary tumors over the life-span of the female Charles River (Sprague Dawley) rat: the influence of ovariectomy, thyroidectomy, and adrenalectomy-ovareictomy." *Cancer Res.* 26(3): 400-411.

24	Mattison, J.A., Lane, M.A., Roth, G.S., Ingram, D.K. Calorie restriction in rhesus monkeys. Experimental Gerontology 38:35-46, 2002.

25	Choi, Charles. *Live Science*. "Monkey DNA points to common human ancestor." Online: www.livescience.com/health/070412_rhesus_monkeys.html

26	G. S. Roth, M. A. Lane, D. K. Ingram, J. A. Mattison, D. Elahi, J. D. Tobin, D. Muller, E. J. Metter, Biomarkers of caloric restriction may predict longevity in humans. Science 297, 811 (2002).

27	Sinclair DA. "Toward a unified theory of caloric restriction and longevity regulation." *Mechanisms of Aging and Development*. 2005 Sep;126(9):987-1002. PMID: 15893363

28	McGlothin, Paul and Averill, Meredith. *The CR Way*. Collins, New York: 2008. Pg 6.

29	Ibid. pg 110.

30	Sinclair DA. "Toward a unified theory of caloric restriction and longevity regulation." *Mechanisms of Aging and Development*. 2005 Sep;126(9):987-1002. PMID: 15893363

31	Cousens, Gabriel. *Spiritual Nutrition*. North Atlantic Books, Berkeley: 2005. Pg 332.

32	Cao, S X, Dhahbi, J M, Mote, P L, and Spindler, S R. "Genomic profiling of short- and long-term caloric restriction effects in the liver of aging mice." *Proc Natl Academy of Sciences*, 98(19):10630–10635. Cited in: Fahy, G, and Kent, S. "Reversing Aging Rapidly with Short-Term Calorie Restriction." *Life Extension*, May 2001.

14

Detoxification and the Healing Process

Brenda Cobb

When I was diagnosed with breast and cervical cancer in 1999 I had no idea just how toxic I was. My doctors said I must have surgery, chemotherapy, and radiation to rid my body of the cancer. I refused those treatments because my own family members who had the same types of cancers tried the surgery and drugs, but either the drug therapy killed them right off or their cancers came back with a vengeance. I did not want to go down that dead-end path.

I set out to find a natural way to help my body heal itself. When I discovered the living and raw-foods lifestyle it just felt like the perfect path for me. In six months the cancer was gone, and so were the symptoms of allergies, arthritis, migraine headaches, fatigue, psoriasis, acid reflux, indigestion, and heartburn. My gray hair even turned back and my eyesight improved. It was a miracle.

As a result of my own healing and transformation, I began teaching others how to heal naturally with raw and living foods. I believe that it is more than the organic raw and living foods that are so important in the healing process: the detoxification of the body, mind, and emotions is just as, if not more, important than the foods. Thousands of people have come to my raw and living foods center with symptoms, illnesses, imbalances, and diseases such as cancer, diabetes, heart disease, depression, multiple sclerosis, lupus, candidiasis, chronic fatigue syndrome, constipation, fibroids, endometriosis, colitis, irritable bowel syndrome, headaches, hypertension, parasitic infections, AIDS, HIV, and a host of other conditions. What I have seen is that if a person will change lifestyle habits, eat organic raw and living foods, and detoxify the body, mind, and emotions, the body can and will heal itself. It is very inspirational to see people completely heal even when mainstream medicine has pronounced them hopeless, terminal, and incurable. There is always the opportunity to heal, if a person is willing to do what it takes.

A toxic world

Today's population is so toxic, and the general health has declined so severely, that people are now sicker than ever. In America we spend more money on health care than any other nation, and yet we are on the bottom of the heap when it comes to good health. Even our brainpower has diminished because of these toxicities. This has nothing to do with not having enough to eat. The quantity of food is there, but the nutrition is gone. People are overeating themselves into toxicity and deficiency. As we become fatter we become weaker. More toxins are stored in fat than in any other part of the body.

We live in a toxic world with chemicals and pollutants manifesting themselves in a variety of symptoms and diseases. Immune and hormonal dysfunction, neurotoxicity, psychological disturbances, cancer, and many other well-known diseases are created in part from toxicity. Industrial and petrochemical toxins continue to accumulate in the human body faster than they can be eliminated. Most people have a lethal mixture of chemicals, pesticides, food additives, heavy metals, anesthetics, pharmaceutical drugs, legal drugs (alcohol, tobacco and caffeine), and illegal drugs (heroin, cocaine, and marijuana) clogging up the body. With the combination of these toxins it is no wonder we are facing more diseases and illnesses than we have ever known before.

We are much more exposed to chemicals than any previous generation. Smog is in virtually every city, and most drinking water contains more than 700 different chemicals and excessive levels of lead, mercury, fluoride, and chlorine. More than 3000 chemicals are added to food, and more than 10,000 chemical solvents, emulsifiers, and preservatives are used in food processing and storage. These toxins remain in the body for years and cause serious damage.

Labels on food are deceiving, because they do not always list every ingredient. Things we cannot even imagine are lurking in our food. We don't realize how toxic food has become. We are ingesting chemicals, pesticides, hormones, and antibiotics by the buckets. Gasoline, paint, household cleansers, cosmetics, pesticides, and dry cleaning fluid pose a serious threat to human health. The body cannot easily break down these pollutant toxins, and the effect is devastating on the kidneys, liver, pancreas, heart, lungs, and other organs and glands.

The human body has not been able to adapt to the fast ecological changes in the environment, and so as the Earth has become more polluted, so has the average person. The body is a filter that "traps" these pollutants and eventually becomes so overloaded with toxins that it manifests devastating diseases. The quality of life of most people has been greatly diminished because of the high level of toxicity that leads to fatigue, headaches, aches and pains, and serious health problems.

If you have a healthy immune system with efficient organs of elimination and detoxification and a sound circulatory and nervous system, you can handle a great deal of toxicity. But if your body has been damaged from chronic exposure to environmental pollutants and is deficient from the lack of real nutrients, then the normal bodily functions are impaired and disease sets in. Excess cooked foods, animal proteins, fats, caffeine, alcohol, sugar, and chemicals inhibit the optimum function of the cells and tissues of the human body. We must cleanse these toxins and waste products out of the body to restore optimum function and vitality. Health cannot be restored to a toxic body. Remove the toxicity and the body will heal itself.

Just changing your diet to eliminate food that you know is not good for you is not enough to restore health. You must also get the toxins out of the body and focus on rebuilding the organs and glands with good nutrition. When a body is toxic it is also acidic, and an acidic body creates disease. Alkalinity must be restored if the body is to heal. Cooked food is acidic. Raw vegetables, fruits, and living sprouted foods are alkaline. Negative thoughts are acidic. Positive thoughts are alkaline. While detoxing the body you are also restoring the alkalinity, and this will help to bring about good health.

Benefits to health

Periodically undertaking some form of detoxification is extremely important. You can clear waste products and dead cells from your body with a good detoxification process. You can revitalize your body's natural functions and healing capacities by detoxifying the body and building it back up with nourishing real food. The body was created by God to heal itself. It can restore health from even the most devastating diseases if it is given what is needed to detoxify and heal.

Some of the benefits of detoxifications are that you will have more energy, greater mental clarity, improved eyesight and hearing, reduction of stress on the immune system, increased vitality, reduced blood pressure and blood fats (cholesterol and triglycerides), and a sense of well-being from the inside out. It is important to detoxify for maintenance of normal bowel function, integrity of the intestinal flora, to enhance the natural ability of the body to resist infections, lower and eliminate allergies, and clear up skin disorders. If you want to reduce and eliminate symptoms and diseases, to feel mentally and physically rejuvenated and energized, then you must detoxify.

How do you know if you need to detoxify? When you feel fatigue, confusion, aggression, mental disorders, and low energy, it's time to detoxify. When you experience headaches, allergy symptoms, joint pain, respiratory problems, back pain, food allergies, insomnia, mood changes, arthritis, constipation, hemorrhoids, sinus congestion, ulcers, psoriasis, and acne, it's time to detoxify. When you are diagnosed with any disease or illness you must detoxify.

You can detoxify your body with a raw and living food diet, colon cleansing and emotional healing. Eating nourishing, cleansing foods is very important, but it is just as important to detoxify the mind and the emotions as it is to detoxify the blood, lymphatic system, and every cell. Negative thinking and emotions buried deep inside create toxicity in the organs that can lead to serious diseases. A toxic mind can create a toxic body. A good detoxification program includes the body, mind, and spirit, and only when you address each of these areas can you truly heal.

Diseases such as diabetes can be virtually eliminated by detoxing the body and adopting a living and raw-food healthy lifestyle that includes good eating and exercise habits. People usually tend to turn to drugs to treat a disease such as diabetes, but drugs do nothing more than add to the toxicity and create more problems. Other diseases such as cancer, arthritis, and heart disease can be improved and eliminated by detoxing and rebuilding the body.

How to cleanse your body
The easiest and most inexpensive and effective methods of detoxification include fasting programs and eating specific raw and living foods. These methods require little cost other than to eat healthy organic food and drink filtered water. When a person begins to detoxify by eating foods like organic greens, vegetables, herbs, and living sprouts, the body will release toxins quickly.

Detoxification remedies in pills, powders, and liquids are not the answer. A true detoxification must be done with real whole foods and fresh juice fasting. The remedies sold in bottles can be very harsh to the body and only get out the surface layer of toxins. Colonics and enemas help tremendously with the detoxification process and with symptoms including headaches, nausea, aches, pains, brain fog, cloudy vision, distorted hearing, stomach pains, diarrhea, insomnia, and depression. It is the toxins in the blood and colon that are creating these symptoms. When you clean out your colon, you will see how these symptoms "magically" disappear.

Sometimes people resist colon cleansing because they are embarrassed, or think it is disgusting. A dirty, impacted colon is one of the main contributors to poor health. We must become more comfortable with cleaning the inside of the body. It is even more important than cleaning the outside. You wouldn't go for years without brushing your teeth, washing your hair, or taking a bath. These are things that most people do every day, but those same people rarely if ever clean out the inside of the body, and this is where disease begins.

It is very important to add pro-biotics back into the body when you do systematic colon cleansing. Enemas and colonics clean out the bad impacted waste but can also clean out the good bacteria. The good bacteria are absolutely necessary to bringing the body back to good health. Fermented foods such as cabbage sauerkraut are full of the beneficial bacteria every person needs. A complete pro-biotic complex, including soil organisms, is necessary to help restore good colon health.

Fasting

Fasting can be very beneficial for detoxification, but most people are too toxic to begin cleansing with a water fast first. This process releases toxins quickly and can be too much for a person with a weakened immune system. I do not recommend that persons who are very sick go on a water-fasting regime unless they are monitored by a doctor or health professional who understands the fasting process and how to help a person through it safely.

However, fasting can be very helpful to healing, and there is really no disease that cannot be healed through fasting and prayer. Many times fasting can leave a person nutritionally depleted and weak. This is why I recommend beginning your detoxification process with green juices and organic raw and living foods such as dark green leafy vegetables blended into cleansing and nourishing smoothies. The blending breaks down the food into the smallest particles possible so they are much easier to digest. Drinking and implanting wheatgrass juice in the colon is also a vital part of any good detoxification plan.

Powerful detoxifiers

There are several detoxifying foods that are very powerful to clean out the body and rebuild it. Kale, collards, mustard greens, and dandelion are some of the most cleansing greens in nature. These dark greens are valuable as an internal body cleanser, and they stimulate the liver and other tissues out of stagnancy. Because of their high water content, these greens are a good cleansing food and useful in ridding the system of poisonous substances.

Asparagus has a substance called asparagine, which is nature's most effective kidney diuretic. It breaks up oxalic and uric acid crystals in the kidneys and muscles and eliminates them through the urine. Asparagus also contains substantial amounts of aspartic acid, an amino acid that neutralizes the excess amounts of ammonia that linger in the body and make us tired. Its high water content and roughage encourage evacuation of the bowels by increasing fecal bulk with undigested fiber.

Celery is a natural diuretic and contains compounds known as coumarins, which appear to be useful in cancer prevention. Celery is very alkaline. It counteracts acidosis, halts digestive fermentation of foods, purifies the bloodstream, aids digestion, and can help clear up skin problems. Celery's rich organic sodium content dislodges calcium deposits from joints and holds them in solution until they can be eliminated through the kidneys.

Beets are one of nature's best bodily cleansers, as they help dissolve and eliminate acid crystals from the kidneys, eliminate blood toxemia (which causes varicose veins), detoxify the liver and gallbladder, and eliminate pockets of acid material in the bowel.

Raw cabbage, both red and green, detoxifies the stomach and upper bowels of putrefactive wastes, thereby improving digestive efficiency and facilitating rapid elimination. It also works to alkalinize the body, stimulate the immune system, kill harmful bacteria and viruses, soothe and heal ulcers, help prevent cancer and clear up the complexion. Raw, saltless cabbage sauerkraut is excellent for cleansing and rejuvenating the digestive tract and promoting better nutrient absorption as well as the growth of healthful (acidophilus) intestinal flora.

Raw sweet potatoes and yams are beneficial for detoxifying the system, because they contain substances called phytochelatins that can bind heavy metals such as cadmium, copper, mercury, and lead, and thus participate in metal detoxification of body tissues.

Wheatgrass juice is extremely cleansing and has almost all vitamins and minerals known to man. It is pure, cleansing chlorophyll, which is a powerhouse when it comes to cleaning out the body and nourishing it at the same time. Wheatgrass truly is a medicine for the body.

Fresh air, deep breathing, and yoga also help detoxify the body. Sunshine is very helpful, especially during the detoxification process. Most people are full of candida, and sunshine is absolutely necessary to help rid the body of this parasitic yeast. Expose the entire body (no clothes if possible) to sun at least 30 minutes each day. Get out in the sun before 11:00 am or after 3:00 pm and feel the warming and healing rays.

While nourishing your body with good nutritional support it is extremely important to think positive uplifting thoughts and give thanks for the opportunity to detoxify your body. Rather than dreading the process, embrace it! It is a sacred and spiritual experience and is nothing to be feared. Learning about your body and what to do to help yourself will boost your confidence. Do not allow fear to hold you back. Fear is a toxin to the body, and it settles in the kidneys, which, in turn, cannot properly detoxify the blood. The emotions and thoughts are as important as the food, water, and sunlight.

Drink a lot of water during the detoxing regime. Most people don't drink enough water on a regular basis, and many diseases are made worse because of dehydration. Drinking purified water will help flush out the toxins quickly.

Emotional healing
All of these things are extremely important in helping the body detoxify, but one of the most important parts of restoring health is the healing of emotional issues that contribute to the creation of disease. There are emotional reasons for every illness. In all of the people I have helped to overcome tremendous health challenges, I have discovered that just changing the diet and cleansing the body is not enough to create a true and complete healing. A person must address the emotional issues that have contributed to the development of the disease and heal these emotions to restore complete health.

This is probably the most challenging part of healing for most people. Many of us have buried our emotional stuff so deep that sometimes we don't even realize what is truly at the root of our issues. We stuff our feelings deep inside because they are too painful for us to face. Not until we face these emotional issues and do the work to heal our feelings and forgive ourselves and others can we achieve the healing we desire.

I have found Bach flower essences and essential oils to be of a tremendous help in the healing of emotional issues. The flower essences and essential oils have a high healing vibration. Oils like frankincense, myrrh, and helichrysum are just a few of the most powerful oils for healing the emotional and physical self. Disease cannot live in a body with a high vibration.

It takes many things to bring about a complete healing, and detoxification is just one very important part of the journey. Start where you are right now. Your journey to better health can be an exciting experience. Give yourself the gift of detoxification and cleansing and see how great you can feel. It is one of the best gifts you could ever give yourself.

About the Author:

Brenda Cobb *founded the Living Foods Institute in Atlanta, Georgia in September 1999, just seven months after she was diagnosed with breast and cervical cancer. What began as the biggest challenge in Brenda's life turned into a wonderful gift for humanity. Brenda amazed her doctors when she completely healed herself by using raw and living foods, detoxification, cleansing, and emotional healing. Since opening the Living Foods Institute, Brenda has expanded her Healthy Lifestyle Course to help people heal on every level. She has trained thousands of people how to restore optimum health from almost any disease. To date, she has written 9 books:* **The Living Foods Lifestyle®; Colon Cleansing For Optimum Health; 101 Raw and Living Food Recipes; Get Started Now For Good Health; The Living Foods Training Manual; Healing Fibroids, Endometriosis, Tumors and Cysts; A Plan For Health; Good Health Now;** *and* **Organic Raw and Living Food Recipes**. *She was awarded an Honorary Cultural Doctorate in Therapeutic Philosophy from the World University in September 2003 and the Phoenix Award by the City of Atlanta for helping its citizens to become healthier.*
The Living Foods Institute, 1530 Dekalb Ave., Atlanta, Ga. 30307. 800-844-9876
www.livingfoodsinstitute.com
Email Brenda at Brenda@livingfoodsinstitute.com

15

Superfoods and Supplements

Jameth Sheridan, ND

The addition of enzyme-active superfoods and whole food supplements is strongly advised.

It's important to differentiate between an isolated supplement and a superfood or other whole foods supplement. Whole food and superfood "supplements" are encouraged; isolated or synthetic supplements are not. A superfood may be defined as a food that is unusually and naturally high in nutrients such as vitamins, minerals, phytonutrients, unique and/or healing elements.

Superfoods include (but are not limited to) the following, whether fresh or dried:

• Spirulina
• Chlorella
• Klamath Algae
• Grasses
• Maca
• Flax Seeds
• Milk Thistle
• Nettles
• Dandelion Greens
• Burdock Root
• Wild edibles
• Miso
• Etc.

Superfruits are a subclass of superfoods and include:

• Goji Berries
• Pomegranate
• Acai
• Etc.

What is and is not a superfood is very loosely defined and is subject to an individual's own determination. Blueberries are every bit as much as a superfruit in my book as any of the above, for example.

Chlorophyll-containing foods

Chlorophyll is what makes plants green, and consuming it in whole-food form from plants is extremely beneficial for us. In fact, it is considered so essential for optimum health, a chapter has been devoted to it earlier in this book. Chlorophyll is one molecule different than hemoglobin. It provides protection from radioactivity, and it alkalizes. Chlorophyll is a powerful detoxifier of many harmful substances. It must come from whole foods for optimum effectiveness.

Spirulina

Spirulina, to me, is the #1 single superfood in the world! Spirulina is a blue-green algae that, along with wheatgrass, is the original superfood. It has several thousand years of use. It was known for giving Aztec and Inca runners endurance and strength. It is 50–60% protein with all essential amino acids. It is an excellent source of B vitamins including B-1 and B-2, iron, and boron (for calcium utilization), etc. It is high in the amino acid phenylalanine for mood elevation and appetite suppression.

The nourishing, detoxifying, regenerating, immune supporting, balancing, and immense benefits of spirulina place it firmly as the #1 superfood in existence.

Unlike an isolated or synthetic vitamin product that may have few carotenoids in it, spirulina naturally contains several hundred carotenoids, including beta carotene, xanthopyll, cryptoxanthin, zeaxanthin, and leutin. Extracts of spirulina have been shown to inhibit AIDS and herpes viruses. Tobacco smokers have shown resistance to cigarettes when taking spirulina. It enhances activity of bone marrow cells, natural killer cells, macrophages, and T-cells. Spirulina specifically feeds friendly bacteria (prebiotic). By taking it alone, your numbers of friendly flora will increase.

The protein content of spirulina is notable due to the fact that, other than chlorella, it is the highest source in the world, including ANY animal product. Many sources mistakenly report that all high protein diets create large amounts of uric acid in the body. Uric acid contributes to general body acidity, osteoporosis, and kidney damage/stones. Vegetable proteins, like spirulina, form very little uric acid. It is the high animal protein in diets that is harmful, not plant proteins. You could have too much protein from the plant kingdom if you took too many isolated plant protein powders, but you would have to take very much more of them! Blue green algaes are the only known source of the pigment phycocyanin. Research shows it helps to protect against kidney failure. So not only is spirulina high in "complete" protein, it is also produces little uric acid and has protective effects.

Small amounts of the essential fatty acids DHA and EPA are found in spirulina and other algaes. Spirulina's primary fat is GLA (Gamma-linolenic acid). GLA is an Omega-6 fatty acid that is also found in evening primrose oil, blackcurrant seed oil, and borage oil. GLA's positive effects include reducing inflammation. Recent research has shown spirulina to be effective at preventing cardiovascular disease and to promote extremely high antioxidant levels, possibly even more so than the metabolic antioxidant enzymes superoxide dismutase and glutathione peroxidase (which milk thistle seed extract can stimulate). Because spirulina has such a balancing and energizing effect on people, some have thought it is a stimulant. This is not true. Spirulina's effects are from the massive array of healing substances it contains.

Spirulina is green in so many ways.
As a source of protein per agricultural resources, spirulina blows away any other food, especially animal proteins. Spirulina yields 200 times more protein per acre than beef. Spirulina does not deplete any topsoil. One kilo of beef protein causes 145 kilos of topsoil loss. As for water savings, spirulina uses only 2% the water required for beef protein. Spirulina uses about six gallons of water for a ten gram serving. Cow milk uses 65 gallons; a chicken's egg uses 136 gallons; and cow flesh/steak/burger, etc, uses a whopping 1,303 gallons of water.

Algae are the largest producers of oxygen on the planet. The growing of spirulina and other algae like Klamath Lake AFA and chlorella contributes to increased oxygen supplies. Algae absorb carbon dioxide and release oxygen, just like land plants, but at a much faster rate.

Spirulina is an incredible source of a wide array of vitamins, minerals, chlorophyll, protein and phytonutrients. It deeply nourishes and cleanses the body at the same time. It can be very grounding in a good way, especially if someone is on a too-low calorie diet, too-high sugar diet, or is on a cleanse. There is such an immense amount of information on spirulina that it could easily fill a whole book. Two species of spirulina are available for human consumption, *Spirulina Platensis* and *Spirulina Azteca*. Platensis is milder in flavor and is far more common at the time of writing. Azteca is stronger in flavor and is the species the Aztecs harvested. Both are awesome. Spirulina *easily* lays claim to the world's #1 superfood! In fact, it would be hard for anything else to challenge it.

Klamath Lake Algae (Afanizomenon Flos Aquae)
Klamath algae, like Spirulina, is a blue-green algae. Many people use the terms "blue-green algae" and "Klamath Lake Algae" (Klamath) to mean the same thing. However, it is not accurate since Spirulina is also blue-green. Klamath Lake Algae, also known as AFA, grows wild in Klamath Lake, Oregon, USA. Being a blue-green algae, Klamath shares many of the nutritional characteristics with spirulina, including having phycocyanin, and is excellent for use as a whole food source of nutrients and cleansing. They are essentially nutritionally equivalent, with each having their stronger areas nutritionally. I use both and love their

effects individually and together. Some people prefer one over the other. I suggest you try them both. Klamath will be discussed in much more detail by a different author elsewhere in this book. I do want to clear up a myth about the two algaes. There is the impression in the raw foods community that Klamath is superior to spirulina, partly due to the fact that Klamath costs considerably more to buy than spirulina, and that spirulina was unfairly bashed in the late 80's and early 90's by a then prominent Klamath proponent. Both of these blue-green algaes are awesome!

Chlorella

Chlorella is a green algae. It does not contain the beneficial blue phycocyanin pigment of the blue-green algae, but as a consequence it has more chlorophyll than any blue-green algae, including Spirulina and Klamath. Much research has shown that chlorella is a particularly potent detoxifier of toxic metals including cadmium, mercury (from the environment, silver fillings, and fish consumption), lead, radioactive uranium, barium, cesium, plutonium, dioxin, etc.

Chlorella stimulates interferon production (which leads to the production of more macrophages and specifically T-cells) for increased immunity. It also contains vitamins B1, B2, B3, B6, B-12, folic acid, biotin, pantothenic acid, PABA, phosphorus, potassium, magnesium, calcium, and zinc (10 times more zinc than pumpkin seeds), copper, manganese, and germanium.

Seaweeds

Seaweeds are very rich in trace minerals not found in land plants. They are particularly high in minerals. Kelp is the highest mineral food I am aware of, at approximately 40%. Kelp has much more potassium than bananas. Kelp also contains vitamin D. It has sodium alginate that removes heavy metals and radioactivity, binds cadmium, mercury, lead, radioactive uranium, barium, cesium, plutonium, dioxin, etc. Kelp also contains non-toxic iodine, which displaces radioactive iodine and helps keep the thyroid healthy. Note that iodine in isolation is LETHAL. There is no known toxicity of iodine from eating kelp. Iodine is not toxic when in a whole food of vegetable origin (see also notes on iron, later in this chapter).

If you soak kelp in pure water for a few minutes and then rinse it off, it can be eaten straight. It can be used as a wrap for vegetables. The inner part of the kelp is thicker and hard to eat without cooking. Eating it raw requires blending it with something. You can even blend it into a smoothie to help balance out the sugar; it will thicken anything you blend with it.

Dulse also rocks when it comes to concentrated nutrition and is really easy to eat. Soak and rinse it and you can eat it straight. It's also great to add to salads in large quantities. Nori is another seaweed that's perfect for rolling veggies and avocado in for vegan sushi. Hijiki and arame are more noodle-like and can be used that way. I have a great recipe for "MacArame and Cheese" (Vegan Cheese) – see *Uncooking With Jameth and Kim*. Sea vegetables are awesome sources of incredibly powerful nutrients. Use them liberally.

Grasses

Grasses, along with spirulina, are the original superfoods. Wheatgrass was popularized by Viktoras Kulvinskas and Ann Wigmore. Grasses are extremely alkaline-forming, more so than other greens, such as algaes. If you have indigestion, grass juice is amazing for curing it fast. It's also very high in chlorophyll. Like all greens, they are loaded with nutrients.

Wheatgrass is the most popular grass. Kamut and Spelt are ancient forms of wheat. Please take note that ALL grasses are gluten-free. When a gluten grain such as wheat, barley, triticale, or rye grows into grass, it loses its gluten. Tray-grown grasses are easiest way to get fresh grasses into your system. You can get this at juice bars and you can relatively easily grow this yourself. Note that not all grains will sprout, and unsprouted grains definitely contain gluten. If you are gluten-sensitive, do NOT harvest or eat the grain. Cut the grasses above the grain, and rinse them. In fact, you should always rinse your grasses.

Tray-grown wheatgrass has a characteristically "sickly sweet" flavor, and some get nauseous when they take it straight. Adding minerals to the soil helps this. There is NO problem mixing grass juice with either fruit or vegetable juices, or with water. This is an excellent way to get more in you.

There in an alternative to 7–10-day-old tray-grown wheatgrass. In many places you can get frozen wheatgrass juice that has been grown in the soil for months. This grass is much easier to take. I have never met anyone who could not palate this. Also, most grass powders are from grasses grown in the soil for months and can taste quite good. I personally use a lot of the dried grasses and feel great benefit from them. Dried whole grass powder need to be ground extremely fine to get the most out of them. Grasses are on the opposite end of the green food spectrum from algaes like spirulina, Klamath Lake, and chlorella. Mature grasses (not usually the tray grown) have a really nice, really nutritive, alkalizing feel to them.

Nettles

Nettles are extremely high in chlorophyll and are actually significantly more nutritious than grasses in many respects. They are very high in minerals (2–3 times mineral content of grasses) and vitamins, including non-toxic iron, vitamin C, and silica. It is much higher in minerals then grasses. The first time I had fresh nettle juice I was amazed at the immense energized feeling I got.
Nettles are a mild diuretic (removes excess water from the body). They are particularly helpful for kidney health, arthritis, gout, allergies, and eczema. Both the root and the greens are beneficial. The root is particularly helpful for prostate health. Nettles are another plant source of vitamin D.

Horsetail

Also very high in minerals and probably the single best source of organic Silica, which is non-toxic and absorbable in whole horsetail. Silica promotes healing and regeneration of cartilage, bone, hair, nails, lungs, skin, and helps prevent scar tissue. Horsetail contains significant amounts of calcium and non-toxic iron (good for anemia) as well as beta carotene, B1, B2, B3, C, E, PABA, selenium, magnesium, phos-phorus, potassium, zinc, manganese, and rhodium. Horsetail is a mild diuretic and promotes kidney detoxification. Unlike drug-based diuretics, horsetail does not cause a harmful loss of minerals – potassium, etc.

There are several types of horsetail available. *Equisetum palustre* is poisonsous and should not be eaten. *Equisetum arvense*, when fresh, has the enzyme thiaminase in it and can destroy vitamin B1 in the body. Horsetail either needs to be dried or heated to remove the thiaminase. Be careful if you gather any herb from the wild.

Weeds, leaves and roots in general
Chickweed, amaranth leaves, moringa, horsetail (*equisetum arvense* only), lamb's quarters, dandelion leaves, blessed thistle, and other weeds are also super-nutritious with their own healing properties. But remember, just because something is a plant does not mean it is a superfood! Some plants are toxic and poisonous.

Superfruits
Superfruits include high ORAC fruits like blueberries, raspberries, goji berries, pomegranates, and acai. Any fruit that is extremely well grown in nutrient-dense soil can be a superfruit.

Maca
Maca is a root that originated in the mountains of Peru. It has been used for thousands of years as a food and a medicine. It has traditionally been known to increase energy, increase libido in both men and women, and balance hormone levels in both men and women, and modern research has show this to be true. Maca is NOT a stimulant, but rather a powerful adaptogenic tonic superfood of the ancients.

Maca is a cruciferous vegetable, and thus contains some of the potent detoxification phytonutrients that all cruciferous vegetables have. However, being a cruciferous vegetable, it can produce gas when taken in raw form. The traditional way the Peruvians consumed it was cooked over a fire, like a potato. No enzymes, but it did release the phytonutrients and eliminate the problem with gas. Maca is a really balancing superfood that I think everyone can benefit from. If you get gastrointestinal distress from it, do one of the following things. 1. Take maca mixed with high-potency probiotics, enzymes, and digestive herbs (much more effective this way too) (best choice). 2. Take a maca extract, which does NOT have the vitamins and minerals of maca but also does NOT have the gas-producing elements (not ideal). It DOES have the main phytonutrients that are *thought* to make maca effective. 3. Eat it the way the Peruvians did. 4. Lower your usage level.

Carob
Carob is an awesome superfood. Unlike cacao, carob actually tastes good. Carob is an amazing bowel moderator. If loose bowels are present, carob can

stop it. If constipation is present, carob can make the bowels move. Regular carob consumption in sufficient quantities can help to produce very clean, regular, and toilet-paper free bowel movements (slippery elm, marshmallow root, and other herbs will also help, but not as much as carob alone). Like apples and pears, carob is high in pectin. Pectin can absorb poisons (including radioactive elements) and cholesterol. Carob, being a whole plant foods, contains many nutrients such as magnesium, potassium, iron, manganese, chromium, copper, etc.

Carob, belonging to the healing family of foods known as legumes, contains lignans. Lignans have been found to be antiviral, antifungal, antibacterial, and anti-inflammatory. They also show strong hormone balancing and anticancer properties. Lignans are a powerful class of phytoestrogens that have been shown to have a protective effect against a wide range of cancers, and to help balance hormones. Flax seed (not the oil) is also very high in lignans, especially when sprouted.

Cacao and other stimulants

Cacao is "all the rage" in the raw foods community as of this writing, similar to yerba mate of years ago. Cacao has replaced carob as the "chocolate of choice" for raw foodists. (Carob is described elsewhere in this chapter). Let's give a little history of cacao. Cacao usually refers to raw chocolate. The ancient Mayans believed that cacao was discovered by the gods and left for the Maya to use. Their mythology states that cacao was given to humans after they where created from maize (corn) by the divine grandmother goddess. They had a cacao god and an annual festival to honor her. Unfortunately, the Maya were into animal sacrifice, and an innocent dog who was cursed with naturally occurring cacao colored markings was sacrificed!

"Cooked" chocolate: Prior to its introduction into the raw food movement, chocolate was considered, on balance, NOT good for you. Chocolate has either theobromine, caffeine, or both in it. Chocolate causes rapid heart rate, an unnatural drug-type stimulant high, followed by a crash, and eventually nervous exhaustion. Chocolate can certainly "jack you up" with energy, but so too can cocaine. If you take sufficient chocolate at night, you can NOT sleep. This is NOT natural. Chocolate is not a superfood but rather a naturally occurring food with drug-like effects to it. Other naturally occurring plants, like kola nut, yerba mate, coffee, and guarana, are also very harsh stimulants. They absolutely have their use in herbal medicine, but regular usage weakens the body.

Enter raw cacao: Then came raw chocolate. It's RAW for god's sake. It must be good for us! This is a dangerous half-truth. The plant oleander will kill you whether it is raw or cooked, and so to will some species of mushrooms (others can save you health), as well as many other poisonous plants. There are many hallucinogenic plants, and they have that effect whether they are raw or cooked.

Regular chocolate is undeniably toxic, as it contains cacao powder, cacao butter, cow milk, refined sugar, pesticides, and, depending on flavor and manufacturer, possibly much more toxic garbage. A vegan, non-raw rice-milk chocolate bar has the following ingredients: "Organic cane sugar, organic cocoa powder, organic rice powder, organic cocoa mass (containing cacao), natural algae, organic vanilla extract, salt". You can see that there is a big difference between the two products. Although they are both chocolate, the vegan milk-chocolate bar is vegan, organic, and has a superior sweetener. BIG advantage. A raw chocolate/cacao bar typically has ingredients such as: organic cacao powder, organic cacao butter, organic agave nectar, organic vanilla beans, organic lucuma powder (superfood), organic yacon syrup (superfood). The raw cacao product has, *by far*, the best ingredients of them all. Superior sweeteners with superior blood-sugar regulation, and in some cases superfoods for sweeteners. These things make the raw cacao product much healthier. However, there is still the cacao.

Cacao as an antioxidant: Cacao is hailed as an amazing antioxidant, and this is one of the things that it is advertised for and consumed. Let's look at how Cacao stacks up to other foods. ORAC listed in TE/g units.

Cloves	3144*
Cinnamon	2675*
Oregano	2001*
Turmeric	1592*
Cocoa/Cacao	809*
Parsley	743*
Cumin	768*

Cacao ranks pretty high on this chart, and that is certainly to its credit. However, the stimulative effect of cacao increases your body's need for antioxidants, so the functional level is lower.

If you are looking for really high ORAC values, plant extracts are extremely high. For example:

Resveratrol – *from:*

Grapes and Japanese knotwood	23,000**
Turmeric	15,500**
Green tea extract	14,000**
Quebracho bark extract	13,480**
Grape seed extract	9,600**
Milk thistle seed extract	6,800**
Cocoa/cacao	809*

*USDA Database for the Oxygen Radical Absorbance Capacity (ORAC) of selected Foods
S. Bhagwat, D.B. Haytowitz, and J.M. Holden

**Brunswick Labs. Norton, MA

My bottom line on cacao
Cacao is a powerful, ceremonial, addictive, whole food medicinal drug that can be of benefit for the very short term. It should be used sparingly, if at all, and with reverence for its easily unbalanced power. The leaders who attended the International Living Foods Summit in April 2007 all agreed that caffeinated and/or addictive substances *(even in their raw form)*, such as cacao/chocolate, coffee, caffeinated teas, etc., if consumed at all, are best to be used only occasionally and consumed in minimal quantities. When cacao is raw, it causes the same drug-like, stimulative, and addictive reactions as when it is cooked! You can mix it with better ingredients, or eat bad tasting cacao nibs by themselves, but you still have drug effects. There is no way around this. Just because something is raw does not make it good for you. *Again, just because something is raw does not make it good for you.*

How I use cacao: I, and many others, have overdone cacao in the past, and have suffered for it. Today, I occasionally use cacao as a sacred medicine, ceremonially, and to stay awake at the wheel on long car trips. If my wife and I want to stay up late and watch a movie, and it is already late, we will occasionally take some cacao. Or I will sometimes take it before exercise when I otherwise do not feel like exercising. A little cacao can give the boost to get moving. Green tea can also be used occasionally for energy. It is super-high ORAC, anti-cancer, and is not addictive. If you can achieve the same effects with non stimulant superfoods, that is better.

Ginger
Ginger is anti-inflammatory, an antioxidant, and an anti-nausea agent. It has been proven to be more effective for motion sickness than a prescription drug. It is not uncommon to come across facts like this when comparing foods and natural medicines to drugs. Ginger also lowers high blood pressure and raises low blood pressure.

Burdock Root
Somehow the ancients knew that Burdock was a blood purifier. Today, we know that it can spread apart clumped blood cells. Burdock is one of the main herbs in the Essiac anti-cancer and herbal purification tea. Burdock is over 40% insulin, which helps balance out blood sugar. Insulin is a pre-biotic and promotes the growth of beneficial bacteria.

Nopal cactus
This is an awesome superfood! It has been used for thousands of years by Mexican natives both as a food and for enhanced health and vitality. Nopal cactus is highly nutritious and contains a unique phytonutrient vitamin and mineral profile that contributes to its beneficial effects. It is helpful to balance blood sugar and insulin levels. So much so that those taking insulin will need to monitor themselves when taking it. It lowers cholesterol. It helps the bowels to move, but it is not a laxative. It is anti-viral (specifically anti-herpes). Research has shown it greatly reduces the effects of hangover from alcohol, indicating its ability to detoxify and support the liver.

Nopal cactus is also high in bulk-forming mucilaginous fiber that assists most foods, herbs, and supplements taken with it to be gently and naturally time-released into the blood stream. This includes the timed-release of sugars into the blood stream to support healthy blood sugar and insulin functions*. It will also time-release other foods/herbs into the blood stream, including unhealthy foods. Slowly releasing less-than-optimally healthy foods into the blood stream, it will allow the body to deal with the resultant toxicity with less difficulty.

Dandelion
Dandelion leaf is extremely high in minerals and vitamins. It is probably the highest in minerals of all land plants. It is much higher in beta-carotene and other carotenes than carrots. Dandelion is a mild diuretic and bowel mover. It is very liver supportive. It increases the flow of bile and is a digestive aid.

Probiotics
Probiotics are definitely superfoods. Probiotics are the healthy bacteria that inhabit our intestines. They are essential to break down our foods properly, create vitamins, for detoxification, and for the immune system. A good, plentiful colony of probiotics inhibit pathogenic bacteria and candida yeast. NON-dairy probiotics are best.

Milk thistle
Milk thistle seed is amazing for detoxification and protection. It is definitely one of my top superfoods. It is an extremely powerful liver superfood. Most of the research on milk thistle has been done on the seed extract, and the comments below refer to this form (unless otherwise stated).

Milk thistle seed extract is a double antioxidant. First of all, it far exceeds cacao in ORAC scores. Cacao is approximately 800 ORAC per gram, and milk thistle seed extract is approximately 6,800 ORAC per gram (seven times higher). In addition, milk thistle provides the raw materials that allow the liver to produce more of the extremely powerful antioxidants superoxide dismutase (SOD) and glutathione peroxidase. These metabolic antioxidants are even more powerful than the superfood antioxidants.

Milk thistle seed promotes powerful liver cleansing of metabolic wastes, environmental poisons, and drugs. This is particularly important if you eat and live unhealthily and if you eat animal products. Animals have their own metabolic wastes in their tissues. The last thing you need is someone else's toxins. Milk thistle is a cleanser, protector, and a regenerator. It actually stimulates liver cells to regenerate and make more co-enzyme Q10. It is so powerful that people have been able to survive what would otherwise be lethal doses of poisons. A group of naturalists were able to survive from deathcap mushroom poisoning (which is usually fatal in a day) by taking enough milk thistle seed. *Caution: Do NOT overdose on lethal poisons.* Other research has shown milk thistle seed to be helpful in preventing skin cancer.

Flax Seed, chia seeds, hemp seeds, Omega-3s

Flax seeds are one of the best sources of Omega-3 fatty acids. Additionally, flax seeds have 27 identified anti-cancer compounds, according to James Duke of USDA. Chia seeds are just as good of a source of fatty acids as flax. Hemp seeds come next. Many other vegetable foods contain omega-3, fatty acids, including purslane, and oats. There is a huge difference between animal-derived omega-3s and plant sources. Animal sources contain preformed EPA and DHA. Vegetable sources contain the pre-cursors of these nutrients. Whereas omega-3s from plant product do NOT have a toxicity, EPA and DHA do have a toxicity. Too much of them can result in bruising easily, prolonged external bleeding, and internal bleeding. I repeat, the toxicity is ONLY from ANIMAL sources of EPA and DHA.

Plant omega-3s that convert are NON-toxic. Elsewhere in this chapter, I write about beta-carotene (plant precursor to vitamin A) and pre-formed vitamin A (only found in animal parts and chemically synthesized). Beta-carotene has NO toxicity, whereas vitamin A HAS toxicity. Can you see the similar pattern? Sprouted seeds are far better sources of Omega-3 than non-sprouted seeds. Oils naturally do NOT have the highly beneficial lignans (unless added back) that whole seeds do. Lignans are anti-cancer, anti-viral, anti-bacterial, and anti-inflammatory.

Miso

I consider unpasteurized Miso to be the #1 superfood condiment. It has thirty-five times the anti-cancer genistein as whole soy beans, has organic sodium, is anti-radiation, etc. Even your condiments can be superfoods. Too little of the right type of sodium can be a huge problem (see Salt chapter), and consuming adequate amounts of healthy salt is essential to good health. *See Salt chapter for more details on Miso.*

Two things you can do with superfoods

Improve your digestion: If you are having trouble digesting food, peppermint, fennel, and ginger (among other herbs), eaten raw or made into a tea, are helpful. *For an antacid*; eat some slippery elm alone, or add marshmallow root to it. I have also found celery juice and fresh or frozen wheatgrass juice to be extremely helpful for acid indigestion (probably due the very high alkalinity of these two foods).

By no means does this chapter constitute a complete list of superfoods, but the above should hopefully send you in the right direction. When deciding if something is a superfood or not, use your own judgment: what is and what is not a superfood is up to the person making the claim.

Superfoods are a gift from nature. They are here to help us heal and live a better life. I am deeply grateful that my mind and body has been exposed to them, and I think you will be too.

When is a supplement a supplement
This is a very important question. A traditional multi-vitamin/mineral product has various vitamins and minerals in it. The vitamins can be obtained in 2 ways. They can be synthesized artificially, or they can be isolated down from a "food" source. Either of these methods makes the vitamin absorb VERY poorly and sometimes causes imbalances. Minerals can not be synthesized, but in supplements they are essentially isolated down from foods or inorganic substances (like chalk and rocks). Isolated vitamin and mineral nutrients can and do have an important role, but most are poorly absorbed and utilized and they can and do have toxicities. There are cases where they can and have been helpful, but they are a double-edged sword in general.

Beta Carotene and Vitamin A
For example, beta-carotene is one of approximately 600 carotenoids found in natural foods. It is one of the pre-cursors of vitamin A. Studies of synthetic beta-carotene have found that it does nothing to enhance our health. Studies of beta-carotene isolated, refined, and purified from a food source does show that it has some beneficial effects. However, beta-carotene when in *actual foods* (like, spirulina, chlorella, carrots, etc.) has been shown to have immense benefits. Vitamin A supplements are either synthetic, or obtained from animals. Vitamin A does NOT occur in the plant kingdom. There is a VERY GOOD reason for this. Pre-formed vitamin A is Toxic!

Intakes of 20,000 IU of either synthetic or animal derived vitamin A during pregnancy may result in (less than 20 percent) of spontaneous abortions, and birth defects (J. Am. Med. Assoc. 257:1292-1297,1987). "Naturally" occurring vitamin A is also toxic. Arctic explorers suffered acute vitamin A toxicity when they ingested the livers of polar bears or seals (which are high in naturally occurring vitamin A). It is not enough to be whole food, it must be vegan as well.

Beta-carotene, on the other hand, is 100% non-toxic at any level of consumption, provided that it is eaten in a whole, vegan food. There is ZERO toxicity of beta-carotene from actual food sources! You might think that if you consumed too much actual food beta-carotene, you would have too much vitamin A. However, this is not the case, as nature has a built-in system for this.

Our livers convert beta-carotene into vitamin A only AS NEEDED. Therefore, there is NO toxicity. You can have all the kale, carrots, broccoli, spinach, dandelion leaves, or spirulina you want, and you will never have a beta-carotene or vitamin A toxicity.

Vitamins and minerals NEVER occur as isolates in natural plant foods
Vitamins and minerals from the plant kingdom are always organically bound to a complex of other materials such as bioflavonoids, enzymes, minerals, amino acids, etc. These complexes are required for the optimum absorption and non-toxicity of the nutrient.

Vitamin C

Ascorbic acid is the base of the vitamin C molecule, not by any means the whole thing. The vast majority of vitamin C supplements are forms of ascorbic acid. Let's look at ascorbic acid supplementation. Ascorbic acid is very acid. If you leave it on your teeth overnight, it will etch them away. And ascorbic acid does not come with any alkaline mineral buffers. 1500 mg of isolated ascorbic acid has been shown to cause anemia in people.

Vitamin C, like all vitamins and minerals from actual food, is always found organically bound with other natural materials, including bioflavonoids and copper. If it has vitamin C in it, is has these elements. When isolated vitamin C is consumed, it tries to re-combine with its natural elements, which includes copper. Vitamin C draws copper from the bloodstream. Copper is required for iron assimilation. Without sufficient copper, you can not assimilate the iron that is in your blood stream. With insufficient iron, you are anemic. However, it gets worse. You have plenty of iron in your blood stream, yet you can not assimilate it. Unassimilated iron is toxic and is a free radical. What is created is a simultaneous deficiency and toxicity of iron at the same time! All this from isolated ascorbic acid. Stop taking the ascorbic acid, and copper and iron levels will return to their previous levels. Ascorbic acid is a supplement.

Some companies mix ascorbic acid with other organic and inorganic chemicals to make less unabsorbable version of vitamin C (like calcium ascorbate) and others dry-mix isolated bioflavonoids with isolated vitamin C. These measures, to a very small degree, move the isolated vitamin C toward being more whole, but are still so far off. What is needed is vitamin C from actual food.

Other companies mix ascorbic acid with tiny amounts of food sources of vitamin C. This is a miniscule step in the right direction, but functionally the same as isolated. Contrast this to getting vitamin C from fruits, vegetables, or herbs by eating those foods. There is NO toxicity of vitamin C in actual food form, at any quantity!

Vitamin C is high in many foods, and if you are eating a variety of whole, vegan foods with lots of fruits and vegetables, being anything other than sufficient in it is virtually impossible. If you need additional vitamin C, I suggest whole food sources like acerola berries, rose hips, amla berries, and camu camu berries. Acerola and rose hips can be taken/eaten straight, but amla and camu camu are usually gross-tasting, so you will have to take a "supplement" of them. In this case, if the "supplement" is just dried camu or amla, it is really not a supplement. It is just dried whole food in a bottle. That does not make it a supplement.

I would like to mention that copper, in its inorganic form, like you might get from copper foodware, and from cooper water pipes, is VERY toxic.

Iron in isolation iron from an animal product is a toxic oxidant. It is a free radical, the opposite of an antioxidant. Isolated iron is so toxic that it has poisoned and killed people. Many years ago, bottles of iron-containing supplements were required to have a warning similar to the following: "Warning, accidental overdose of iron-containing supplements is chief cause of fatal poisoning in children under 6". This statement is true. Isolated iron is a toxic supplement. Iron from foods such as greens has no toxicity at any level of usage.

Calcium, for example, requires boron, magnesium, manganese, silica, sodium, vitamin K, phosphorus, vitamins, hormones, enzymes, etc. for absorption. All these nutrients need other nutrients as well. Calcium can calcify arteries and soft tissues of the body if taken as a supplement.

The bottom line is that all vitamins and minerals require a great deal of organic co-factors for absorption and assimilation without toxicity. Superfoods provide these. Supplements do not.

Warning and caution regarding NOT taking isolated supplements

When given a choice between a natural plant food source of a vitamin or mineral, or an isolated or synthetic one, the natural whole food is always better. However, isolated vitamins and minerals can and do have benefits in certain circumstances. For example, if someone is starving, they will benefit from an isolated multivitamin/mineral product if they do not have a superfood product available. If someone has severe low blood sugar or diabetes, they don't know about natural things to control blood sugar such as Nopal Cactus, cinnamon, and Actual Food™ Chromium, they will benefit from taking isolated chromium far more than it will hurt them. If someone has heart disease and they are not a whole foods vegan taking superfoods, they will benefit from taking isolated B-6 and B-12 to lower homocysteine levels. I don't take ANY of these isolated nutrients at present, but I would if the need arose. Compared to drugs, isolated vitamins and minerals are immensely beneficial with few side effects. I have seen individuals NOT take any supplements, superfoods, or herbs and die of deficiency diseases, including many raw food "purists". There are things that I would die for, like defending my life partner, but saying that I never took a single isolated supplement is not one of them! That is crazy! My point is to NOT THROW THE BABY OUT WITH THE BATHWATER, in ANY area of your life! Please!

I wish you great health and happiness, always!

About the Author:

Jameth Sheridan, N.D. is a longtime Vegan, Raw Fooder, Herbalist, and hard-core holistic medicine researcher. He is an outspoken perfectionist on a deeply driven, on-going mission to uncover and spread truth, ethics, and full-spectrum health. He walks his talk and fully embraces as many aspects of a holistic lifestyle as he can, including non-toxic building. Dr. Sheridan is the single most recognized pioneer in bio-compatible nutritional superfoods. He brings a unique blend of scientific, yet vastly open-minded, deeply thorough approach, and an understanding of life force, whole foods, and mother nature to all that he does, with a deep reverence for all life. Dr. Sheridan researches, grows, and provides the highest quality superfoods under his own label, HealthForce Nutritionals, private labels, as well as makes custom formulas for other hard-core companies worldwide. Jameth is one of those unique people who is deeply caring, compassionate, introspective, and humble, while at the same time he is not afraid to call upon his Warrior spirit to challenge the status quo or go against the grain, if, upon reflection, that is what he truly believes is right. He lives his life as a modern follower of codes of honor such as Bushido and Chivalry.

Dr. Sheridan's websites: www.HealthForce.com   www.RawFoodResearch.com

"The quality, therapeutic concentration, and affordability of a nutritional product can, and often does, mean the difference between lethargy and energy, sickness and health, and, quite literally, life and death. I don't want anyone to be tired, sick or dead because they could not obtain or afford the best possible product. If someone does not feel this same way, they should not be in the nutritional product business. I live and breathe this philosophy in both my personal and professional life and constantly strive to evolve HealthForce products and offer them at the best possible values. I would rather die than compromise these principles" – Jameth Sheridan, N.D.

16

The Importance of
Vitamin B12

Gabriel Cousens, MD, MD(H) and
Brian Clement, PhD, NMD, LNC

The authors of this chapter at their respective organizations, Tree of Life and Hippocrates, have a strong base of experience in seeing thousands of people who are B_{12} deficient and who get better with natural B_{12} supplementation. Our commitment is to provide optimal information to enable people to be successful in living a live-food plant-source only lifestyle. As scientists, we are committed to "do no harm". With the addition of B_{12} supplementation in a person with B_{12} deficiencies we see a greater sense of well being, better neurological and mental functioning, agility and stamina.

Brian Clement's work, using a special intracellular assay for human active B_{12}, suggests that heavy meat and dairy users may actually have more deficiencies than plant-source only people. B_{12} is used more rapidly in conditions of high mental and physical stress, which is abundant in today's world. Whatever are the actual percentages of human active B_{12} deficiencies, they are high.

Digestive devolution
Clement has made some fascinating discoveries about the devolution of the human digestive tract. At the Harvard and NYU medical libraries he studied medical sketching of the GI tract at 50-year intervals from 1700 through 2005. As he examined sketches of the ascending colon, which is connected by a valve to the small intestine, he found that, at the base, the shape tended to elongate inward like the front of a round boot. This "boot" became progressively smaller between 1700 and 2000. By 1950 it had disappeared and in its place was an appendix. The latest pictures show a small appendix and the complete

absence of this "boot". Somehow in this biological transformation we make the hypothesis that perhaps the B_{12} bacteria dropped from the small intestine where they produced B_{12}, which was actively absorbed in the ileum of the small intestine into the ascending colon where it was minimally absorbed through the hepatic-entero circulation. Depending on how much this part of the anatomy devolved may explain why some people can go for 30 or more years without B_{12} supplementation and why others can barely go a year, with the majority becoming deficient in B_{12} by six years.

An important thing to keep in mind is that there has been a devolution of the human anatomy over the years, and humans have adapted to the situation by taking a biologically active living B_{12} supplement. In the allopathic world the only viable source for B_{12} is by eating meat and dairy products. Animal flesh and secretions are filled with B_{12}-producing bacteria; so also is the non-purified water in India. The bacteria in the Indian water actually supplied sufficient B_{12} to the vegans – along with other parasites and viruses – but is not a reason to keep drinking contaminated water. When Indians moved to England they started to develop B_{12} deficiencies because their water was purified. Possibly in the next few years we will find B_{12}- producing bacteria that grow in the small intestine, or some combinations of some superfoods that will supply enough B_{12}. In the meantime it is important to understand the importance of B_{12} in maintaining well-being. We recommend this out of respect for your own health and for the growth of the plant-based live-food movement in the world. The health disasters and deaths that have resulted in ignoring B_{12} supplementation need not continue.

B_{12}

B_{12} acts as a co-enzyme whose job is primarily connected to the methylation process needed for the production of phosphatidylcholine, myelin, melatonin, catecholamines, DNA, RNA, cysteine, and normal red blood cells. There are several forms of active B_{12} that work as co-enzymes in the body: adenosylcobalamin, methylocobalamin, cyancobalamin (found in supplements and fortified foods because it is the most stable form of B_{12}), and hydroxocobalamin. There are many natural B_{12} analogues in food, but they do not work as active co-enzymes in the body and may actually block the active B_{12} co-enzyme function.

Understanding B_{12} Absorption

Understanding B_{12} absorption pathways in humans gives additional weight into the B_{12} question. The only organisms known to manufacture B_{12} are bacteria, which are found in water, soil, and the digestive tracts of animals and consequently in their tissues or milk. B_{12} is not in honey. In flesh foods the B_{12} is usually attached to a carrier protein for transport or storage. When this protein-bound B_{12} reaches the stomach, the acids and enzymes that are secreted in the stomach free up the B_{12} from the protein it was bound to, and it becomes attached to a specific protein called R-protein, which transports it through the stomach into the small intestine. Intrinsic factor, a protein complex that transports B_{12}, is also made in the stomach. In the small intestine, the B_{12} is separated from the R-protein via pancreatic enzymes and becomes attached to the intrinsic factor (IF). The IF then takes it to the ileum, which is the last part of the small intestine where it is absorbed by special receptor cells designed to receive the IF-cobalamin complex. The IF-cobalamin complex protects the B_{12} against bacteria and digestive enzyme degradation. It makes sure the ileum cells absorb it in priority over the B_{12} analogues. B_{12} absorption may also happen by passive diffusion which accounts for 1–3% of the B_{12} absorbed. B_{12} from supplements is not bound to protein, so it does not need to go through this complicated process. When large amounts of B_{12} are taken in from supplements, it can overcome IF defects and be absorbed by passive diffusion. It can also be absorbed sublingually (under the tongue) at higher rates than passive diffusion in the ileum.

The average non-vegetarian stores between 2,000 and 3,000 picograms (pg, same as micrograms) of B_{12} and loses about 3 pg per day. About 60% of the total amount of the B_{12} in the body is stored in the liver, and 30% is stored in the muscle.[1] The body has a special circulation pattern between the digestive tract and the liver. Through the bile, we secrete 1.4 pg per day of B_{12} into the small intestine, and healthy people reabsorb about 0.7 pg. Research suggests that if people have a low B_{12} intake, the absorption increases to draw even more B_{12} into the system. However, there is still a general potential for slow loss, depending on the variation in this special, what is known as enterohepatic circulation, before we develop the potential of B_{12} deficiency symptoms.[2] Slight differences in enterohepatic circulation may determine how long one can go before developing a B_{12} deficiency.[3] All this is taking place above the large intestine and has nothing to do with how clean the colon is.

Importance of B_{12}

To understand the significance of this issue, we need to understand a little about the importance of B_{12} in the diet. B_{12} has two main functions. One is that methylocobalamin is catalyzed by the enzyme methionine synthase to change homocysteine into methionine. When this enzyme is not working or deficient, the homocysteine in our system increases. Elevated homocysteine also happens with deficiencies in B-6 or folic acid. Recent research has associated this increase with the increased potentiality of heart disease, deterioration of the arteries and nerves, increased hearing loss with age, and a 170% increase in having two or more pregnancy losses in the first trimester.[4] Other diseases associated with an elevated homocysteine are: Alzheimer's, neural tube defects, and increased mortality. When the homocysteine is elevated, it appears to be a nerve toxin, as well as a blood vessel toxin. The second major function of B_{12} is as a coenzyme using 5'-deoxyadenosylcobalamin in the enzyme methyl malonyl-CoA mutase in the conversion of methyl malonyl-CoA to succinyl-CoA.

One of the major symptoms of B_{12} or folic acid deficiency is macrocytic anemia. Folate, also called folic acid, is needed to turn the uracil into thymidine, an essential building block of DNA.[5] This DNA is needed for production of new red blood cells and for red blood cell division. B_{12} is involved in the pathway that creates methyl cobalamin. This B_{12} also produces a form of folate needed to make DNA. So if there is no B_{12}, folate can become depleted and DNA production slows down.

Accurate measurement of B_{12} levels

Another little side-part of the methyl malonyl-CoA to succinyl-CoA conversion is that when the B_{12} is not available, the methyl malonyl-CoA levels increase and are converted to methyl malonic acid, which accumulates in the blood and urine.

Since the B_{12} is the only co-enzyme required in this pathway, methyl malonic acid levels (MMA) in the urine are considered the new gold standard as an indicator of B_{12} deficiency.

Other causes of high methyl malonic acid are genetic defects, kidney failure, low blood volume, dysbiosis, pregnancy, and hypothyroid. The MMA test is important because the progressive medical community no longer considers serum B_{12} levels an accurate measurement of appropriate amounts of B_{12}. In other words, a normal serum B_{12} may not mean that B_{12} levels are healthy. We need a urinary assay of methyl malonic acid really to determine the answer. This is an important point, because when the author first wrote about this issue in *Conscious Eating*, the establishment of the methyl malonic acid assay as the gold standard had not taken place yet. Some of the author's statements at that time were based on the world research, which was using serum B_{12}. A serum B_{12} of 200 pg or more was considered adequate. As a result of the new gold standard and what we know about MMA and homocysteine, the B_{12} serum levels should be around 340–405 pg. In some cases, as high as 450 pg is needed to maintain a normal homocysteine level. Therefore, serum B_{12} levels less than the optimal of 450 pg may be considered as indicating a B_{12} deficiency.

B_{12} Deficiency

There are a variety of symptoms of B_{12} deficiency, which are important to vegans and live-foodists. The first is low energy. It could be a reason why some people just don't feel well on these diets, besides not getting the right protein/carbohydrate/fat mix for their constitutional type. There are specific neurological symptoms, often described as "subacute combined degeneration". Some of this damage can be almost irreversible if it becomes chronic. This nerve system degeneration affects peripheral nerves and the spinal cord. Some of the typical neurological feelings include depression, numbness and tingling in the hands and feet, nervousness, paranoia, hyperactive reflexes, impotence, impaired memory, and behavioral changes. These B_{12} deficiency symptoms are consistent with those suffered by the famous fruitarian Johnny Lovewisdom, who lead a short-lived, vegan community in Ecuador. He suffered from weakness, partial paralysis, and after a few years was unable to stand or walk. Similar symptoms happened in another short-lived fruitarian community in Australia. Other B_{12} deficiency symptoms include: diarrhea, fever, frequent upper respiratory infections, infertility, sore tongue, enlargement of the mucous membranes of the mouth, vagina, and stomach, macrocytic anemia, and low white blood cell and platelet count. These symptoms should not be confused with a "healing crisis". Two of the major possible causes of nerve damage caused by B_{12} deficiency are: (1) a lack of methionine available for conversion into S-adenosylmethionine (SAM) because of lack of sufficient B_{12}. This causes a lack of SAM, which is needed for production of phosphatidyl choline, which is needed to make myelin sheaths (coating for the nerves);[6] (2) the accumulation of propioyl-CoA (a 3 carbon molecule) resulting from the inability to convert methyl malonyl Co-A to succinal Co-A (4 carbon). The result of the excess of propionyl-CoA creates an excess of 15 and 17 carbon chains fatty acids, which are incorporated into nerve structure and which alter nerve function.[7] Some of the causes of B_{12} deficiency are low dietary intake of B_{12} and/or poor absorption, which usually comes through loss of intrinsic factor and/or a lack of stomach acid.

Consistent research over the last decade has shown that vegans and live-food people of all ages and sexes have a much higher risk of becoming B_{12} deficient.[8,9,10,11,12,13,14,15,16,17,18,19,20,21] There are more than 15 studies on vegans and an additional three studies on live-food vegans. The most dramatic was a study done by Dong and Scott on 83 subjects at a Natural Hygiene Society conference. Ninety-two percent of the non-B_{12}-supplementing, primarily live-food vegans were B_{12} deficient. This seems to increase with the amount of time as a vegan. There are no studies that show that vegans do not get deficient over time. This does not mean that everyone becomes B_{12} deficient within six years as previously thought. The problem may not show up for many years. One case study reported by Bernstein[22] in 2000 describes a man in his eighties who had been vegan for 38 years and reported excellent health. Over a period of a few weeks he began to be emotionally erratic, depressed, confused, incontinent, and lost motor skills so significantly he could barely stand without help. Although diagnosed as "senile dementia" his B_{12} was so low it was not detectable. Fortunately, after one B_{12} injection he could sit without help by the next morning. The incontinence stopped within 48 hours, and by the end of one week his mental state returned close to normal.

B_{12} deficiency is particularly hazardous for newborn babies, especially babies of vegan live-food nursing mothers who are not using B_{12} supplementation. Since 1980 there have been 130 reports of serious B_{12} deficiency in the infants of vegan mothers whose primary food was breast milk and the mothers did not supplement their own or the babies' diets with B_{12}. Lack of B_{12} in the mother's diet has been shown to cause a severe lack of myelin in nerve tissue.[23] B_{12} supplementation in infants has shown a rapid increase in B_{12} values, but the question is if there are some long-term developmental problems, even if the B_{12} values are returned to normal. Von Schenck, in a review of 27 cases of infant B_{12} deficiency done in 1997, suggested that in many there was permanent damage. Seven were followed for twelve years after diagnosis. Five of these seven had abnormal neurological development twelve years later. Vegan pregnant mothers need to supplement with B_{12} during pregnancy and while breastfeeding. Goraya, in 1998 in India, reported many infants had a B_{12} deficiency in breastfed infants in low socio-economic status. Some, but not all, responded to B_{12} therapy.[24] The conclusion is obvious: prevention is the key concept. In contrast to the average adult storage of 2,000–3,000 pg of B_{12}, newborns of mothers with normal B_{12} have about 25 pg. Studies have shown that the milk during the first week of life does contain large amounts of B_{12}.[25] The B_{12} storage in infants at birth is normally adequate to last the first few weeks of life.[26] Afterwards, they must get it from breast-milk or other sources. If a vegan or live-food mother is already B_{12}

deficient during pregnancy, the baby may be born with seriously low B_{12} levels and develop clinical signs of deficiency as soon as two weeks.[27] The general research suggests that even among non-vegetarians, B_{12} can be insufficient in infants, and that perhaps *all* breastfeeding mothers should consider B_{12} supplements for themselves and their infants during the time of breastfeeding. This lack of B_{12} in the mother's diet during pregnancy has been associated with a lack of myelin production, which is the coating of the nerves.[28] A B_{12} deficiency in a baby takes somewhere between one to twelve months to develop. It often manifests as failure to thrive and slow developmental progression. The babies are often lethargic, lose their ability to use muscle adequately, have tremors, and even their sensory attunement decreases; they also have irregular macrocytic anemia.[29,30] There is some question, even though the values return to normal, that children with a sustained B_{12} deficiency before starting B_{12} supplementation may have sustained abnormal neurological development.

The good news, as supported by at least one major study in the United Kingdom in 1988, which showed, in studying 37 vegan children, that there was normal growth and development in children who were breastfed for six months at a minimum, when there was B_{12} supplementation.[31] Other studies have shown that young and teenage children who were supplemented with B_{12} were found to grow normally.[32,33]

Adults who were vegetarian without B_{12} supplementation for greater than six years usually had lower B_{12} than non-vegetarian adults in the general research. In one study of adults by Crane et al[34] in 1994, 81% of the vegan adults had a B_{12} lower than 200 pg and 19% of those were less than 100 pg. That is approximately the percentage of adults who are low in B_{12} in most vegan and live-food studies. In the author's clinical experience, meat eaters as well as vegans and live-fooders tend to have a fairly high percentage of B_{12} deficiency, although the incidence is less in meat eaters. In vegetarians and vegans, there is also a high percentage under 200 pg. In one study there were 62% under 200 pg and 19% under 100 pg.[35] As mentioned previously, a study in 1982 by Dong and Scott[36] of live-food vegans with 83 subjects from the Natural Hygiene Society showed that 92% of the vegans had a B_{12} less than 200 pg, and in 53% it was less than 100 pg. The World Health Organization (WHO) considers B_{12} deficiency to be less than 200 pg using the old criteria. The percentages of B_{12} deficiency tend to increase over time on a natural hygiene diet. Another study in Finland in 1995 Rauma et al[37] that examined B_{12} status of long-term 100% live-food vegans found that 66% of the people had a B_{12} lower than 200 pg. One study done in 2000 by Donaldson[38] at Hallelujah Acres on primarily live-food practitioners, but with some B_{12} supplementation via nutritional yeast, showed only about 15% of the people were less than 200, and none of them less than 160. The supplementation with nutritional yeast was 5 pg of B_{12} from one tablespoon of Red Star Vegetarian Support. Repeated studies on vegans in a variety of different world regions all showed a significant B_{12} deficiency in vegans who did no B_{12} supplementation, especially if they were vegan for six years or more. Some of these studies included: in Australia with Seventh Day Adventist ministers by Hokin and Butler in 1995[39]; in Thailand in 1988 by Areekul et al[40]; in

1990 in Israel by Bar-Sella et al[41]; by Tungtrongchitrat et al in 1993[42]; Crane et al in 1994[43]; and in China in 1998 by Woo et al[44]. There seemed to be an increase in B_{12} deficiency over time. When vegans took B_{12} supplements, there was no significant difference between the vegan and non-vegetarian B_{12} levels.[45,46] This is also true with elderly B_{12} supplemented lacto-ovo vegetarians versus non-vegetarians.[47,48]

Many non-vegetarians also have a poor B_{12} status because there are many other factors that can cause B_{12} deficiency. They include: malabsorption or inadequate intake of protein, calories, or B_{12}, radiation exposure, drugs, and a variety of toxins, paraminosalicylic acid, alcohol, pancreatic tumors, failure of the small intestine to contract and move food associated with bacterial overgrowth, oral contraceptives, fungal infections, liver and kidney disease, tobacco smoking, B_6 or iron deficiency, and mental stress.

B_{12} in Food
Up until this time, many of us have felt that additional supplementation for live-food practitioners, with sea vegetables or probiotic formulas, was sufficient for protection against B_{12} deficiency. This does not seem to be the case according to research. In macrobiotics practitioners, who primarily cook their food, we see a very high percentage of children actually having growth retardation due to low B_{12} intake. Many of us have felt that spirulina, aphazonimom-flo-aque (AFA), and all the sea vegetables had enough active B_{12} to avoid a B_{12} deficiency. Although the research is not fully in, we do know that, as pointed out in *Conscious Eating*, these substances do have human active B_{12}. The problem is they also have a significant amount of analog B_{12} that competes with the human active B_{12}. This analog amount was not measured in the author's studies that were presented in *Conscious Eating*. Using the methyl malonic acid excretion approach, which is now the gold standard, research showed that when people used dry-roasted and raw nori from Japan, the dry-roasted nori actually made the methyl malonic acid (MMA) status worse; it actually reduced the B_{12} status. Therefore dry-roasted nori could possibly worsen a B_{12} deficiency. Raw nori seemed to keep the methyl malonic acid at the same level, meaning it did not harm the B_{12} status, but the research showed it did not particularly help it either. No food in Europe or the US that has been tested shows that it lowers methyl malonic acid. Research absolutely has to be done to answer this question fully. The author is hopeful that the gold-standard level of research in the future will reveal an authentic, natural, B_{12}, vegan food. Already, Vision Industries, Inc., is interested in doing this level of B_{12} research with AFA.

There are many ideas of vegan foods that may have active B_{12}, but few are proving to actually raise B_{12} levels or prevent its loss.[49,50,51,52] The research has shown, for example, that tempeh (cultured soy) does not supply human active B_{12}. Research in both the US and the Netherlands has confirmed this.[53,54] There was one paper by Areekul et al. in Thailand in 1990[55] that showed that tempeh from one particular source in Thailand did have some B_{12} analog, but what they basically found was that fermented soybean did not contain B_{12} but that *Klebsiella pneumoniae* was isolated from the commercial tempeh starter. Other foods such as barley, malted syrup, sourdough bread, parsley, shitake mushrooms, tofu, and soybean paste, had some B_{12} in them but did not seem to alter B_{12} status. Amazake rice, barley miso, miso, natto, rice miso, shoyu, tamari, umeboshi, and a variety of nuts, seeds, and grains did not contain any elements or even any detectable B_{12} analog. The author's study using the earlier gold-standard test of using B_{12} active bacteria to determine human active B_{12} did show indeed that arame, dulse, kelp, kombu, and wakame had significant human active B_{12}. But research suggests they have higher analog concentrations which may cancel their human B_{12} effect. A study done in 1991 by Miller found that serum B_{12} appeared to be unrelated to consumption of wakame, kombu, and other sea vegetables or tempeh in macrobiotic children. Other researchers feel that it is possible that raw nori, not dry-roasted nori, is a source of active B_{12}. Other studies have shown that dulse did have a certain amount of B_{12} analogue per serving.

Until research is done to see if these actually lower the methyl malonic acid levels, the issue we raise is, we cannot assume that because a food has human active B_{12} it will help avoid B_{12} deficiency, because the actual non-human active analogs may be blocking the human active B_{12}. The same question arises now with the aphanizomenon flos-aqua (AFA), spirulina, as well as chlorella. So, until we actually do the gold standard test of these, with the urine methyl malonic test, to see if it actually lowers the methyl malonic acid, it is reasonable to eat these foods, but not count that they are actually going to raise your human active B_{12}.

Getting B_{12} in less tasteful ways
There is one exception to this lack of vegetarian B_{12}, which is that we do produce B_{12} from bacteria in our large intestine, but since this B_{12} is produced in the area below where B_{12} is reabsorbed, it is really not available for absorption. Some people have argued that a lot of species of lower mammals do not need B_{12}. The reason why this is true is that a lot of species that are primarily vegetarian animals eat their feces. Human research also has shown if you eat your feces, you will get enough B_{12} (The author does not recommend this practice). Dr. Herbert sponsored research in England where vegan volunteers with a documented B_{12} deficiency were fed B_{12} extractions made from their own feces.[56] It cured their B_{12} deficiency. So, there is a natural vegan way to do it. It may not be the most tasteful way, however. The issue is not about clean bowels. B_{12} producing bacteria were growing in their bowels, but humans do not normally absorb B_{12} from the large intestine.

Some have theorized that organic foods, in various regions, would improve the B_{12} tests by lowering the MMA levels. Unfortunately, there has been no research to show that washed or unwashed organic food has made a difference in lowering the MMA. One study by Mozafar[57] in 1994 has shown that when B_{12} analogs are placed in the soil with cow or human manure, the plants do absorb them. Unfortunately, many soils in the US and around the world are deficient in B_{12}. Many animals, aside from eating their own feces, will ingest a variety of eggs, insects, small vertebrates, or soils. For example, gorillas, who are the closest to vegan of all the species, will eat insects and sometimes their feces.

So there are ways to do this for vegans, but again, they may not be the most aesthetic or tasteful. The author would love, at this point, to come up with an alternative to this, however it doesn't seem to be the case.

The need for more research

The author's serum B_{12} of 600 pg may have thrown off his conclusions when he wrote his summary in *Conscious Eating* in 1990. The author's body may have been within that 20% of vegans and live-food practitioners that don't seem to be affected within the first six to ten years. But he remains more concerned about the other 80% that are B_{12} deficient and the approximately 50% whose B_{12} levels go down to less than 100 pg over six years. These overall conclusions are not finalized. Although there is not enough research to prove there is absolutely no vegan food that increases human B_{12} in the system, there is enough to suggest a preventative approach of supplementation. It is a possible suggestion that large amounts of dulse, raw nori, and an algae called cocolithophorid algae, also known as pleurochritias cartera, may provide sufficient human active B_{12}. Unfortunately, they have not been fully tested with the gold standard. It took 30 years to prove smoking cigarettes causes cancer, but why wait 30 years to find out?

Healthy levels of B_{12}

The next question is, what is a healthy level of B_{12} in the blood serum? The answer is that a serum level of 340–405 pg keeps the homocysteine level down within normal levels, and 450 pg may give optimal coverage for most everyone. The normal serum homocysteine level is 2.2–13.2 micromoles/liter. The normal adult urine MMA is .58–3.56 micromoles/mmol/cr. The normal level of B_{12} for breast milk is 180–300 pg per ml. The normal urine level for children is 820–11,200 micromoles/mmol/cr of MMA. The normal serum B_{12} level of children is 160–1300 pg per ml.

Using the methyl malonic acid test as the gold standard, elevated methyl malonic acid was found in subjects with a B_{12} up to 486 pg. This is a really important statement, because up until this time, most of the studies in the world health basically say that 200 pg and above is not considered deficient. That was somewhat why *Conscious Eating* suggested that B_{12} in many vegans and raw foodists was low-normal, but still within normal. Using the gold standard urine methyl malonic acid test, studies show that without supplementing with B_{12}, vegans have higher homocysteine levels than lacto-ovo vegetarians and non-vegetarians, which means they are deficient in B_{12}. The good news, of course, is that B_{12} supplementation will decrease these high homocysteine levels back to normal range.

Supplementation of B_{12}

The research conclusion is that: it is a reasonably safe bet that about 80% of the vegan and live-food population, within six to ten years, runs the risk of a subclinical or clinical B_{12} deficiency and increased homocysteine levels. Perhaps over a 30-to-50-year span it may reach 100%. An even higher percentage of newborns run this risk. Out of concern for all, particularly for the author's fellow live-food practitioners and vegans, it is well advised to supplement with an actual B_{12} human active supplement, especially during pregnancy and while breastfeeding. There are vegan B_{12} supplements, which allow us to be fully successful vegan, live-food practitioners.

The author's general recommendation is that if you have symptoms of B_{12} deficiency, you can even start with a 1,000 pg injection, or according to the research, an oral administration of 1,000 pg per day for two to four weeks, which is equal to repeated monthly injections. After about a month of the oral, the dose can be cut in half. One can even cut that in half, too. Nutritional Red Star yeast is a B_{12} fortified food that significantly cuts the B_{12} deficiency rate down to 15% in one study, but as a yeast it can activate candida. The safest and healthiest approach is to do the supplementation approach with a B_{12} living extract.

The art of supplementation for B_{12} is relatively simple. The minimal need is about 6 pg or micrograms per day. We lose 3 pg per day. At the Tree of Life we have an activated high-cellular resonance B_{12} supplement that has 6 pg per ½ teaspoon. The author recommends a minimum of ½ teaspoon two times per day in water. This liquid form is ideal for children. The author feels that a smaller daily intake better mimics how the body assimilates B_{12}. Chewing a B_{12} tablet or letting it dissolve in the mouth is also a simple way. Crane *et al.* in 1994 suggested a 100–500 mg tablet a minimum of one time per week if the tablet was chewed. Those who chewed a 100 mg tablet one time per week for six weeks brought their B_{12} from a below normal of 116 up to 291. Those who swallowed it without chewing, raised it from 123 to 139. B_{12} supplements made of cyanocobalamin are damaged by prolonged light exposure.[58,59] Because of vulnerability of smokers to cyanocobalamin, oral supplementation with methylcobalamin (dibencozide) and adeosyl cobalamin (co-enzyme B_{12}) can be used. Hydroxy cobalamin is also a good form of supplement but is primarily in the injectible form. The Tree of Life uses this form for injection. Research shows that it is retained in the body more than cyanocobalamin. Methylcobalamin and adenosylcobalmin requires 1000–2000 mg per day for adequate supplementation.

Another question that is relevant to B_{12} supplementation is how much is safe? The Institute of Medicine has not set an upper limit on what is unsafe for B_{12} intake. Other researchers suggest that B_{12} intake of 500–1000 mg per day is completely safe and that the cobalt and cyanide contribution in 1000 mg of cyanocobalamin are toxicologically insignificant.[60] However, people with cyanide metabolism defects, chronic kidney failure, and smokers are safest to use another form than cyanocobalamin. This is because they may have a compromised cyanide detoxification system. There is not, at this time, any significant evidence that cyanocobalamin has been shown to be harmful to vegan smokers. It is more of a theoretical consideration.

Some people eat according to their philosophy and belief of what they feel is natural. This may cause problems. For example, the black Hebrews, a group of African-Americans who have migrated to Israel, have horrendously high levels of infant B_{12} deficiency, with a certain amount of B_{12} deficient deaths, as well as adult B_{12} deficiency. They did not believe in taking supplements. Data in a 1982 study by Shinwell and Gorodischer [61]showed that of the infants who were breastfed for three months, and then were given diluted homemade soymilk for three months to one year, 25 of them (a significant percentage) had protein deficiency, iron and B_{12} anemia, as well as zinc deficiency. In the 1982 study, three of the infants were dead on arrival, five more died within a few hours of hospital admission, despite treatment. Serum levels were low in nine of 15 cases and undetectable in three. This is a not very good example to show the world how we want to treat our children. We can make those choices. There is a theory of what it means to be natural, but there is also a theory of what it means to be healthy.

What we mean by "being successful" is in being completely healthy, which includes having no B_{12} deficiency and no elevated homocysteine levels. It is the author's medical opinion as a holistic physician, nutritionist, vegan since 1973, live-food vegan since 1983, and as a person committed to supporting all those who choose to become healthy live-food vegans, that it would be wise to incorporate some B_{12} supplementation in your diet. It is more natural to be healthy than it is to be anything less than that. It may be the first time in history since the Garden of Eden that as a culture we have the capacity to healthfully follow the vegan teaching of Genesis 1:29.

Summary

- B_{12} is critical for optimum health and well being.
- Approximately 80% of children and adult vegans and live-food practitioners become B_{12} deficient after 6–10 years without B_{12} supplementation.
- Infants with B_{12} deficient breastfeeding mothers may become deficient in as short as two weeks and suffer irreparable damage.
- The author strongly recommends B_{12} supplementation for all vegan and live-food practitioners to maintain optimal health and well being.

About the Authors:
Gabriel Cousens, M.D., M.D. (H) Diplomat American Board of Holistic Medicine, Diplomat Ayurveda. Dr. Cousens is an internationally celebrated healer, spiritual facilitator, peace-worker, author and lecturer. The founder and director of the Tree of Life Rejuvenation Center in Arizona, USA, Dr. Cousens is also a best-selling author whose titles include Spiritual Nutrition, Rainbow Green Live Food Cuisine, Conscious Eating, Depression-Free for Life and There Is A Cure for Diabetes. Currently the Tree of Life 21 Day program is being offered in two locations, Tree of Life US and Tree of Life by the Dead Sea.

To Reach Us in the US
For more information on our programs or for reservations, fill in the "Call-Me-Now" form at www.treeoflife.nu, or call toll-free 1-866-394-2520 (local 1-520-394-2520).
Tree of Life Rejuvenation Center

P.O. Box 778 (mail)
686 Harshaw Road (shipping)
Patagonia, AZ 85624 USA
Toll-free 1-866-394-2520; local 1-520-394-2520
E-mail: info@treeoflife.nu
Website: www.treeoflife.nu

To Reach us at The Tree of Life at the Dead Sea

Serving Israel and European communities. The Center is located thirty minutes from the holy city of Jerusalem and forty-five minutes from Tel Aviv International Airport. For further information, international air and road travel, and registration, please call Ya'ara at +972-50-226-7596.
E-mail treeoflife.israel@gmail.com.
Website at http://www.treeoflife.org.il

Dr. Brian Clement, *PhD, NMD, LNC, has spearheaded the International progressive health movement for more than three decades. By conducting daily clinical research as the director of the renowned Hippocrates Health Institute, the world's foremost complementary residential health Mecca, he and his team have developed a state-of-the-art program for health maintenance and recovery. His Florida (U.S.A.) center has pioneered a program and established training in active aging and disease prevention. With hundreds of thousands of people participating in this program over the last half-century, volumes of data have been accrued, giving Clement a privileged insight into the lifestyle required to maintain youth, vitality, and stamina. Among Dr. Clement's many publications are Living Foods for Optimum Health and Longevity and Lifeforce. His latest book, Longevity, delivers cutting-edge knowledge coupled with a common sense practical approach that will raise your level of health and happiness.*

Dr. Clement is first and foremost a devoted husband and a caring father of four. In addition to daily counseling and research studies, Clement conducts conferences worldwide on attaining health and creating longevity, giving delegates a roadmap for redirecting, enriching and extending their lives.

www.hippocratesinst.org

(Endnotes)

1   Messina M, Messina V. The Dietician's Guide to Vegetarian Diets. Gaithersburg, MD: Aspen Publishers, Inc., 1996

2   Donaldson MS. Metabolic vitamin B-12 status on a mostly raw vegan diet with follow-up using tablets, nutritional yeast, or probiotic supplements. Ann Nutr Metab. 2000;44(5-6):229-34. And personal communication with author Jan 31, 2002.

3   Kuhne T, Bubl R, Baumgartner R. Maternal vegan diet causing a serious infantile neurological disorder due to vitamin B12 deficiency. Eur J Pediatr 1991 Jan;150(3):205-8

4   Nelen WL, Blom HJ, Steegers EA, denHeijer M, Eskes TK. Hyperhomocysteinemia and recurrent early pregnancy loss: a meta-analysis. Fertil Steril. 2000 Dec;74(6):1196-9

5   Guyton AC, Hall JE. Textbook of Medical Physiology, 9th ed. Philadelphia, PA: W.B.

Saunders, Co: 1996. p. 845-7.
6   Grattan-Smith PJ, Wilcken B, Procopis PG, Wise GA. The neurological syndrome of infantile cobalamin deficiency: developmental regression and involuntary movements. Mov Disord 1997 Jan;12(1):39-46.
7   von Schenck U, Bender-Gotze C, Koletzko B. Persistence of neurological damage induced by dietary vitamin B-12 deficiency in infancy. Arch Dis Child 1997Aug;77(2):137-9.
8   Ashkenazi S, Weitz R, Varsano I, Mimouni M. Vitamin B-12 deficiency due to a strictly vegetarian diet in adolescence. Clinical Pediatrics 1987;26(Dec):662-663.
9   Sanders TA, Purves R. An anthropometric and dietary assessment of the nutritional status of vegan preschool children. J Hum Nutr 1981 Oct;35(5):349-57.
10   Hokin BD, Butler T. Cyanocobalamin (vitamin B-12) status in Seventh-day Adventist ministers in Australia. Am J Clin Nutr 1999 Sep;70(3 Suppl):576S-578S.
11   Areekul S, Pattanamatum S, Cheeramakara C, Churdchue K, Nitayapabskoon S, Chongsanguan M. The source and content of vitamin B-12 in the tempehs. J Med Assoc Thai 1990 Mar;73(3):152-6.
12   Bar-Sella P, Rakover Y, Ratner D. Vitamin B12 and folate levels in long-term vegans. Isr J Med Sci 1990;26:309-312.
13   Tungtrongchitr R, Pongpaew P, Prayurahong B, Changbumrung S, Vudhivai N, Migasena P, Schelp FP. Vitamin B12, folic acid and haematological status of 132 Thai vegetarians. Int J Vitam Nutr Res 1993;63(3):201-7.
14   Campbell M, Lofters WS, Gibbs WN. Rastafarianism and the vegans syndrome. BMJ (Clin Res Ed) 1982 Dec 4;285(6355):1617-8.
15   Crane MG, Sample C, Pathcett S, Register UD. Vitamin B12 studies in total vegetarians (vegans). Journal of Nutritional Medicine 1994;4:419-430.
16   Crane MG, Register UD, Lukens RH, Gregory R. Cobalamin (CBL) studies on two total vegetarian (vegan) families. Vegetarian Nutrition 1998;2(3):87-92.
17   Haddad EH, Berk LS, Kettering JD, Hubbard RW, Peters WR. Dietary intake and biochemical, hematologic, and immune status of vegans compared with non-vegetarians. Am J Clin Nutr 1999;70(suppl):586S-93S.
18   Woo J, Kwok T, Ho SC, Sham A, Lau E. Nutritional status of elderly Chinese vegetarians. Age Ageing 1998 Jul;27(4):455-61.
19   Dong A, Scott SC. Serum vitamin B12 and blood cell values in vegetarians. Ann Nutr Metab 1982;26(4):209-16.
20   Rauma AL, Torronen R, Henninen O, MykkanaenH. Vitamin B-12 status of long-term adherents of a strict uncooked vegan diet ("living food diet") is compromised. J Nutr 1995 Oct;125(10):2511-5.
21   Donaldson MS. Op. cit.
22   Bernstein, L. Dementia without a cause. Discover February 2003:31
23   Lovblad Kirlian, Ramelli Genes, Remonda L, Nirkko AC, Ozdoba C, Schroth G. Retardationof myelination due to dietary B12 deficiency: cranial MRI findings. Pediatr Radiol 1997 Feb;27(2):155-8.
24   Goraya J. letter about Persistence of neurological damage induced by dietary vitamin B12 deficiency. Arch Dis Child 1998;78(4):398-9.
25   Specker BL, Miller D, Norman EJ, Greene H, Hayes KC. Increased urinary methylmalonic acid excretion in breast-fed infants of vegetarian mothers and identification of an acceptable dietary source of vitamin B-12. Am J Clin Nutr 1988 Jan;47(1):89-92.
26   Kuhne T, Bubl R, Baumgartner R. Maternal vegan diet causing a serious infantile neurological disorder due to vitamin B12 deficiency. Eur J Pediatr 1991 Jan;150(3):205-8.
27   Drogari E, Liakopoulou-Tsitsipi T, Xypolyta-Zachariadi A, Papadellis F, Kattamis C. Transient methylmalonic aciduria in four breast fed neonates of strict vegetarian mothers in Greece. Journal of inherited metabolic disease. 1996 19S:A84. Abstract.
28   Lovblad K, Ramelli G, Remonda L, Nirkko AC, Oxdoba C, Schroth G. Retardation of myelination due to dietary vitamin B12 deficiency: cranial MRI findings. Pediatr Radiol 1997 Feb;27(2):155-8.
29   Davis JR, Goldenring J, Lubin B. Nutritional vitamin B12 deficiency in infants. Am J Dis Child 1981(Jun);135:566-7.
30   Lovblad K, et. al. Op. cit.
31   Sanders TA. Vegetarian diets and children. Pediatr Clin North Am 1995 Aug;42(4):955-65.
32   Sanders and Purves. Op. cit.
33   Fulton JR, Hutton CW, Stitt KR. Preschool vegetarian children. Dietary and anthropometric

data. J Am Diet Assoc 1980 Apr;76(4):360-5.
34   Crane et. al. 1994 Op. cit.
35   Ibid.
36   Dong and Scott. Op. cit.
37   Rauma AL, Torronen R, Hanninen O, Mykkanen H. Vitamin B-12 status of long-term adherents of a strict uncooked vegan diet ("living food diet") is compromised. J Nutr 1995 Oct;125(10):2511-5.
Donaldson MS. Op. cit.
38   Hokin and Butler. Op. cit.
39   Areekul S, Churdchu K, Pungpapong V. Serum folate, vitamin B12 and vitamin B12 binding protein in vegetarians. J Med Assoc Thai 1988 May;71(5):253-7.
40   Bar-Sella, et. al. Op. cit.
41   Tungtrongchitr, et. al. Op. cit.
42   Crane, et. al. 1994. Op. cit.
43   Woo, et. al. Op. cit.
44   Harman SK, Parnell WR. The nutritional health of New Zealand vegetarian and non-vegetarian Seventh-day Adventists: selected vitamin, mineral and lipid levels. NZ Med J 1998 Mar 27;111(1062):91-4.
45   Alexander D, Ball MJ, Mann J. Nutrient intake and haematological status of vegetarians and age-sex matched omnivores. European Journal of Clinical Nutrition 1994;48:538-546.
46   Brants HA, Lowik MR, Westenbrink S, Hulshof KF, Kistemaker C. Adequacy of a vegetarian diet at old age (Dutch Nutrition Surveillance System). J Am Coll Nutr 1990 Aug;9(4):292-302.
47   Campbell et. al. Op. cit.
48   Herbert V. Vitamin B-12: plant sources, requirements, and assay. Am J Clin Nutr 1988;48: 852-8.
49   Areekul et. al. 1990 Op. cit.
50   van den Berg H, Dagnelie PC van Stveren WA. Vitamin B-12 and Seaweed. Lancet Jan 30, 1988.
51   Specker et. al. Op. cit.
52   Ibid.
53   van den Berg et. al. Op. cit.
54   Areekul et. al. 1990 Op. cit.
55   Shinwell ED, Gorodischer R. Totally vegetarian diets and infant nutrition. Pediatrics 1982 Oct;70(4):582-6.
56   Mozafar A. Enrichment of some B vitamins in plants with application of organic fertilizers. Plant & Soil 1994;167:305-311.
57   Areekul et. al. 1988 Op. cit.
58   Sneider Zinc, Stroinski A. Comprehensive B12. New York: Walter de Gruyter, 1987.
59   Libidium Kirlian, McKay G. Images in clinical medicine. Ischemic retinopathy caused by severe megaloblastic anemia. N Engl J Med 2000 Mar 23;342(12):860
60   Hathcock JN, Troendle GJ. Oral cobalamin for treatment of pernicious anemia? JAMA 1991 Jan 2;265(1):96-7

17

Dark Field Microscopy

Anna Maria Clement, PhD, NMD, LNC

For half a century we have explored human health and the components that promote disease prevention and elimination, as well as prevent premature aging. Twenty-five years ago we began to use microscopic blood research to determine the best course of action for those aspiring to superior health. This tool has afforded us significant insight into the workings of the human body and mind. We have discovered that every experience, be it physical, emotional or mental, impacts human cells, which of course are the structure of our total anatomy. After conducting tens of thousands of studies, a clear pattern has emerged, and now we can apply this finding in the quest to guide people in every aspect of their lives. Hippocrates Institute is blessed to have had so many pioneers in the study of dark field microscopy that we thank them for all of their efforts, sincerity, and scientific contributions.

The nature of disease
The history around the nature of disease is well described by The Body Therapy Wellness Center: "The argument about the nature of disease became more divided in 19th-century France. Louis Pasteur was a French chemist who lived between 1822 and 1895. He described the scientific basis for fermentation, the process used to make beer and wine, showing that it is carried out by microorganisms, called germs. Pasteur learned that these germs are also responsible for spreading contagious disease, at least infectious disease that came from outside the body as an invader.

Claude Bernard was a French physiologist who first discovered that the body makes every effort to maintain a steady internal state (the internal environment). He included the immune system as part of that finding.

Antoine Be'champ was a French microbiologist and medical school professor who was often at odds with Pasteur. Pasteur believed that bacteria were the significant players in infectious disease. Be'champ believed that the internal environment described by Bernard was the significant player. He attempted to prove this at a medical meeting by drinking a glass of water containing a large quantity of cholera germs. He was not affected by the deadly cholera, proving that his system was more important than his encounter with the bacteria.

In addition to his debate with Pasteur about the internal or external cause of infectious disease, Be'champ identified tiny biological particles that he called microzymes. He found microzymes in all cells, dead or alive, and in ancient chalk deposits. He found that these fundamental biological units could change into pathological bacteria. This was the beginning of the concept of pleomorphism (many forms, described below). This means that something can change into many different things.

On his deathbed, Pasteur conceded that he was wrong and Be'champ was correct. However, this had very little effect on Pasteur's disciples. The concept of Pasteur that infectious disease is caused by coming into contact with pathogenic bacteria became the standard belief of most physicians today. Lost for many years, the concept of Be'champ (pleomorphism) was that the pathogen came from within the body when the internal environment was out of balance.

> **The concept of pasteur that infectious disease is caused by coming into contact with pathogenic bacteria became the standard belief of most physicians today.**

Pleomorphism
Be'champ's pleomorphism theory of a basic building unit of the universe (which he called microzymes) was ignored for many years. German physician and bacteriologist Gunther Enderlein described the life cycle of bacteria in 1916. He found tiny particles in blood that he called protits. Under normal conditions, he found the protits to work symbiotically with the immune system. However, when the pH of the blood changed, the protits changed into pathogenic bacteria. The protit merge to form rudimentary nuclei called symprotits. The symprotits then add a tail to form a sperm-shaped unit called a spermit. The spermits enter the red blood cells (RBC) and one can see multiple tails sticking out of the cells as they enter. Once inside the red blood cells they begin to multiply and mature. They consume the red blood cells as they grow. As the volume of red blood cells decreases, the maturing forms look like barnacles on a ship. However, the forms are really inside the transparent cell membrane of the red blood cell. The form gradually matures and then exits the red blood cells as bacteria without cell walls

– mycoplasma. When mycoplasma enters other cells they are called rickettsia. Mycoplasma and rickettsia are the major cause of chronic diseases. One of the forms that can exit the RBC's is Proprionbacteria acne. This bacterial form is often found in the mouth around the teeth. It is also the precursor of the fungus which is present in all cancer, Mucor Racemos fresen.

It is likely that the microzyme of Be'champ and the protit of Enderlein are the same thing. Certainly they both reached the same startling conclusion. They discovered that an element normally present in all cells could become pathogenic bacteria from inside the body. Thus it is not necessary that the body be externally exposed to pathogenic bacteria to become ill. Enderlein discovered that all cancer cells contain the same fungus, Mucor racemes fresen.

In the 1940s and early 1950s Enderlein developed biological remedies from plants and fungal extracts, which he found capable of changing pathogenic bacteria back into harmless protits by changing the tissues' pH back to normal. In the 1920s and 1930s Royal Raymond Rife, a bacteriologist in San Diego was trying to find the cause for cancer. He discovered that a cancer-causing organism was found to have four forms, which he called the BX (associated with carcinoma), Virus BY (associated with sarcomas), Monoccoid forms (found in more that 90% of cancer patients), and crytomices fungi. He found that these forms could change in the laboratory from one form to another in 36 hours. Note the finding of those similar to Enderlein. Rife discovered that these pathogens could be killed with a radio frequency of 2127 or 2128 Hz, which was used at the University of California School of Medicine with documented success. All 16 terminal cancer patients were successfully treated under the observance of a team of doctors from various universities. However, he was later accused of quackery and taken to court. He was found guilty, but his work had been burned and his equipment destroyed by corporate forces.

In 1946, a French scientist named Gaston Naessen noted some unusual particles in blood samples he was studying. Because they are barely visible with standard light microscopes, he set out to develop a different type of microscope. He developed a special type of "Dark Field" microscope in which one could see the interior of living cells in their live state. (Light microscopes require that the tissues be killed and dyed with stain to reveal their internal parts) Using this high powered dark field he defined the particles, which he called somatids (small bodies). Naessen found that these somatids were capable of pleomorphism. They could change from particles the size of viruses to bacteria, yeast, and fungal forms. He also noted that chronic diseases such as rheumatoid arthritis, multiple sclerosis, lupus, and cancer showed fungal forms in the blood cells."

Another view I have gained insight from is that of Norman Alan. "A second approach to live-blood analysis has been assembled from many sources of Professor Lida Mattman of the Wayne State University and her colleague, Dr. Phil Hockstra. Micro-organisms, when challenged, shed their cell walls. While this leaves them less virulent, it also makes them less vulnerable. Shedding their skins, they lose most of the markers that identify them as foreign bodies to our immune systems. They can also now change their shape – this simple change of shape is also called pleomorphism – and this means they can easily invade and hide in the body's own cells.

In live blood analysis as taught by Dr. Hoskstra, attention is paid to the microbes, to the shape and activity of the white blood cells and red blood cells. By observing the red cells we can tell a lot about the state of metabolism in general and of the liver in particular. Meanwhile, observing the white cells gives us a reading on the state of the immune system, and the pattern of microbes tells us if disease is overwhelming the body's defense. Note that while we call this "live-blood" analysis, it is really dying blood that we are observing. In a sense we are watching how quickly decay sets in after we take the drop of blood out of the body and this tells us how much resilience and vitality there is in the body. It is a measure of the body's health."

Live blood testing

Live blood testing is a way to screen hematological status by using phase contrast and dark field microscopy. We use phase contrast in viewing fungus, bacteria and crystallized structure living cells and to see details that we could not see otherwise. Dark field illuminates reflex on slide, especially low-contrast crystallized forms that phase contrast would hardly pick up. It is of invaluable help at Hippocrates in choosing supplements and therapies for our individual programs. It is not a conventional diagnostic tool. What we observe in dried blood (we use droplets of capillary blood from the top of the pinkie finger) is biochemical reactions that leave cellular patterns that correlate with an anatomical and emotional history. From this, one can gain extraordinary insight into the current functions and dysfunctions of the total individual.

> **Every experience, be it physical, mental or emotional, impacts human cells.**

One of the consistent observations gleaned from repeat testing of those who adopt a living food diet is the evidence of greatly reduced stress and widely enhanced nutritional gains. This is exceptionally true when one maintains the raw/living lifestyle, as it can dramatically reduce negative patterns that have impacted the cellular system throughout the body. Most interesting in the observation of live blood is the consistent increase of electrical frequency in and around the cells after a person continues a green live-food diet over a period of time. This phenomenon is significant, because this electrical shield prevents free radicals from killing healthy red blood cells. It is free radical damage that causes all premature aging and disease. Anti-oxidants, phyto-chemicals, proteins, vitamins, minerals, hormones, oxygen, and enzymes inherent to living food are the contributing factors to this high frequency savior of the cells. When food is cooked it is either void or greatly lacking in these essential elements.

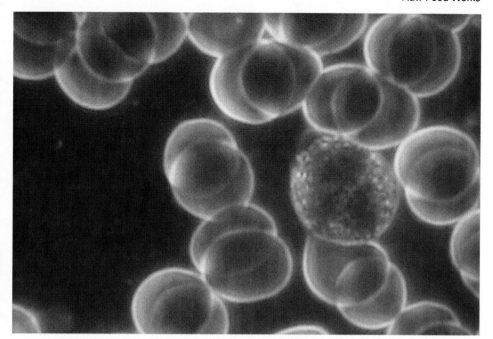

Figure 1: Healthy red blood cells with one leukocyte (white blood cell)

After seeing multitudes of people's blood microscopically, the most common sight is *rouleaux* which is sticking and stacking of red blood cells. This is an indication of the lack of life and oxygen that these cells suffer, in great part due to the absence of protein and the presence of excessive fats, sugars, and prescription medications.

One of the most common maladies today is accumulated plaque. Throughout the ventrical system this reflects in the live cells as large crystals. This plaque reduces blood flow, preventing full nourishment and oxygenation of the organs throughout the body. Additionally, it greatly increases the possibility of cardiovascular disease, heart attack, strokes, phlebitis, etc.

Platelets made in bone marrow have a lifespan of 11 days. They circulate in the blood and form a plug if vascular damage has occurred. They also promote coagulation. Seen under the microscope, they appear to be 1/3 the size of blood cells (small discs). When platelets have been mutated they look like spider webs under the microscope. It is usually an indication of liver stress, infections, alcohol, medications, etc. Nowadays this is a much more frequent event due to increasingly poor diets, air and water pollution, pharmaceuticals, lack of exercise, and emotional stress. Problems with excess fat in the blood stream may cause platelets to stick together, promoting capillary blockage, and may be the cause of strokes or heart attacks.

Nutritional deficiencies are also exposed in both live and dried blood tests. These deficiencies either reflect as chronic (long-term) or recent. When the cells lack essential nutrients their structure is impaired and their abilities to function are reduced and at times are dependent upon the magnitude of the deficiency.

Magnificence of the immune system
One of the most revealing aspects of microscopic observation is the magnificence of the immune system, when observed in its on-going quest to protect the body and eliminate health-robbing invaders. Most important are T-cells and B-cells (lymphocytes), and leucocytes. Leucocytes are reminiscent of rabbits foraging for food on an open field; they rapidly surround the fare and consume it. This process begins with the head rabbit (T-cells) directing them to consume, quickly and effectively, all that they can, clearing the field (plasma). During this time, B-cells are acting as assistants of the active rabbits, making sure that they find every morsel. The immune system also protects them by secreting protective cells (antibodies), so that the rabbits (leucocytes) can focus on their food consumption (debris, bacteria, yeast cancer, parasites, etc.)

Efficiency and deficiency
My ongoing research at Hippocrates Health Institute has afforded me the understanding of how living foods increase lifespan and diminish the potential and reality of disease. In observing cells, one of the greatest and most common deficiencies is that of B12. Without this vital bacteria nutrient your red blood cells (the building blocks and the main means of transport within the body) are not able to absorb other nutrients and carry oxygen, leading to anemia. Anemic conditions are troublesome, because they affect everything from the skeletal structure to each and every organ. One's anatomy will become weakened and ultimately far more vulnerable to opportunistic disease. We have found through thousands of investigative studies that bodies containing the highest amount of saturated fat contract the greatest B12 deficiency. Ironically, it is so-called common knowledge that animal food source consumption prevents this deficiency. On the contrary, we have proven this wrong over decades.

Today there is much talk about acid/alkaline concerns in human health. There is a lot of good information being dispensed so that the general public is now privy to information that natural health care professionals have known for years. After observing multitudes of blood tests we have observed that disease and acidity are often synonymous. There are those who make unsubstantiated claims that disorder cannot exist in an alkaline environment. We have found this to be false in many cases. There are several reasons that the international public generally has too little alkalinity and high acidity. Environmental toxins, stress, dairy and meat consumption, unripened fruit, flour products, coffee, and other lesser elements all vastly contribute to acid conditions. It is interesting to observe the erosion that acid and its crystals conduct on the cell and physiology. This culprit plays a major role in breaking down hard tissue (bones) and their adjoining cartilage. Osteoporosis, arthritis, and neuropathy are the major diseases manifested by acid.

The right environment
Cardiovascular disease, phlebitis, diabetes, and even cancer thrive in an acid

pH. One's immune system flourishes in an 80% alkaline/20% acid environment when consuming a balanced living food diet. It is almost unanimous that within two to three weeks one can transform an acid condition to a balanced pH. In this way the bodily systems, beginning with the cells (red blood cells, white blood cells and immune system cells), all function at their maximum level and provide the foundation for superior health.

There are also, of course, more specific things we can tell at times, including signs of free radical damage and oxidation. With yeasts and candida we can see some indication of how prevalent these are in the whole body. Further, we always get a lot of information about the degree and the types of anemia that may be present. Primarily we find that dark field live blood analysis is a way of monitoring general health. It is particularly useful in tracking a person's response over time to the treatments they employ. This reveals signs so that one can alter those treatments depending upon the findings. In certain conditions, especially cancer or other life-threatening diseases where time is a crucial factor, dark field microscopy can possibly be of help in choosing and monitoring the effect of therapy.

History of health
Out of all the remarkable discoveries I personally have made by researching blood cells of each and every participant that has attended Hippocrates program, it is a stunning fact that our health history (body and mind) is reflected in a clear pattern of calendar blocks. This is achieved by blotting blood droplets on a microscope glass slide, dried and viewed under a high-definition microscope. The first droplet contains the greatest amount of blood cells. The remaining five droplets naturally decrease blood cell contribution as you blot down the line. After the first two specimens, the remainder reflects five-year intervals. The first shows current circumstance, whereas the second reviews last year's history. The third regressively reveals two through seven years, whereas the third shows years eight to fourteen, etc. This blood chemistry observation works by a simple biological principle, infraction. The first droplet exposes current concerns, yet does not reveal if the given problem has a history. If the second droplet reflects the same structural problem as the first, it unveils the reality that the body has been dealing with the disorder for at least a year. When moving on to the third study and finding the same disruptive pattern, we are sure that it has been there long term, potentially chronic. This elevates or dismisses the relevance of any known concern. It also allows the subject and me to understand the origins, history, and severity of a given concern. What is remarkable is that you can see that a 60-year-old broke their leg 20 years ago or that a 20-year-old has been developing a disease for a decade. Equally astounding is what I discover in the cell structure on how the emotions impact blood cells. This is not a surprise to quantum biologists who understand that every cell thinks independently and equally acts as a unified participant in the anatomical framework.

All life forms experience memory
All life forms experience memory, although certainly not in the same way that the human mind works. This memory is no less valid, as the universe systematically

works at many subtle levels, requiring its future to be fueled by the past. It often shocks the research participant when we ask if they had an emotional upset with either a female or male in their past. You can literally pinpoint the hormonal impact that the cells suffered by any given trauma. Many boundaries would be broken if conservative and closed science worked at the most intricate levels. This would permit them to determine the root and foundational cause of disease. What is best about all of these seeming faults is that they can be altered and even erased when one commits themselves to a change of mind, diet, and spiritual landscape. Hippocrates Life Change Program in full is 21 days. Within this time I have been given the opportunity to view thousands and thousands of entry microscopic panels, which are then retaken upon departure. When the individuals face their irregularities (mind, body) there is scientific evidence that the healing and functionality of the body's cells is abundantly possible. Cells, like humans, at their core seek maximum function and total balance. This intent mandates their direction, rendering them fully responsible to reach complete health. The human mind, with its adoption of fragile and negative thoughts, tricks us into believing that compromise in moderation is acceptable. By pursuing this skewed perception the person impairs their biology and shortens their life. Observing cells impacted by these renegade thoughts reveals the scars of such disorder, although unlike the human mind, they do not permit them to become inherent. Individual cells completely submit themselves to a continuum of service at the highest level. When we release them to pursue that noble and essential work by living with integrity, our bodies become vehicles for positive outcome.

One aspect of conducting ongoing investigation of human blood cells that touches me daily is to observe the positive effect it has on the people being researched. The vast majority have never had the opportunity to see what they are made of, so they visibly appear like a child who sees Santa Claus for the first time. When their higher consciousness presents itself they embrace the fact that they are a gathering of living elements that make up one individual. When they understand that in total they are made of up trillions of cells, they begin to feel privileged and filled with the grandeur of their enormity. This is an enriching educational experience that is unsurpassed in its permanent, mind-changing ability.

About the Author:
Anna Maria Gahns Clement, Ph.D., N.M.D., L.N.C. embarked on her vocation as a practitioner of natural health care when she assumed the directorship of Sweden's BRANDAL CLINIC in Stockholm, an internationally recognized and well-respected center for health recovery. Her single-minded mastery of skills as a naturopathic medical doctor, Ph.D., nutritionist, iridologist, bodywork therapist, touch-for-health facilitator, and nursing health care provider served to enhance the instinctive qualities she possesses. She founded the first living-food organization in Scandinavia and was a member of the Natural Health Care Coalition, a government-supported effort in unifying the field of complementary health care in her native Sweden. For twenty-five years she has been co-director and chief health administrator of Hippocrates Health Institute situated originally in Boston, Massachusetts and now located in West Palm Beach, Florida. Dr.

Clement is considered to be one of the leading experts in live blood cell analysis, a revolutionary research tool pertaining to a person's state of health. Anna Maria Gahns Clement is the author of three books on the application of natural health methods in family and children's care. She addresses groups globally on the importance of taking responsibility for all realms of life.

As multi-faceted as her life is, the one role Anna Maria considers to be the most important, most challenging and, undoubtedly, the most enjoyable of all is her role as mother to her four children, whose exemplary health is a tribute to her and the Hippocrates lifestyle.

www.hippocratesinst.org

Dark Field Microscopy

18

How to Make the Change Easily, Joyfully and Successfully

Karen Knowler

Switching to eating raw foods, or more raw foods, is easy and truly exciting when you know how! It's the "know-how" part that people sometimes lack, and when they do figure out what to eat then there's the "sticking with it" part that inevitably will come up, as with all lifestyle changes. Through my work as a coach, and a raw-food coach specifically, I have created recipes, solutions, and maps suitable for anyone wishing to eat more raw foods. And the best bit about it? It's really fun! I'd like to begin by introducing you to what I call "The Successfully Raw Pyramid". This is what all of my work and coaching is based on, and as you will see from the diagram below it comprises of the following areas:

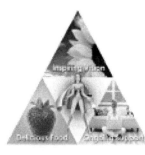

- Delicious Food
- Ongoing Support
- Inspiring Vision
- The fourth area in the middle represents the "you" that you have always wanted to be and the "you" that you can and will become when you start working proactively with the information I'm about to share with you. So if you're ready to find out how you can go raw easily, joyfully and successfully, then let's go!

Delicious food

It goes without saying, I hope, that the food you eat needs to taste delicious – otherwise you wouldn't want to eat it, right? Well, with raw food it's no different. It's about finding foods, recipes, and ingredients that make your taste buds sing and that bring you a whole new experience and appreciation of food. Having grown up on a diet of junk food and very little raw and living food, when I first got into raw foods in 1993 I was amazed at how quickly and excitedly my body and taste buds responded to the new living foods I was introducing. It was really an amazing experience, and to this day I am still in love with the new world that opened up to me.

One of the things I got right from the start and which I want to encourage you to do too is to eat only foods you truly love. No forcing, no "this is supposed to be good for me so I'll grin and bear it" kind of approach. That won't feel like fun at all! This is about being very honest and loving with yourself and trying new things with an open mind and open taste buds but it being okay if you don't like them... chances are you'll love most of the new foods anyway.

When I am coaching clients for the first time, I take a lot of time to find out from each client what their own personal preferences are within the diet they currently eat; from there I can create a raw-food menu for them that "ticks all the boxes" as far as taste, volume, portability, "mouth feel", and comfort are concerned. There is absolutely no need to think that choosing raw means sacrificing or "giving up" anything. All we let go of when we choose raw is dead health-diminishing foods that can never gift us with vibrant health. Clients' initial reservations quickly become replaced by a new, living reality whereby not only do the foods taste great, but they look great, feel great and guess what? They deliver great benefits to whoever eats them – including you!

So where to start in finding raw foods you love? Start where it's easiest: with the foods you already know and love. These foods are likely going to be the fruits and vegetables, and maybe nuts and seeds, that you've been used to eating before. Certainly there are going to be some fruits and vegetables you love in their fresh, raw state, whether they be the humble apple or something more exotic like a mango, papaya, or passion fruit; or perhaps you love raw carrots more than cooked, or adore munching on fresh spinach or watercress? Make a list of all the raw foods you know you love already. List as many as you can think of from each of the following genres; these will give you a foundation on which to build:

- Fresh fruits
- Vegetables
- Salad vegetables
- Leafy green vegetables
- Herbs and wild greens
- Nuts
- Dried fruits
- Beans, pulses, and legumes
- Grains
- Seeds
- Sprouting seeds
- Indoor greens

- Vegetable seeds
- Edible flowers
- Mushrooms
- Sea vegetables
- Algaes
- Oils
- "Stimulants" (garlic, cayenne pepper, etc.)
- Spices
- Flavorings and sweeteners
- Superfoods
- Other handy additions

Now while when you transition to more raw foods the focus should not necessarily be on "how much raw?" (this will usually take care of itself naturally and increase as you feel more alive). It is wise to start thinking about the cooked foods you are eating and see how you can upgrade those. This is actually much easier than you may think. Perhaps bread and cheese are a couple of your everyday mainstays? Well, as luck would have it, you can have both bread and cheese raw (as well as most, if not all everyday favorites), and the cheese can be dairy or non-dairy as you desire. Raw bread and other starchy crunchy carbs can be recreated in a dehydrator or low-temperature oven, as well as cookies, snack bars, pizza bases, and a whole assortment of delicious foods that you may never have believed possible! You can also buy them ready-made from some health food shops, which is how I started. Add to this my own personal favorite – ice-creams of all consistencies, colors and flavors, and you will discover that when you choose live raw foods you choose greater variety as well as vitality – not less!

As you will find, the more you look the more you see. The world of raw foods is vibrant, colorful, energetic and exciting! When you start to dip your toe in the water you'll find that both you and your body will love what starts to happen, and when you're ready for more, there's plenty more waiting for you!

Here's the rundown of your coaching assignments for Corner 1 of the Successfully Raw Pyramid.

First steps you can take to make sure the delicious food corner is secured in your Successfully Raw pyramid:

1. List all the raw foods you currently eat that you love, using the Raw Food Groups checklist to cover all the bases
2. List all the cooked foods you currently eat that you love and find raw or healthier equivalents for them, whether they are recipes you make yourself or pre-prepared foods you buy in stores
3. Create a menu plan for yourself, including all your current favorite raw foods – and filling in the gaps with your favorite cooked foods, but the healthier versions of them
4. Follow your menu for a few days and see how you feel. Consider adding in a

juice per day or a fruit smoothie to bring more life into your diet through your drinks as well as your food

5. Commit to trying one new raw food recipe or ingredient per week in order to keep bringing new tastes, flavors, and experiences to your live-food diet

If you'd like an introductory step-by-step program to follow for three days, including delicious recipes, then you can download yours free at www. successfullyraw.com, where I've done all the thinking for you!

Ongoing support
It's no secret that at this time in our history raw food is still considered "strange" by many. Indeed I know that a few years prior to trying raw food I would have thought it was extreme to say the least, as well as totally unachievable and "unrealistic". How wrong I was proved to be! Thinking that raw food eating is "odd" is both ironic and a bit of a giggle as raw food has been the *only* constant in our diet since the beginning of time, and yet we've become so conditioned to eat pre-packaged food in the past couple of generations that we've completely lost sight of what's "normal".

So, as you begin to bring more raw foods into your world it shouldn't come as a surprise that other people may not be quite as supportive or open-minded as you! Not that this is a "given". Many people I meet these days actually find it fascinating, intriguing, or inspiring. This is a brave new world you're entering, and once you step inside, the chances are that you won't want to go back! At the same time you'll still want to live your life and spend time with your friends and family as you've always done, but things may look or feel different now. For this reason, finding and securing support is imperative. The support side of things has two aspects to it: internal and external. It's vital that before you move along your raw-food journey too far that you get clear inside yourself that this is really what you want to do – no "shoulding" on yourself! I have found that those who succeed on raw foods embrace a living foods lifestyle from their *hearts,* and in many respects it becomes part of who they are, a choice that represents many values that they hold dear. This will need to be the same for you, and we'll be looking more at values in a moment.

As far as the external side of things go, you'll want to make sure that on a very practical level your kitchen is set up to support you. This means making sure that you have the right foods and equipment and enough space to prepare meals for yourself in a way that feels good. Even if you're not someone who loves cooking or prepping food, you'll still want to have the space to lay out all your raw bits and pieces and create a meal, drink, or dessert for yourself. All of this can be done in just a few minutes when you've found the quick and easy recipes that you love (which is another of my secrets!).

Beyond the kitchen you may well find that as you start to eat more raw and living foods you will begin taking a closer look at your home and addressing any issues relating to clutter. It is practically a given that as you start to bring more raw foods into your diet and clean up your body that you'll automatically start doing the same to your home! It's simply a case of wanting to clean up your world on every level. It happens so subconsciously that you could easily miss it, but I'm willing to bet that it won't be long before you find yourself addressing all those old jobs and piles of paper that you've been hoarding or ignoring for quite possibly years... it's fascinating but so true!

Moving beyond your home, on a wider scale it's really important, actually VITAL, that you find like-minded people to connect with. This may be online or locally; it doesn't matter; what matters is that you have people who are thinking and feeling like you to share experiences, tips, and resources. This journey is a thousand times richer for the amazing people that it can, and will, bring into your life. In fact it's another reason why I love eating this way so much – the people that are attracted to it are truly some of the most wonderful people on the planet, and it's been incredible to meet and learn with them and from them.
There are indeed many things you can do to support yourself as you experiment and bring more raw foods into your world. What matters most is that you feel happy about what you're doing at every stage, and this is where possibly the most exciting aspect comes into play – the inspiring vision.

The next steps you can take to make sure the ongoing support corner is secured in your Successfully Raw pyramid:

1. Ask yourself, "are my mind, body, heart, and soul all eager and excited by this raw food journey?" – if yes, then great; if no, you'll need to find out what's blocking you and why.
2. Organize your kitchen in such a way that you have plenty of raw foods, including lots of diversity, an array of exciting raw food recipes, and the equipment you need to start experimenting. You can purchase a blender, juicer, and food processor very cheaply if you buy well known brands or visit eBay.
3. Spend time organizing your home so that it feels like a place you really want to spend time in. You'll be changing in ways you cannot currently predict as you detoxify physically, so it's important that your home feels like your castle and provides a lovely retreat for you as you transform on all four levels.
4. Find like-minded people online or locally. There are lots of ways to do this, and you can find a list on my website in the support section.

Should you find yourself wanting to make changes in your life as you eat more raw food (the raw energy can make you realize what's not serving you), then give yourself permission to transform. Raw food naturally puts you back in touch with what matters to you; this might sound a bit kooky now, but trust me; you'll find out that it happens as you let go of foods that block your awareness.

Inspiring vision
What is it about raw-food eating that attracts you? Is it the promise of weight loss, more energy or stamina, a leaner, cleaner body, or something less physical like clarity of mind and great concentration? It doesn't matter why you choose to go raw; what matters is making what I call "your big why" something that really

speaks to you – the highest, most inspired version of you that you've discovered to date. When I first got into raw foods it was for two reasons: First, to lose weight that I had struggled to lose since age 14, and second, because I wanted to be a super-healthy vegetarian. Quite simply the more I cleaned up my diet, even with cooked foods, the more I realized the impact that our food choices have on us on every level, and I wanted to see how good I could feel.

So with raw food my original inspiring vision was to lose weight and find a body shape and size that I was happy with – and this I did, more quickly than I expected as it happens! I was thrilled to find that it was the most enjoyable and genuinely satisfying way to lose weight I had ever come across, and that's because I was eating as much as I wanted, just cleaner leaner foods that I adored. However, after the weight-loss target was reached there was the question: Now that my goal has been met, what was there waiting for me next? Thankfully by this time my raw diet had opened up so many new doors that I simply wanted to "follow the yellow brick road" and see where raw foods would lead me. The journey had become so exciting and compelling that I wanted to see how good I could look and feel if I carried on.

Looking back now, I realize that raw food absolutely played into my key values, another reason why it was a joy for me and easy too. Values are those things that really mean a lot to you, such as honesty, integrity, love, creativity, imagination, potential, bliss, and so forth. When you get clear on your values, which you can do by making a list of those things that inspire you and impress you in others, then you can proactively find a way to "do" raw food that supports you in living your values and reaching your brightest and highest life goals. When you align raw food with your values the journey becomes truly exciting and rewarding in unimaginable yet nonetheless truly life-changing ways. Creating an inspiring vision for yourself is therefore not only important for staying raw but also an invitation to step into a new more alive and pro-active way of living on every level. For me this has been the most unexpected yet wonderful aspect of raw food eating that I never would have expected, but it has ultimately delivered so much more than a slim body; my energy that has gone through the roof!

The steps you can take to make sure the inspiring vision corner is secured in your Successfully Raw pyramid:

1. Make a list of all your reasons for wanting to go raw – these can be many and varied, or few yet highly specific and meaningful.
2. Make a list of your core values and next to each one write how going raw will help you live your value to its highest potential.
3. Create a vision board using magazines, scissors, and glue. Simply collect images, words, and phrases of the things you would most like to do, be, or have and arrange them on a large sheet of paper or card – this will make your vision come alive and give you something to aspire to on a daily basis, until you make all those dreams come true and can then create another!
4. To stay inspired, keep reading uplifting books, websites, or attending seminars; it is always helpful and life-changing to connect with those who

have already made these changes and are living their bliss because of it. As you can see, there is more to going raw than simply changing what you eat, but it's with the food that we all have to start. So long as you keep the food easy, quick and delicious you will find in no time that the raw food journey has plenty more to offer you than healthy meals and a new perspective on food – it will quite literally change you from the cellular level out.

About the Author:

Karen Knowler has been dubbed "the world's premier raw food coach" and is known for her quick, easy, and delicious raw food recipes as much as her deep insight, compassion, and wisdom. Former Managing Director of **The Fresh Network**, the UK's Raw and Living Foods organisation, founder and former editor of Get Fresh! magazine, and author of a multitude of life-changing books, eBooks, and articles, Karen has more than 15 years of personal experience of eating a raw food diet and has been teaching, writing, and coaching professionally on raw foods for a decade. Karen is well-known internationally, has lectured in England, the US, Holland, Germany, and Wales, has been seen by over 6 million viewers live on national TV, appears frequently in the national press and has coached and worked with people from all backgrounds, including well-known celebrities. Within the raw food movement, Karen's most powerful work includes the development of a unique set of "Raw Coaching Models", which outline the raw food journey inside and out and which form the basis of all Karen's work. Karen's central philosophy is that raw food is a potent tool for bringing us home to ourselves and living life to the full on every level. Find Karen at www.TheRawFoodCoach.com.

19

It's Not Just What You Eat - Lifestyle and Beyond

Jameth Sheridan, ND

Diet is a critical part of a healthy lifestyle, yet not the entire picture. A full-spectrum, health-supporting lifestyle is encouraged. This includes physical exercise and exposure to sunshine, as well as psychological health. Avoiding environmental toxins and toxic products is essential. Paramount is pure water (for consumption and bathing), the use of natural fiber clothing, and non-toxic personal-care products. Also consider healthy options in home furnishings/ building materials and related items.

It tends to be human nature to put your all eggs in one basket; to rely on the "magic bullet" to cure all of your ills. Following the dietary suggestions in this book can make an immense difference in your health, but there is a holistic lifestyle that, when applied as a synergistic whole, will take your health and life to new heights.

I've been athletic and conscious of what I eat for most of my life, and too may times I have heard people saying things like "I burn off toxins by exercising". I like to point out to those people that the running guru in the 1980s (Jim Fixx) said the same thing and dropped dead of a heart attack while running! The same principle applies to those who believe they are eating a very healthy diet. They often think that they can ignore their psychology, their air quality, their water quality, their personal care products, their clothing, what type of building they live in, etc. They *can* ignore these things, but they will fall short of fulfilling their entire potential of health and happiness. Below I will address some non-raw aspects of health.

Psychological health

If your psychology is not healthy, you are not either. Let me give you an example. Years ago my wife and I were attending a beautiful event in the mountains called the "Whole Being Weekend". It was a great event with massage, loving music, and all sorts of spiritual, personal growth, and health-related events. The atmosphere was one of non-judgment, peace, and brotherly/sisterly love. The food served was vegan and organic. As my wife and I walked through the food hall, we noticed that nothing was raw! We became annoyed and judgmental. So much so that we left! We left this awesome event just because they had the gall to serve 100% organic and vegan food, but nothing raw. As I look back on that now, I realize how judgmental we were. *We* created these negative, non-spiritual emotions in ourselves and denied ourselves the weekend. That was crazy and was not a good example of a healthy psychology. I am glad I am not that way now. It is important to address any and all other areas of your psychological being. You are what you eat, but also what you think and feel.

Exercise

Exercise is a BIG issue. It is next most important to being on a whole-foods vegan diet with lots of raw foods. Without it, you cannot be fully healthy. Exercise can take any form you want. Hiking, weights, gym, aerobics, pilates, swimming, biking, exercise videos, sports, whatever you will actually do. But do *something*! I have been an "on and off" athlete all of my life. I know that the difference when I am "off" is dramatic. Everything gets worse – my metabolism, my circulation, my brain functioning, my drive, and my emotions.

Personally, I love physical exertion. I love to move rocks to build walls and to work hard in the garden. I also love to "go into battle" in my gym that fills my entire garage. After all the sweating, breathing, and exerting, I feel awesome, for days! It has been proven that exercise positively affects your ability to feel good and to sleep well at night. Let's put it this way: If I had a choice between the following:

1. Eat 100% healthy (vegan, mostly raw, organic, etc) with *no* exercise
2. Eat 50% healthy (vegan, 50% raw, with regular processed foods and health food junk foods) with *lots* of exercise,

overwhelmingly I would pick option 2! This might shock some of you, but I have lived and breathed both experiences many times over. Exercise is so transformational for your health. I suggest you eat well and exercise.

Air

Air quality is essential. The fresher your air, the better off you are, all other factors being equal. So does that mean that everyone wanting a healthy life should move out far into the wilderness? No it doesn't, and that is not practical. Here is what I suggest you do. Keep a steady stream of outside air coming into your living space at all times. This could be keeping a window opened, even a little bit, all of the time. Indoor environments accumulate pollution in the air at a rate far greater than outside air. We breathe in oxygen (O_2) and breathe out carbon dioxide (CO_2). If O_2 levels get too low, and/or CO_2 levels get too high, all mammalian life dies! Unless you live in an indoor jungle that includes a running waterfall, inside air has far less O2, far more CO2, and far more pollution in it. I grew up in Connecticut, on the northeast coast of the United States. Cold winters where you need heat to survive are a reality there. At 10 degrees Fahrenheit/-12 degrees Celsius, or lower, you certainly do not want to keep a window wide open. However, even the smallest opening will allow fresh air to come in. In fact the greater the difference in temperature between inside and outside air, the less of an opening you need. If it is 30 degrees outside and 60 degrees inside (30 degrees difference), outside air will rush inside and *vice versa*. If it is 0 outside and 60 inside (60 degrees difference), air will rush in and out twice as fast. The bottom line is to try and get some sort of air exchange at all times.

You can install a fresh air system in your HVAC system (heating, ventilation, air conditioning) that automatically brings fresh air into your home. I have this at my home. Check into this, or have a HVAC professional do it for you. Otherwise, use the window method. Note: Do not compromise your safety from intruders by leaving windows and or doors open in such a way that you could be harmed.

For your information, parking your car in the garage is *not* healthy. Cars give off pollutants; keeping them cooped up in the garage concentrates these toxins, and you get a highly toxic whiff of them when you use your car. Let you car air out in the open. Do something that benefits your health in your garage (convert it to a gym, exercise studio, study, creative space, etc.).

The indoor environment

Having plants in your indoor environment is absolutely awesome! My wife and I once lived in a 340 sq ft. studio apartment. One day we decided to get a bunch of plants for it. We got bigger ones for the floor and smaller ones for shelves. We put a plant anywhere we could afford to give up the space, and we also hung some from the ceiling. What a difference this made in our tiny little home. We felt like we lived in a jungle! We also added a small fountain. It felt physically, emotionally and spiritually better.

Air purifiers

I highly recommend getting an indoor air purifier. There are various types, and each has its pros and cons. I use a super hyper HEPA filter when I am not around. These units have a fan and are very effective but also make noise, which bothers me. At night, I use silent, fan-less purifiers/filters. They are not nearly as effective, but they are quiet and can be on all night without disturbing you. I personally think that sleep is much deeper and more restorative in complete silence. I program the HEPA types to come on and crank up to maximum speed when I'm out and to be off when I am home.

Ozone air purifiers have been popular. Ozone is an amazing oxidizer of a wide variety of substances. If you douse a room with enough ozone after someone has smoked in there, any evidence of the smoke and smell will be gone. It's amazing for mold too. Ozone is an oxidant, the opposite of an antioxidant, but too much can oxidize your lungs and temporarily impair you ability to breathe. Be cautious of ozone air purifiers for that reason. I use them only for period purges, when neither I nor any living creature is in the space! You could kill your animals if they are left behind with high concentrations. I almost killed myself once with an ozone accident.

I have various types of air filters and purifiers all over my house and office. Another option is to install air-cleaning equipment right into your HVAC system. Then, every time you turn on the heat, air, or circulation fan, your air will be purified. It's great, if you have the ability to do this. I would also add a very strong UV tube and a negative ionizer to the stream.

Sunshine and light
Full-spectrum light is essential to our health. The sun is full-spectrum light. Regardless of how good of a diet you are on, too much sun exposure creates free radicals and suppresses the immune system. However, too little does the same thing. The right amount of sunlight greatly enhances the immune system, balances many hormones, creates vitamin D and strengthens your bones, and puts you in a much better mood! Try to get at least some exposure to the sun daily on as much of your body as is appropriate. If you are fair-skinned, you need less; and more if you're dark-skinned.

Regarding indoor light, the ideal would be glass skylights (without UV protection if you can get them). Next best would be the "full spectrum" types of lights that have been available for decades. None of these is as good as the actual sun, but they are far better than regular lights. There have been dramatic positive changes in people's health, mood, energy, and learning ability just by changing the lights to full spectrum. They come in fluorescent, incandescent (screw-in), and LED forms. LED (light emitting diode) are the most eco-friendly and last the longest. Get the best lights you can.

Note: At night, most people do not like completely full-spectrum lights and the "cooler" type of light that they cast. I think that this is because as the sun sets, it has a "warmer", more yellow hue. I do not suggest "cool" full-spectrum lights for nighttime mood lighting. It just does not feel right. But in the day, bring on the daylight, "cooler" looking sunlight and full-spectrum bulbs.

Water
Pure water is also essential. The "old school" way to purify water is by steam distillation. Distillation produces water without any minerals and usually not any contaminants. It is very effective in making pure water without chemicals. The down side is that the water is not nearly as "wet" as it could be. Water not wet – what the heck does that mean?

Different waters have different abilities to hydrate, and this is related to the "surface tension". Surface tension is a measure of how much force it takes to break the surface of water. The greater the surface tension, the harder it is to break the surface. For example, if water has high surface tension, particles will float easily on top of it. High surface tension water is *less* wet. With low surface tension water, particles dropped on the top will sink more easily. Low surface tension water is *more* wet.

Here is a low-tech test you can do to check surface tension: Take distilled water and drop a tea bag into an exact quantity of it. Take another water (bottles, purified, etc) and drop the same type of tea bag into the same exact quantity of it. Pick a tea that has a really distinct color to it. See which glass gets darker from the tea. You can check in 30 minutes and overnight. The one that is darker has lower surface tension and is wetter.

Distilling water increases the surface tension substantially, making it less wet. Reverse-osmosis-treated water is just as pure as distilled, but it does not become less wet (has a lower surface tension). This is the primary reason I prefer reverse osmosis system water to distilled. There are energetic devices you can buy to lower the surface tension of any water, and in general I think these are good, and I use them myself. There are always greater and lesser things in life, the real and the fake, which is also the case with water devices.

Wetter water is better able to hydrate and cleanse. The best-quality water in the world is that which is found in high-water content fruits and vegetables. It is a very low-surface-tension water, and it is also "structured" or "clustered", both of which are very good. I am a huge proponent of juicing and high-water-content foods. Coconut water is great anytime and as the base for smoothies or powdered green drinks.

Distilled water proponents look down on water from natural springs and rivers, and in some cases, this is not good for you. These waters contain inorganic minerals, too much of which in your system can harm your health. However, there are some natural springs in which, because of the way the water flows, the surface tension gets very low (is really wet). In this case, the minerals stay in suspension and in my experience they don't cause problems: in fact they are a very significant improvement over distilled. When I am out somewhere, I drink the best bottled water I can find. When home, I drink out of my reverse osmosis system, with various energetic devices attached to it.

What about the water you do your dishes in, your laundry, brush your teeth in, bathe and shower in? For this, I suggest a whole-house filter installed at your main water line, before any water gets to your house. This way, the water you use that you do not drink will also be pure.

Personal care products
If you wouldn't eat it, you probably should not put it on your body. Whatever you put on your body will end up in your bloodstream, and it will do so directly, without having the chance to be detoxified by your liver first. That is why personal care products are so important.

Try to use only non-toxic shampoos, toothpastes, makeups, deodorants, skin care, and any other product that you might put on or near your body, or that may enter your body through scent. Regular perfumes are very toxic just from smelling them. I sometimes cannot stand to be near someone if they have heavy perfume on. Essential oils from plants not only smell better, but also are therapeutic. You can use individual oils that you like or buy pre-made mixes. There is a non-toxic alternative to everything toxic. If you can find it, use it.

The clothes you wear are also important. Try to emphasize natural fibers like organic cotton, hemp, soy fibers, and bamboo. Regular cotton is not as good as organic cotton, because commercially grown cotton may be the most heavily sprayed crop in the world, due to the fact that no one is eating the cotton. Then the cotton is bleached with chlorine or other chemicals. Commercial cotton is not nearly as soft as organic, and it contributes massive amounts of chemicals to the world. I don't want this on my body, on my planet, or on my conscience. Vote with your dollars.

Natural fiber clothes also tend to be much more comfortable. As with anything, don't throw the good out with the bad and be so purist that it backfires. Let me make it clear that by no means am I a "moderation in everything" type of guy. Not in the least! I say bring on huge quantities of the good stuff and zero quantities of the bad stuff. However, if some yoga or workout pants, for example, are 90% organic cotton (or less for that matter), and 10% synthetic fiber, yet they are so well fitting that they inspire you actually to use them to work out, and the 100% organic product un-inspires you and you are unable to make the adjustment, then you are better off with the non-organic pants, in this case. All other factors being equal, organic is better. I think you get the idea.

Electromagnetic radiation

Electromagnetic radiation is a blanket term that refers to radiation from electricity. There is electrical, magnetic, radio frequency, and microwave radiation. Electrical and magnetic radiation comes from power lines (overhead, underground) as well as from the wires that run through houses, businesses, and appliances. Radio frequency and microwave radiation comes from cell phones, microwaves, and wireless Internet. All of these have negative health ramifications. All but the electrical radiation goes right through walls.

Here is what to look for and what to do. When sleeping, keep clocks and anything plugged in as far away from your body as possible (minimum one foot). The best solution would be to get a battery-powered alarm clock. Do not sleep near a circuit breaker panel. Try to get at least four feet away from it, preferably farther. Be aware of what is on the other side of a wall. A circuit breaker panel might be right on the other side of the wall. Any motors create large electromagnetic fields. This includes refrigerators. Try to not sleep on the other side of a wall of a refrigerator. Old CRT TVs also have a large field. Watch out for bedrooms on the other side of them. Flat panel TVs have much less radiation.

Huge amounts of radiation come from transformers. Transformers are found on the telephone poles at various places. They take the super-high-voltage power and transform it to household currents. If you can easily see one of these outside of your home, you are probably being affected by it. For underground power lines, the transformers are typically green boxes on the ground. Stay away from these.

Transformers are also on many appliances we use and are attached as a "box" to the cord. They take the alternating current (AC) power from the wall plug and convert it to direct current (DC) that powers lots of appliances. These transformers, just like the ones on the power lines, put out a lot of EMF. Keep these transformers as far away from your personal space as is reasonably possible.

Juicers, blenders, dehydrators, and everything that is electrically powered produce fields. We cannot get completely away from this. I would never want someone not to juice because of EMF concerns. That would be counter-productive. Just don't sleep with a juicer running next to your body. There are lots of "harmonizers" that claim to help reverse the negative effects of EMFs. I have been using these types of devices for more than 20 years, and I suggest you do too. Some work, others do not. I have a list of what I think may work on www. HealthForce.com.

Regarding cell phones, they sure are convenient! But they sure are harmful. Get a harmonizer(s) for your cell phone as well and hope it works. I have several on mine. Try to use your cell as little as possible. Call people back from landlines when you can. Use an earpiece with an AIR tube right near your ear. Regular headsets can act as antennae and make the problem worse. Use your speakerphone and give some distance between you and the phone. If your car supports Bluetooth, use it. Bluetooth is not good either, but it only goes about 30 feet, so I think it is much less bad.

I personally know 2 people who each carried 2 cell phones on their belt for about 1 year. They both got kidney cancer on the same side of the body where they carried their cell phones (which was right next to the affected kidney)! And one of them was a raw fooder who had had cell phone harmonizers all over his phones! The "average" person had his kidney removed. The raw fooder stopped carrying the phones on his body, went on a hard core, superfood, juice and herbal healing program (including other healthy actions in lifestyle and healing), and completely reversed the tumor!

Wireless Internet networks are becoming more and more prevalent and are not healthy. You may not be able to eliminate this from public buildings, but you can eliminate it in your own home. If you can use hard-wired Internet, you are much better off. If you are a provider of Wi-Fi services and it brings customers to your stores, I strongly suggest you investigate and utilize as many harmonizers as you can—and hope that they work. If you can get a whole-house surge protector with electromagnetic interference reduction, this can also help too.

Advanced EMF
In many cases there is a better way to run wires in homes to lower the EMFs,

and I suggest you search the Internet for the best. For you electricians, I will say that when doing wiring you should not share neutrals from different circuits, and no neutrals from different circuits should be joined in junctions. This creates huge fields. Neutrals joined in junctions from different circuits can be fixed at any time, but sharing a neutral on a wire must be done while the house is being wired or re-wired. You can get inexpensive electromagnetic field (EMF) meters online. They measure in milligauss. The best reading is 0, especially in your bed with the lights out. This may not be realistically obtainable. If you can't get 0, go for less than one or even less than three. Just do the best you can. It may be as easy as replacing your alarm clock with a battery-powered one or moving your bed. In my bedroom, I needed to gut the entire room down to studs and re-wire it to get to 0.

Home furnishings

If you are redecorating, building, or remodeling a space, look for green (eco) and non-toxic options. Do your research and you can do way better than normal building. Know that "green" and "non-toxic" are not always the same. Recycled wood shavings mixed with formaldehyde glue are "green" but not non-toxic. Look for both. A great resource for this information is www.NaturalHomeMagazine. com and www.EcoVelopments.com. There are non-toxic and eco green paints, glues, caulking, stains, window blinds, you name it! I suggest you buy from companies that only make non-toxic eco products. Some "regular" companies have jumped on the green bandwagon, but some of their products are suspect. I want to support the companies that truly get it. There are so many truly non-toxic eco green companies out there now that there is no reason to give the bad companies your business simply because they provide a few products that are less bad than what the conventional companies provide. There is no reason to choose this kind of "lesser evil." By supporting companies that are truly green, you can have it all. Just do what your budget or situation allows.

About the Author:

Jameth Sheridan, N.D. is a longtime Vegan, Raw Fooder, Herbalist, and hard-core holistic medicine researcher. He is an outspoken perfectionist on a deeply driven, on-going mission to uncover and spread truth, ethics, and full-spectrum health. He walks his talk and fully embraces as many aspects of a holistic lifestyle as he can, including non-toxic building. Dr. Sheridan is the single most recognized pioneer in bio-compatible nutritional superfoods. He brings a unique blend of scientific, yet vastly open-minded, deeply thorough approach, and an understanding of life force, whole foods, and mother nature to all that he does, with a deep reverence for all life. Dr. Sheridan researches, grows, and provides the highest quality superfoods under his own label, HealthForce Nutritionals, private labels, as well as makes custom formulas for other hard-core companies worldwide. Jameth is one of those unique people who is deeply caring, compassionate, introspective, and humble, while at the same time he is not afraid to call upon his Warrior spirit to challenge the status quo or go against the grain, if, upon reflection, that is what he truly believes is right. He lives his life as a modern follower of codes of honor such as Bushido and Chivalry.

Dr. Sheridan's websites: www.HealthForce.com www.RawFoodResearch.com

"The quality, therapeutic concentration, and affordability of a nutritional product can, and often does, mean the difference between lethargy and energy, sickness and health, and, quite literally, life and death. I don't want anyone to be tired, sick or dead because they could not obtain or afford the best possible product. If someone does not feel this same way, they should not be in the nutritional product business. I live and breathe this philosophy in both my personal and professional life and constantly strive to evolve HealthForce products and offer them at the best possible values. I would rather die than compromise these principles" – Jameth Sheridan, N.D.

PART 2

The Principles in Practice

Part 2

Healing Diabetes Requires a Shift in Consciousness

Gabriel Cousens MD, MD(H)

> *"Society is always taken by surprise by any new example of common sense."*
>
> *– Ralph Waldo Emerson*

> *"No physician can ever say that any disease is incurable. To say so blasphemes God, blasphemes Nature, and depreciates the great architect of Creation. The disease does not exist, regardless of how terrible it may be, for which God has not provided the corresponding cure."*
>
> *– Paracelsus*

Healing diabetes requires a shift in consciousness. To liberate ourselves from the cultural, nutritional, and personal habits that contribute to the manifestation of diabetes is not only to heal ourselves and realize better health than persons who are not diabetic, but is also is an Act of Love that contributes to a multi-level positive transformation of society. Yes – the fact that Type-2 diabetes is a curable disease has been common knowledge in the live-food community since the 1920s when Max Gerson, MD healed Albert Schweitzer of diabetes with live foods. I know, from my own 35 years of clinical experience as a holistic medical doctor, together with that of live-food therapeutic centers, that diabetes is not a fixed sentence. It is not our natural condition and has only become a problem of pandemic proportions since the 1940s. The word *pandemic* comes from the Greek *pan-*, meaning "all", plus *demos,* meaning "people or population". A pandemic is an epidemic that becomes very widespread and affects a whole region, a continent, or the world. This article looks deeply at the underlying causes of diabetes on both the pandemic-global and the personal level, and informs readers how they may achieve rapid reversal from the misery of diabetes and move toward a joyous and healthy life.

Although many people have a genetic susceptibility to Type-2 diabetes, the true causes (which activate the genetic potential physiology of diabetes) lie in a personal and world lifestyle and diet that pull the trigger on the diabetes gun. This *diabetogenic* profile includes, on the level of the individual, a diet high in refined carbohydrates such as white sugar and white flour; high amounts of cooked animal saturated fats; trans fatty acids produced from cooking (and especially frying oils at high temperatures); low-fiber food; coffee, caffeinated beverages and nicotine; insufficient exercise; high levels of stress; and emotional emptiness. Contributory factors on a planetary level include a degraded environment in which the air, earth, and water are, according to the Environmental Protection Agency, filled with 70,000 different toxic chemicals, heavy metals, agrochemicals, and other toxic substances—65,000 of which are potentially hazardous to our health. In addition, we live in a mental and emotional environment filled with messages of stress and death from the media, including news of constant wars and terrorism affecting the planet. The degenerate conditions, lifestyle, and diet that create diabetes emanate from these modern human-created realities, which, taken together, we are calling the Culture of Death.

Data published in December 2006 in the International Diabetes Federation's Diabetes Atlas show that the disease now affects a staggering 246 million people worldwide, with 46% of all those affected in the 40–59 age group. There is clear hope for Type-2 diabetes being completely reversed in a relatively short time. This means that Type-2 diabetes is not necessarily a death sentence; rather, it is a *benign* disease if it is appropriately addressed. Uncontrolled diabetes is a forced death march for those who are not willing to make the effort to heal themselves and a disaster in progress for the cultures and economies of nations worldwide. Obesity is a measurable sign of this trend, as up to 90% of Type-2 diabetics are overweight.

The cure, on the most profound level, is to move away from a global and personal Culture of Death, and to embrace the Culture of Life. On a personal level this means choosing to live in a way that promotes life and well-being for oneself as well as for the planet. It means creating a diet and lifestyle in which there is minimal or no incidence of diabetes. Individually, this means a diet that is organic, vegan, at least 80% live-food, high in mineral content, 15–20% plant-only fat (no animal fat), high-fiber, and with low-glycemic and low-insulin index. Food, in modest intake and individualized, should be well hydrated, sustainable for the duration of one's life, and prepared and eaten with love. Collectively, it means creating a world culture where all people have access to healthy, organic food and water, decent shelter, and an environment free of chemicals and pollutants. Healing diabetes in this personal and global context is an act of love for oneself and for the living planet. It is an expression of the Culture of Life.

The 21-day plus program

The teaching of this chapter is that humanity is created to be vibrant, alive, and healthy. As it says in Deuteronomy 30:19 from 3,400 years ago: *"Today, I have set before you life and death and a blessing and a curse. You must choose life in order that you and your children shall live."* Things have not changed. We still have that choice. This book is about empowering you, health professionals, and national and global policymakers to have that choice. Even in the most adverse circumstances, it still is possible for motivated individuals and nations to heal on the Tree of Life 21-Day Plus program as an act of love and consciousness.

This program includes a minimum seven-day Green Juice Fast in the first week, which greatly accelerates the reversing of the diabetic degenerative physiological process. Based on research by Dr. Stephen Spindler, it is our theory that calorie restriction turns on the anti-aging and theoretically the anti-diabetic genes. In our dietary approach, there is actually no restriction, but the participant is invited to enjoy a delicious, healthy cuisine. This is the powerful secret of the success of this program. In the second week, a four-day course shows people how to let go of their belief that diabetes is incurable. It also shows people how to let go of all the psychological programming and habits that create the diabetes lifestyle. In the third week, people learn how to prepare low-glycemic foods and a healthy healing cuisine. We then have a one-year follow-up that supports people in staying on the program, which includes, if needed, supervised Juice Feasting, a powerful at-home practice for those who need to continue to lose weight and heal the complications associated with a diabetic physiology that may take some time to reverse.

Diabetic lifestyle habits and risk factors

When we break the natural laws, they break us. In this section you are going to read about some things that you may hold very dear as part of what you see as your identity. It is very important that you acknowledge the healthy part of yourself that does not want diabetes or the diet and lifestyle that creates it. Any attachment to the former diet and lifestyle needs to be transformed. *"My precious burdens,"* Walt Whitman said, *"My precious burdens I carry them wherever I go."* In healing from diabetes, we have to let go of our precious burdens.

The personal lifestyle habits, choices, and predisposing diseases that are diabetogenic include:

* High sugar intake
* Flesh food eating
* Overweight and obesity

- Inactivity, especially television watching
- Dairy consumption
- Blood cholesterol
- High-stress lifestyle and hypertension
- Candida
- Depression
- Metabolic syndrome (Syndrome X)
- Toxicity of heavy metals and drinking water
- Vaccinations
- Coffee and caffeinated beverages
- Smoking
- Environmental Toxicity in Foods air, earth, and water

Dairy consumption
Children with diabetic genetic tendencies who drink cow's milk have an 11–13 times higher rate of juvenile diabetes than children who are breastfed by their own mothers for at least three months. Although many are not aware of it, milk consumption is directly associated with juvenile diabetes. The American Academy of Pediatrics made a decision, based on this data in 1994, to strongly encourage families with a diabetic history not to give their children cow's milk or cow's milk products for at least two years. The key to understanding this is that there are more than 100 antigens found in milk. The reason for the increase in juvenile diabetes is that the children have much higher formation of antibodies to the cow's milk antigens.

High-stress lifestyle and hypertension
When the body is under stress, many hormones are released that indirectly increase insulin excretion and indirectly create insulin resistance, a precursor to a diabetic physiology. In the US, 62.5% of adults with diabetes reported having **hypertension** (source: CDC). Hypertension is part of the basket of symptoms seen in Syndrome X, discussed below.

Candida
Candida is also commonly associated with diabetes and is a larger symptom of a Culture of Death diabetogenic diet and lifestyle. Candida is a fungal parasite that excretes toxic waste that can get into the bloodstream and cause symptoms of bloating, clouded thinking, depression, exhaustion, halitosis (bad breath), menstrual pains, thrush, unclear memory recall, recurring vaginal or bladder infections, anxiety, constipation, diarrhea (or both), environmental sensitivities, fatigue, feeling worse on damp or muggy days or in moldy places, food sensitivities, insomnia, low blood sugar, mood swings, premenstrual syndrome, ringing in the ears, and sensitivities to perfume, cigarettes, or fabric odors. Diabetes with its higher blood sugar levels makes people good candidates for candida.

Depression
According to an evaluation of 20 studies over the past ten years, the prevalence rate of diabetics with major depression is three to four times greater than in the general population. While depression affects 3–5% of the population at any given

time, the rate is 15–20% in patients with diabetes, according to the American Diabetic Association. More recent research, however, points to depression as a possible cause or trigger for diabetes.

Metabolic Syndrome (Syndrome X)

Syndrome X was first coined as a term by Gerald Reaven, MD at Stanford University to describe a group of symptoms that arise from an overall metabolic disorder. These symptoms may include Type-2 diabetes, obesity with an inability to lose weight, high cholesterol, high blood pressure, high triglycerides, low HDL cholesterol, and coronary heart disease. Some 655,000 people are newly diagnosed each year, and it is estimated that an equal 655,000 cases are not diagnosed. Some estimates cite some 47 million people with the basket of symptoms known as Syndrome X. A classic symptom and hint of the metabolic syndrome is the accumulation of fat in the abdomen and the inability to lose fat and weight. The metabolic disorder that we've created through unnatural ways of living from the lifestyle and diet of the Culture of Death has a significant effect on people's health. Some researchers estimate that we age one-third faster when blood sugar levels are high.

Toxicity of heavy metals and drinking water

The development of insulin-dependent diabetes mellitus is thought to be accelerated by the interaction of environmental agents with the pancreatic beta cells. Just as consuming organic foods is a way to avoid ingesting toxins, becoming aware of the quality of water one drinks and uses is increasingly essential in today's polluted world, where water can be a major source of toxins. According to *Diet for a Poisoned Planet,* less than 1% of the Earth's surface water is safe to drink. In some places in the United States and other countries, the term "drinking water" for tap water should be considered nothing more than a nostalgic euphemism.

Medical science has discovered how sensitive the insulin receptor sites are to chemical poisoning. Metals such as cadmium, mercury, arsenic, lead, fluoride, and possibly aluminum may play a role in the actual destruction of beta cells through stimulating an auto-immune reaction to them after they have bonded to these cells in the pancreas. It is because mercury and lead attach themselves at highly vulnerable junctures of proteins that they find their great capacity to provoke morphological changes in the body. Changes in pancreatic function are among the pathogenic mechanisms observable during lead intoxication.

According to Fluoride in Drinking Water: A Scientific Review of EPA's Standards, made public by the National Research Council in 2006: The conclusion from the available studies is that sufficient fluoride exposure appears to bring about increases in blood glucose or impaired glucose tolerance in some individuals and to increase the severity of some types of diabetes. In general, impaired glucose metabolism appears to be associated with serum or plasma fluoride concentrations of about 0.1 mg/L or greater in both animals and humans.

Vaccinations and increased juvenile diabetes rates
In the May 24, 1996 *New Zealand Medical Journal*, J. Bart Classen, MD, a former researcher at the National Institute of Health, reported a 60% increase in Type-1 diabetes following a massive campaign in New Zealand from 1988 to 1991 to vaccinate babies six weeks of age or older with hepatitis B vaccine. In the October 22, 1997 *Infectious Diseases in Clinical Practice*, Dr. Classen presented more data further substantiating his findings of a vaccine-diabetes connection. With the hepatitis B vaccine or meningococcal vaccine there was a 64% increase in the incidence of Type-1 diabetes in Finland. The introduction of new vaccines in Finland, including the DPT and MMR vaccines, was accompanied by a 62% rise in the incidence of diabetes in the 0-to-four-years age group and a 19% rise of diabetes in the five-to-nine-years age group between the years 1980–1982 and 1987–1989.

Coffee and caffeinated beverages
According to Hal Huggins in *It's All in Your Head*, one cup of coffee can elevate the glucose level enough to need three units of insulin to counteract it. Caffeine ingestion was associated with a significant reduction in insulin sensitivity by a similar magnitude in the lean (33%), obese (33%), and diabetic (37%) groups in comparison with those given placebo. Caffeine intake significantly reduced insulin sensitivity in all three groups.

Smoking
According to the CDC, 17.7% of US adults with diabetes smoke, and the dangers are very real for diabetics. Smoking affects both carbohydrate and lipid metabolism. Smokers had a 15–20% higher insulin requirement and serum triglyceride concentration. In heavy smokers the insulin requirement was 30% higher.

Diabetes as an accelerated aging reality
Often diabetes doesn't get diagnosed until its complications begin to arise. Major chronic complications include: retinopathy, which leads to blindness; neuropathy, infection of the nervous system; nephropathy, or kidney disease; atherosclerotic coronary disease; and atherosclerotic vascular disease. About 85% of all diabetics develop retinopathy, 20–50% develop kidney disease, and 60–70% have mild to severe forms of nerve damage. Diabetics are two to four times more likely to develop cardiovascular disease (which is a factor in 75% of diabetes-related deaths) and two to four times more likely to suffer stroke. Multiple studies show that insulin resistance doubles the risk of heart attack as early as 15 years before diabetes is diagnosed, along with risk of stroke. Middle-age people with diabetes have death rates and a heart disease rate two times higher than those without diabetes. Diabetics are also three times more likely to develop clinical depression than non-diabetics.

The National Institute of Diabetes and Digestive and Kidney Diseases (NIDDK) reported in 1993 that diabetes is the leading cause of new cases of blindness among adults 20 to 74. About 60–70% of the people with diabetes have mild symptoms to severe forms of diabetic nerve damage. Neuropathy is the major cause of non-trauma lower limb amputation, and studies suggest that as many as

70% of amputees die within five years.

Diabetes, in essence, is an accelerated aging. So hyperinsulinemia becomes a part of the continuum of developing diabetes. It is a tip-off point before we get to diagnosable diabetes and the accelerated aging pattern known as chronic disease. Hyperinsulinemia is telling us that we have a higher risk of developing chronic degenerative diseases. Our carbohydrate metabolism requires attention and is one of the most important life extension factors.

Proper management of carbohydrate metabolism is key to a healthy life and longevity. A normal fasting blood sugar, according to ADA data, is 100. However, as we have already pointed out, the latest research shows that if you have a blood sugar of 86 or higher you are already entering into the first stages of an abnormal metabolism, an accelerated aging process, and are beginning to lose control of a healthy carbohydrate metabolism.

Hyperinsulinemia, is a metabolic time bomb and is associated with a whole series of chronic degenerative diseases. Not only is it a major risk factor for coronary heart disease, but is also linked with the rise in plasma free radicals associated with oxidative stress, which contributes to heart disease and decreased brain function. Cell damage resulting from elevated insulin and blood sugar levels can lead to degenerative diseases such as hypertension and cancer.

Chronically elevated blood sugar contributes also to the formation of advanced glycation end products, also known as AGEs. These result from the non-enzymatic glycosylation of proteins. Once the proteins become glycosylated, they lose their function and contribute further to chronic disease including atherosclerotic cardiovascular disease (ASCVD) and renal failure. They cause part of what we call cross linkages, which are, in essence, an accelerated aging process. This glycosylation also produces sugar alcohols. The AGEs in sugar alcohols are associated with nerve damage to blood vessels, kidneys, lenses of the eyes, and the pancreas, and generally accelerate the aging process. The sugar alcohol formation is associated with cataract development and diminished nerve function. Therefore at a minimum, what we want to do is to try to control the high blood sugar.

Insulin resistance
The diagnosis of insulin resistance is not the same as diabetes. It is associated with pre-diabetes and exists in many Type-2 diabetics. Insulin resistance starts before diabetes and is a whole metabolic shift. About 25 to 35% of the population have a degree of insulin resistance and suffer from the health consequences of hyperglycemia. Magnesium deficiency is very common in my clinical experience and is found in about 90% of people with diabetes. Insulin resistance is also associated with hypertension. Experimental work with magnesium deficiency showed that giving magnesium reduces tissue sensitivity to insulin. If the diet is depleted in potassium, it can also lead to insulin resistance at post-receptor sites. Zinc and chromium play a role in decreasing insulin resistance, as well as does vanadium. Biotin does appear to decrease insulin resistance according to

research.1 Just 600 mg of vitamin E has also been shown to decrease insulin resistance.

Stress also plays a role at the insulin resistance level. Acute stress seems to be clearly associated with severe, although reversible, insulin resistance. We should pay attention to stress, and the treatment of stress. A study by Nelson showed that psychosocial stress played a role in the chronic elevation of cortisol, which results in increased plasma insulin levels.

In summary, factors that may contribute to insulin resistance and thus to diabetes include: high-fat diet; low-protein diet; deficiencies of the omega-3 and omega-6 fatty acids; a diet high in simple carbohydrates; high-glycemic meals filled with refined sugar and starches; stress; low fiber intake; deficiencies of the minerals calcium, magnesium, chromium, vanadium, potassium, and zinc; deficiency of carotenoids; low intake of vegetables; lack of exercise; watching television; and nicotine.

Genetics

Type-2 has a much stronger genetic component than Type-1. A lot of research on diabetes was done in England, where there are 1.9 million diabetics. Findings explain up to 70% of the genetics involved. In Type-2 diabetes, family histories and obesity are major risk factors for the condition.

Type-1 diabetes can run in families, but there is a weak association. About 85% of people who develop Type-1 diabetes do not have an immediate family member who is diabetic.

Diabetes in children

Type-1 diabetes is rising alarmingly worldwide, at a rate of 3% per year. About 25% of the diabetic children now have Type-2, compared with just 4% ten years ago. Type-2 diabetes has changed from a disease of our grandparents and parents to a disease of our children. Part of the problem is that, unconscionably, eight to twelve-year-olds see, on average, more than 7,600 food commercials a year—the vast majority for candy, snacks, cereals, and fast food.

Gestational diabetes

Gestational diabetes is a third major category of diabetes that needs to be addressed. It occurs in five to 14% of pregnant women. It is important to diagnose this effectively and treat it because it plays a big role in the onset of Type-2 diabetes five to ten years later. Half of women who've had gestational diabetes eventually develop Type-2. It is associated with the metabolic changes that take place during a normal pregnancy. To conserve sugar for the baby, the mom's placenta produces hormones that naturally increase insulin resistance, thus rerouting some of the sugar to her fetus that before pregnancy would have gone to her cells.

Gestational diabetes is the most common medical complication in pregnancy. Women who have it face a significantly greater risk of developing diabetes later in their life. Studies have documented Type-2 diabetes at three to five years post-partum in 30 to 50% of the women. Repeated insulin resistance physiologies, due to additional pregnancies, lead to an increase in the rate of developing Type-2 diabetes later. The relative risk for Type-2 diabetes was 1.95 for each ten pounds gained during pregnancy. One study showed a fourfold increase in perinatal mortality in pregnancies complicated by improperly managed GDM. Other studies have suggested an increased rate in stillbirths associated with GDM. Maternal hyperglycemia leads to fetal hyperglycemia and fetal hyperinsulinemia with increases in fetal growth. Growth is bigger in the fatty and the liver tissues.

Alzheimer's associated diabetes

Approximately 4.5 million Americans have Alzheimer's disease, and that figure may triple in less than 50 years, according to the Alzheimer's Association. More than 65% of Americans are overweight or obese, and the Center for Disease Control and Prevention (CDC) estimates that some 21 million people are considered pre-diabetic (the ADA estimates 54 million pre-diabetics). Pre-diabetes and diabetes mean high blood sugar, greatly increasing the chance of developing diabetes, obesity, heart disease, and, according to new research, Alzheimer's. This link could foretell a dramatic increase in Alzheimer's cases, unless dietary and lifestyle interventions are made now.

Researchers are beginning to connect Alzheimer's with diabetes, obesity, and heart disease. It is such a strong connection that Alzheimer's is being referred to by scientists at Brown Medical School as Type-3 diabetes. A variety of studies have shown that people with Type-2 diabetes have about double the average incidence of Alzheimer's.

A comprehensive theory of diabetes

When Roger Bannister broke the four-minute mile in 1954, no one believed that humans had the physiological capacity to run that fast that far. Bannister clocked 3:59.4; the glass ceiling was shattered, and with it the conventional paradigm and conventional wisdom. Now it is commonplace for high school milers to run a mile in less than four minutes. *There is a Cure for Diabetes, and this chapter announces that the four-minute mile of diabetes has been broken and that we have the capacity, if we so choose, to completely reverse Type-2 diabetes.*
By developing a comprehensive theory of the causative level of diabetes we become significantly empowered to develop an overall approach for its reversal. The word *reversing* is different from ameliorating, modifying, or decreasing the amount of medication needed. We are not talking about the old paradigm of managing Type-2 diabetes as exemplified by a belief-system stated in the *New York Times* and backed by most doctors treating diabetes: "Diabetes has no cure. It is progressive and fatal." We have the knowledge, clinical know-how, and experience to completely reverse Type-2 diabetes. All that is needed is to let go of our belief that diabetes cannot be reversed. Then we are free to cultivate the understanding of what is possible.

The allopathic approach, which has indeed not been particularly successful, is that diabetes is a one-way, downhill road to death involving multiple complications. The statistics show that diabetes, as currently treated, will take ten to 19 years from a person's life. When we free ourselves from the lifestyle of the Culture of Death and transition to the Culture of Life, the current pattern of irreversibility shifts to one of reversibility. Type-2 diabetes is a disease of both a complex and simple etiology. The breakthrough in understanding diabetes was found in Dr. Thomas Cleave's 1975 book, *The Saccharine Disease: Conditions Caused by the Taking of Refined Carbohydrates such as Sugar and White Flour,* showing that within 20 years after processed white flour and sugar is introduced into a culture, there is an "outbreak" of diabetes. His statistical analysis showed processed sugar rather than fat as the primary cause.

Dr. Cleave showed that when diabetes mortality was charted against the consumption of refined carbohydrates—white sugar and white flour—rather than total consumption of carbohydrates (both complex and refined), there was a much closer statistical correlation between refined carbohydrate consumption and diabetes mortality. This point was made clearer by the fact that in communities where refined carbohydrates were not introduced, and where a high consumption of complex carbohydrates was maintained, there was not a significant increase in diabetes. Therefore Dr. Cleave concluded, as we have, that the introduction of refined carbohydrates into a culture was the primary, but not sole, cause of the dramatic increase in diabetes. Other underlying causes include increased consumption of cooked animal fats and trans fats, heavy metals, agrochemicals, vitamin D deficiencies, mineral and vitamin deficiencies in general, resulting from a diet of nutrient-poor processed foods, and hormonal imbalances and deficiencies such as a deficiency in testosterone. Dr. Cleave's cross-cultural work, however, highlighted the main issue, which was an excess increase in the consumption of white sugar.

> It is obvious that a successful program for healing diabetes must eliminate all refined carbohydrates from the diet as the primary step in dietary change.

The main dietary cause of diabetes is processed sugar. In my clinical experience we have found that even moderate- to high-glycemic fruits in the diet raise the blood glucose levels of those with pre-diabetes and diabetes. While limited amounts of these foods may be acceptable for those not in a pre-diabetic or diabetic physiology, we do not recommend them until people are maintained in a healthy physiology (fasting blood sugar of 70–85 for at least six months to a year). At that time, it is most prudent to introduce only low-glycemic berries, cherries, and citrus to maintain a healthy physiology.

The second major contributor to the onset of diabetes is a diet high in cooked animal fat and trans fatty acids. An excess of saturated animal fats and trans fatty acids is associated with increased diabetes. The basic research evidence shows that meat eaters have a 400% greater incidence of diabetes. Not all fats are harmful, however. I have observed different things in relationship to different amounts of fat. One of the possible problems that I have seen in long-term use of a 10%-fat diet is the possibility of omega-3 deficiencies. Omega-3 deficiency means less effective cell membrane function, less effective nerve transmission, less effective serotonin and other neurotransmitter production, transmission, and neuroreceptor site function in the cells. Ten percent or less fat in the diet also creates the possibility of omega-6 deficiencies. *The nature of the fat is far more important than the amount of fat*, although both are important. Studies by Dr. Edward Howell on the Inuit showed that when they ate high amounts of raw blubber they did not develop heart disease, high blood pressure, or any significant morbidity. When they began cooking their blubber, they began to develop heart disease and high blood pressure. Specific data on diabetes before and after the change from raw blubber to cooked is not available, but since the switch to the Western cooked-animal-fat diet, as well as to using white sugar and white flour, there certainly has been an increase in Type-2 diabetes. The additional message here is that cooking destroys enzymes and alters the structure of the fat. When you cook or fry saturated fat, it becomes unhealthy. In addition, the processing of fats through hydrogenation changes them from a cis- structure to a trans- structure. There is actually a physical change in the structure.

At the Tree of Life Rejuvenation Center we have found dramatic positive results in healing diabetes by putting people on live foods with a live-moderate-fat diet. We recommend 15 to 20% uncooked fat, depending on a person's constitution. This is still moderately low. Plant-source food has no cholesterol, so all blood lipid levels tend to go to normal. Because of this, we are not convinced that it is fat only that is the problem so much as whether the fat is cooked (or animal-based), and in which the actual structures have changed, and therefore the cell membrane has changed with a consequent compromise in cell signaling. Plant-source-only live-food fats, such as those in almonds and walnuts, have actually been shown to lower cholesterol and help with the healing of diabetes. For example, the people in our study experienced a 44% average decrease in their LDL cholesterol in 21–30 days. Most of these people went to an LDL of approximately 80, which is the minimal cut-off point for the prevention of heart disease.

The omega-3 fatty acids and monounsaturated fats improve insulin function. One study of 86,000 women followed over 16 years, in the Nurses' Health Study, found that those who consumed one ounce of nuts five times per week decreased their risk of Type-2 diabetes by 27%. Evidence suggests that a raw vegan diet, moderately high in walnuts, almonds, and sunflower seeds may be helpful in the prevention of diabetes and in regulating glycemic control.

Achieving Normal Blood Sugar Levels

Blood Glucose Levels
What are conventionally considered "normal" glucose levels are actually unhealthy. It now appears that the optimal fasting blood sugar (FBS), which is one's blood glucose first thing in the morning, should be at 85. The normal range of healthy glucose is between 70 and 85. Accelerated aging occurs with an FBS of 86 or greater and with that an increased risk of premature death. We have just begun to recognize that even a high normal glucose can eventually become a

serious threat to our health. The issue we need to understand is the complex toxic effects that high blood sugar or hyperglycemia create in the body. It should be clear at this point that high blood sugar damages cells and tissues through multiple mechanisms and accelerates all elements of aging. When one wants to lower blood sugar, one of the obvious things to do is to stop the intake of all forms of simple sugars.

A critical key to healing diabetes is eating and living in a way that creates an FBS of 85 and below. A potent means of achieving this is associated with caloric restriction. This information comes from animal studies and our clinical experience, where caloric restriction induced significant reductions in blood glucose levels. The message is: The less we eat, the longer we live, and the better control we have over blood glucose. By decreasing caloric intake, our risk of age-related diseases is diminished and a slowing of aging is activated. When people eat too much in general, their blood sugar often rises. On a calorie-restricted diet, their blood sugar is more likely to stay at normal levels. This observation is from my clinical experience in watching people we call the "canaries in the mine." These are people with Type-1 diabetes or sensitive Type-2s. I would ask them to try a particular food or try overeating and observe their blood glucose levels. This is not as scientifically accurate as double-blind studies, but it certainly pointed me in the right direction. Overeating, even of low glycemic foods may, raise the blood sugar.

To further illustrate this point, a study of 2,000 men over a 20-year period showed that those with fasting glucose levels over 85 had a 40% increased risk of death from cardiovascular disease. With this kind of data, one should not be surprised that the author would define an FBS above 85 as glucose toxicity. The researchers concluded *"fasting blood glucose values in upper normal range appeared to be an important independent predictor of cardiovascular death in non-diabetic middle aged men"*.

In some instances a food has a low glycemic index rating but a high insulin index rating, which is another vantage point in understanding how diet affects insulin levels. The insulin index is based upon the insulin response to various foods, and certain foods (such as lean meats or animal, chicken, fish, or dairy proteins) seem to cause an increased insulin response despite there being no carbohydrates present.

The satiety index (SI) is a relatively new concept that measures how full or satiated people feel after consuming a given calorie load from a variety of foods. It is measured by asking people to rate how satiated they feel after a meal and by how much food they eat after a two-hour delay after consuming the test food. Thus, a high-SI food would leave people more satisfied after eating a set amount of calories, and they would also eat less two hours later when given something else to eat, presumably because they are still less hungry. It seems likely that a diet made up of higher-SI foods would likely lead to less hunger and a lower calorie intake. High-fructose corn syrup is a concern, because it brings high amounts of sugar into the system but does not activate a feeling of being satiated; thus people are more likely to keep eating. The high-fructose corn syrup sweeteners that have been implicated in the epidemic of obesity are an interesting example of a low-SI food, as it does not turn on the natural satiety response.

Oxidative stress

Higher blood glucose also creates oxidative stress. Research has clearly shown that the antioxidants vitamin C and E inhibit the formation of AGEs, and have been shown to reduce protein glycosylation both *in vivo* and *in vitro*, with beneficial results in the treatment of Type-2 diabetes. Vitamins C and E also act as scavengers of free radicals generated by the glycosylated proteins.

Most foods high on the glycemic and insulin indices greatly accelerate metabolic imbalance. If you have a blood sugar that is 200 mg/dl after eating, or actually any time of day, that is considered diagnostic of diabetes. If your fasting blood sugar is 126 or higher on two separate occasions it supports a presumptive diagnosis of diabetes and merits further testing.

Type-1 Diabetes (IDDM)

The cause of Type-1 diabetes is somewhat different than Type-2. The genetic research does suggest that if a first-degree relative has IDDM, a child has a 5 to 10% chance of developing it. The main cause of type-1 diabetes is an inflammatory insult. These insults create an inflammation response, called insulinitis. What happens is that the activated T-lymphocytes infiltrate the islet cells in the pancreas. Macrophages and T-cells appear to be involved in the destructive cycle as they release cytokines that create free radical damage. This free-radical induced islet beta cell death involves breaks in the DNA strands. Type-1 is primarily an inflammatory response from an autoimmune reaction from antibodies being made against the beta cells. Certain viruses seem to attack and destroy the pancreatic beta cells directly, rather than through an auto-immune reaction. Mumps, prior to the onset of diabetes, was found in 42.5% of the subjects versus 12.5% in the control group. There are elevated levels of Coxsackie virus IGM antibodies. Exposure to virus infections *in utero* or during childhood may initiate beta cell damage. Rubella and chickenpox didn't seem to make any significant difference. Some research suggests that routine vaccinations may be linked with inflammation of the beta cells of the pancreas, but it isn't enough data for us to make a definitive statement.

There is a significant correlation between antibodies to cow's milk protein, particularly to bovine serum albumin, in the onset of IDDM. Some studies have suggested that somewhere between 75 and 90% of the cases of Type-1 have antibodies against the beta cells of the pancreas compared to 0.5 to 2% of normal. Cow's milk seems to be strongly linked to the onset of Type-1. Those with Type-1 diabetes were more likely to have been breastfed for less than three months and exposed to cow's milk before four months. Research has also shown that children who consumed pasteurized cow's milk before the age of three were eleven times more likely to develop Type-1 diabetes. In children with Type-1 diabetes, a high percentage had antibodies against certain proteins in cow's milk. These antibodies cross-reacted with beta cells of the pancreas. In 1994, the American

Academy of Pediatrics issued a report after looking into the matter of antibodies to cow's milk protein in association with the onset of Type-1 diabetes in children. Based on more than 90 studies, the American Academy of Pediatrics agreed that, indeed, the risk of diabetes could most likely be reduced if infants are not exposed to cow's milk protein early in life. So if we really want to protect our kids, we must not expose them to cow's dairy directly by drinking or through mothers drinking cow's milk. The good news here is multifold: mother's breast milk is best; and we can also feed our children nut and seed milks made at home to provide superior nutrition *at no risk to their health.*

Type-2 Diabetes (NIDDM)
In Type-2 diabetes, also called non-insulin-dependent diabetes mellitus (NIDDM), obese people in the early diabetic stages secrete an average of 114 units of insulin, which is more than three times the normal 31 units of insulin, and lean Type-2 individuals produce between 14 and 31 units daily. The great variation for Type-2s is determined by the stage of the disease. Again, this is relative, as there seem to be two major stages in Type-2 diabetes. First, we have a hyperinsulin stage for the majority, and then as the beta cells of the pancreas begin to inflame, they get exhausted, scar, and create a shift from hyperinsulinemia to a state of insulin dependence. Therefore, it is very important to maintain an FBS of 85 or lower to keep pancreatic cells from wearing out and creating a hypoinsulin stage.

Living enzymes
Enzymes are substances that make life possible. No mineral, vitamin, or hormone can do any work without enzymes. They are the manual workers that build the body from proteins, carbohydrates, and fats. The body may have the raw building materials, but without the workers, it cannot begin. Included in the Culture of Life anti-diabetogenic diet is a significant benefit we derive from the living enzymes present in uncooked foods. Detailed information on enzymes is presented in Viktoras Kulvinskas' chapter earlier in this work.

In research at George Washington University Hospital, Dr. Rosenthol found that when 50 grams of raw starch was administered to patients their blood sugar rose only 1 mg and then decreased, but when the starch was cooked, there was a dramatic increase of 56 mg in one half-hour. This significant difference in raw versus cooked foods in terms of blood sugar regulation implies that the enzymes in the raw starch might be important. Also, heating activates the breakdown of complex carbohydrates to simple sugars more rapidly, thus raising the glycemic index of the food. My clinical experience has been that a raw-food, low-fat diet with the use of food enzymes and supplemental digestive enzymes has been very effective in the treatment of adult Type-2 diabetes. Cooking affects weight gain as well. Research has found that if raw potatoes are fed to hogs they won't gain weight, but when fed cooked potatoes they gain weight.

Generally speaking, the amount of amylase (needed to digest carbohydrates) in diabetics is about 50% of normal. It has been shown that the amylase content of liver and spleen was raised from two to 17 times over the original when digestive enzymes containing amylase were given. There is some suggestion that the external excretion of the pancreas becomes deficient in enzymes in diabetes and that oral administration of enzymes had a beneficial effect. Dr. Bassler reported a deficiency in amylase in the duodenum in more than 86% of cases of diabetes he studied. Drs. Harrison and Laurent, in 29 cases of Type-2, reported 14 cases with a significantly lower blood amylase and 13 cases with values from the low to lowest limits of the normal range. We need again to distinguish between cooked, saturated, and animal fats, versus raw fats with their natural high lipase content, such as we see in the Inuit diet, along with cold-pressed unrefined olive oil, avocado, as well as predigested raw nuts and seeds soaked overnight, and even sprouted grains, which are healthy sources of fat.

Proteolytic enzymes

Our program uses proteolytic enzymes, lipases, and general combinations of proteolytic lipase and amylase. Proteolytic enzymes seem to be associated with a tendency to clotting, appear to help decrease the inflammation effect of the disease process in Type-1 and Type-2, and seem to help unclog arteries. In Type-2, there is a constant overstimulation of the beta cells of the pancreas, eventually moving to hyperinsulinemia, inflammation, and fibrosis. The fibrosis blocks the ducts of the pancreas and appears to kill the beta cells of the pancreas. There is also inflammation and fibrosis in the glomeruli of the kidneys and fibrin, causing atherosclerosis. The proteolytic enzymes create a lysis of the fibrin plugs in the microcirculation, in the matrix of the plaque. What we see is a significant opening of peripheral circulation and therefore a decrease in the secondary degenerative symptoms. This, of course, is a theoretical explanation for why we feel the proteolytic enzymes work to reverse the diabetic degenerative process. We don't have explicit evidence to prove this theory beyond the three examples.

Minerals play a very important role, and we see specific deficiencies of magnesium, manganese, zinc, chromium, vanadium, and potassium in diabetic patients. These deficiencies could be a result of the blood hyperosmolality and the minerals being lost with excessive urination, in an attempt to get the sugar out of the system. There may be other reasons as well.

A unifying theoretical approach to healing diabetes

In summary, there is a degenerative metabolic process that arises from a diet high in sugar, cooked animal fat, and trans fatty acids, and low in fiber, combined with a lifestyle of stress, lack of exercise, and general toxicity that interfaces with and activates the diabetes-producing genes in both Type-1 and Type-2. We need a theory that includes these genetic realities. Genes play a greater role in Type-2. Diabetes affects the metabolism on many levels of fat metabolism, protein metabolism, and glucose carbohydrate metabolism. The theory must also include hormone balance and enzyme levels, as the degenerative metabolic process affects the hormone flow and is affected by it. In addition, it is affected by our enzyme levels and function, as diabetics have significantly less lipase, amylase, and proteases. The theory needs to include the process of inflammation advancing to fibrosis, which seems to be reversed by proteolytic enzymes, which also minimize and reverse the degenerative process of heart disease, kidney disease, retinopathy, and neuropathy that are the long-term complications of diabetes.

We are looking for a comprehensive understanding that can cut through the complexity of diabetes. The unifying theory and healing approach of the Tree of Life 21-Day Plus program is based on the following principle:

> **What we eat and how we live speaks to our genes. We, by what we eat and how we live, can either degrade our phenotypic expression and activate the diabetic process or improve our phenotypic expression for the prevention and reversal of diabetes.**

Genotype means the actual genes that were given genetically. In essence, genotype is analogous to a computer's hard drive. *Phenotype* is the way the genes express themselves, which can vary according to the signaling systems that we give them through our diet and lifestyle. Phenotypic expression is analogous to our software programs. Put a healthy program in, and we get a healthy response.

Since 1922, when Frederick Banting and Charles H. Best discovered insulin, which was a great contribution and saved many lives, we have taken a more medical or drug-based approach to the treatment of diabetes. Genes are polymorphic (slightly variable), and they can have multiple activators. Diet is a primary activator, and exercise and lifestyle are secondary activators. The Tree of Life diet—which starts out initially as a 100% live-food, high-complex-carbohydrate, low-glycemic and insulin-index, 15 to 20%-plant-source fat (depending on our individual constitution), and low-calorie diet—is specifically designed to upgrade the phenotypic gene expression. It results in turning off the phenotypic diabetic expression and turning on the anti-diabetogenic phenotypic expression.

Calories with Purpose

Key research, carried out in 2001 by Dr. Stephen Spindler supports this holistic theory. He underfed rats by 40%. Within a month they had a 400% increase in the expression of the anti-aging genes, and showed also an increase in the anti-inflammation genes, antioxidant genes, and anti-cancer genes. Why a live-food diet is so successful is that it turns on anti-aging genes, anti-inflammatory genes, and theoretically the anti-diabetic genes. This is because a live-food diet is a natural form of calorie restriction. When you cook your food, according to the Max Planck Institute, you coagulate 50% of your protein, 70 to 90% of your vitamins and minerals, and up to 100% of your phytonutrients. On a live-food diet properly eaten, we actually eat 50% fewer calories as compared to a Standard American Diet (SAD) but maintain a very high level of nutrition. The reason for this is that we are consuming *nutrient-dense foods*, not just calorie-dense foods such as those offered in restaurants and fast-food dispensaries all over the Westernized world. We are becoming nations of overfed, undernourished individuals. Our bodies are rebelling through the metabolic degeneration process called diabetes. They are asking us for nutrients that are not provided through the cooked, processed diet typically found in the Culture of Death.

When we say "calorie restriction," in the Tree of Life context, which is a plant-source-only, live, organic diet, it should not be misunderstood that we are denying ourselves the fuel we need. Nor are we in a cycle of deprivation. On the Tree of Life Rainbow Green and anti-diabetic Live-Food Cuisine we are eating a delicious, filling, natural, and appropriate amount of calories that are nutrient-dense enough to activate an *aliesthetic taste change*. The aliesthetic change is experienced as when we feel pleasurably satisfied from eating. It is also known as the "stop eating" signal we get from our body.

A consciously eaten live-food diet turns on the anti-aging and anti-diabetic genes. On a live-food, plant-only diet people naturally tend to go to their optimal weight. Because of this you automatically lose weight on our program if you are overweight. The people featured in a movie filmed at Tree of Life had an average weight loss (with the exception of the two Type-1 diabetics who were very thin to begin with) of 25 pounds in the first month. Often we see people who are obese lose 100-plus pounds in a year on a live-food diet without doing anything but eating live foods. Since up to 90% of diabetics are overweight, and diabetes is related to obesity, the natural weight loss down to optimal weight on a live-food diet in this context is a powerful plus. A live-food diet creates just the opposite effect of the high-refined-sugar, high-cooked-animal-fat, low-fiber diet that is creating the pandemic today. The pandemic gets worse as we go more into industrialized foods. A 100% live-food Phase 1.0 diet combined with green juice fasting is the most powerful way to upgrade the phenotypic expression and turn off the diabetic genes. A Phase 1.0 diet as described in *Rainbow Green Live-Food Cuisine* is a low-glycemic, green diet with no fruits. This is the diet that a person stays on for the first three months until fasting blood sugar has stabilized at around 85 and the glycosylated hemoglobin (HgbA1c) reaches 6.0 or less. Once we have stabilized into a healthy non-diabetic physiology, then we add low-glycemic fruits found in Phase 1.5 and give people the option of shifting to a diet of 80% live foods, which is the minimum definition of being on live foods according to the 2006 *International Living Foods Summit.*

Ayurvedic principles

On this diet there are some variations, but a general pattern is needed to activate healing. The general pattern, according to Ayurvedic principles, is that diabetes is a *kapha* disorder, although it can happen in any of the three *doshas*. The corrective diet for a kapha disorder is a low-fat, low-sugar diet with more of a focus on bitter, pungent, and astringent foods. Kapha imbalances are made worse by a high amount of oil, a high amount of sugar, and low exercise. Kaphas tend to have constipation, and they are made better by a high-fiber diet. This has been a mode of treatment for several thousand years. The treatment program in this book is based on not only current research, but on thousands of years of effective treatment and understanding. We have simply added a unified theory that enables a very rapid approach to healing and for reversing diabetes naturally. The rapid moving to normal blood sugar levels without any medications encourages people to stay with the program because they get immediate tangible results. Therefore, even in ancient times we already had the answer: an anti-kapha diet, low in sugar, low in fat, high in complex carbohydrates, plant-only and live-food based, and naturally high in fiber. As long as we stay on this diet, we will be diabetes-free.

This is an ongoing protective diet, no matter what your genetic predisposition is. *This is the breakthrough.* Although we have shared a holistic theory, results based on its application are what are most important. Our results speak louder than theory: 100% of Type-2 participants come off medications in four days and many have an FBS of 85 in a few weeks. The average FBS among the participants began at 260 on medications, and ended at an average 86.6, with everyone off all medications. LDL cholesterol dropped an average of 67 points, or 44%, with an ending average level of 82. The rapid reversal is accelerated by green juice fasting and natural supplements of herbs, minerals, high-protease enzymes and digestive enzymes with our food to build up the amylase, and liquid zeolite (Natural Cellular Defense, or NCD) when combined with the green juice fasting to help pull out the heavy metals and 65,000 environmental toxins. We have also found that the NCD seemed to help in decreasing the FBS. With this integrated approach the results of the Tree of Life 21-Day Plus program are rapid and consistent. The quicker the healing, the more encouragement people have and the happier they are.

This approach, based on my clinical experience of over 35 years and guided by a unifying theory of turning on the anti-diabetes genes and turning off the diabetes-producing genes with green juice fasting and live foods, has helped us to break the traditionally held view of diabetes. It is supported by a lifestyle that creates life and not death. The Tree of Life program is a complete holistic approach with the Culture of Life plant-source only live-food cuisine and lifestyle as its foundation.

> *"A truly good physician first finds out the cause of the illness, and having found that, first tries to cure it by food. Only when food fails does he prescribe medication."*
>
> *– Sun Ssu-mo, Tang Dynasty Taoist physician in Precious Recipes*

> *"Let nothing which can be treated by diet be treated by other means."*
>
> *– Maimonides, Jewish rabbi, philosopher and master holistic physician to Egyptian sultan*

The first principle of the Tree of Life 2-Day Plus program to heal diabetes naturally is the Culture of Life anti-diabetogenic diet: organic, plant-source only, live (raw) food, relatively high complex carbohydrates, 15–20% (low to moderate) plant-based fats, moderate protein, low glycemic index, low insulin index, high minerals, no refined carbohydrates (especially white flour and white sugar), high fiber, moderate caloric intake, and all of it prepared with love.

The Culture of Life diet, updated with the concept of individualization as explained in detail in *Conscious Eating*, is best known as the Genesis 1:29 Garden of Eden diet.

The work done by Dr. Stephen Spindler, professor of biochemistry at the University of California-Riverside was a significant breakthrough. Using gene technologies, Spindler studied the expression of 11,000 genes in the livers of young normally fed and calorie-restricted mice, and found that 60% of the age-related changes in gene expression from calorie-restricted mice occurred within a few weeks after they started the diet. The full effects of caloric restriction on the genetic profile for anti-aging develop quickly. Spindler found that caloric restriction results in a specifically produced genetic anti-aging profile and in reversal of the majority of age-related degenerative changes that showed up in the gene expression. As diabetes is an age-related degenerative process, so it follows that a general anti-aging effect should have an anti-diabetogenic effect. Spindler found a fourfold increase in the expression of the anti-aging genes in short-term caloric restrictions, and a 2.5-fold increase in the expression of rejuvenating genes in long-term caloric restriction. He was able to reproduce this with a 95% success rate.

Spindler noted that caloric restriction not only prevented deterioration or genetic change gradually over the lifespan of the animal, but actually reversed most of the aging changes in a short period of time. His research lasted only a month with the rats. In another study, he found that the most rapid change from a genetic aging profile to an anti-aging profile occurred in older animals as well as young and middle-age ones, thus making the point that it doesn't matter at what age you begin. Caloric restriction does appear to turn on the expression of the anti-aging genes and turn off the expression of the aging genes, and it most likely turns off the expression of diabetic genes. We have a full memory of all our gene expression in our chromosomes; all we have to do is push the right dietary button to get a healthy expression.

Returning to Spindler, an important part of his research is that the short-term caloric restriction can turn on the majority of the anti-aging genes. He found that weight loss from caloric restriction improves insulin sensitivity, improves blood glucose values, decreases blood insulin levels, decreases heart rate, and improves blood pressure. In summary, Spindler's results, published in the proceedings of the National Academy of Sciences, showed:

- No matter what age you are, you still get an anti-aging effect with calorie restriction
- Anti-aging effects can happen quickly on a low-calorie diet

- Caloric restriction of only four weeks in mice seems to partially restore the liver's ability for metabolizing drugs and for detoxification
- Caloric restriction seems to quickly decrease the amount of inflammation and stress even in older animals. We see these same positive results in our one-week green juice fasting retreats at the Tree of Life in the US and Israel.

What we eat feeds our genes as well as what we do not eat. It is our choice. This is the key to understanding the diet for reversing diabetes. We will take it one step farther, so that it is very clear. The Tree of Life 21-Day Plus program starts with green juice fasting for seven days, because that is the most powerful form of caloric restriction and therefore has the most potential effect on balancing the insulin messages to our genes to turn off the diabetogenic process. We begin to see positive effects within four to seven days. When we cut through the metabolic complexities of diabetes, and we simply see it as an accelerated form of aging, which it is, then we can apply an approach that gets to the core of reversing the diabetic process—turning on the anti-aging genes and the anti-diabetic genes through the Culture of Life anti-diabetogenic world cuisine.

Client Results
Below is a summary of the fasting blood sugar (FBS) results that we achieved for our pilot study of eleven participants, all off their oral hypoglycemics or insulin. The initial FBS results were achieved with all on oral hypoglycemics and insulin. Everyone was off these medications within four days of beginning the program.

CLIENT	INITIAL FBS	ENDING FBS	FBS POINT DROP	% CHANGE
Client 1	293	88	205	70%
Client 2	287	74	213	74%
Client 3	400	85	315	79%
Client 4	400	109	291	73%
Client 5	248	83	165	67%
Client 6	130	82	48	37%
Client 7	111	87	24	22%
Client 8	300	70	230	77%
Client 9	144	82	62	43%
Client 10	120	65	55	46%
Client 11	279	126	153	55%
AVERAGES	**247**	**86**	**161**	**65%**

Weight
The results summarized in the success stories that follow are occurring in people who are dramatically overweight. We are not operating a weight loss clinic, but our observation is that 82% of people will come into a normal weight within two years of adopting a Culture of Life anti-diabetogenic cuisine and lifestyle. In all cases people felt stronger and healthier. Five people featured in the movie *Simply Raw: Reversing Diabetes in 30 Days*, which was made at Tree of Life, felt so much better by all their indicators that they were able to climb Red Mountain, a 1,000-ft-plus climb over difficult terrain. For many diabetics, even those in a

post-diabetes physiology, weight loss may need to continue to further reduce the risk of the complications of overweight, including increased insulin resistance and the temptation to return to a diabetogenic lifestyle. The average weight loss after one month was 25 pounds for those who were overweight at the beginning of the program.

Eleven Success Stories

Client 1
This 59-year-old male had a health history of Type-2 diabetes for ten years and an FBS near 300 before starting the program. Additional chronic conditions included heart disease with pacemaker, hypertension, obesity, and stroke.

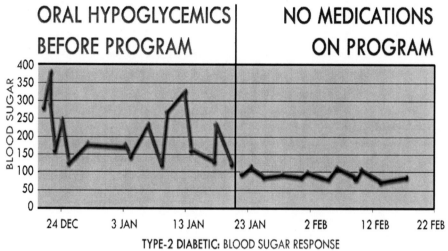

TYPE-2 DIABETIC: BLOOD SUGAR RESPONSE
TREE OF LIFE 21 DAY PLUS REVERSING DIABETES NATURALLY PROGRAM

This client came to the Tree of Life with a history of blood sugar levels near 500, and at the start of the program his blood sugar before lunch on the January 14 was 330. Within a few days of officially beginning the program, on the January 22, his FBS had already dropped to 123, and by the 27th, just five days later, he reached an FBS of 88, close to a normal, non-diabetic FBS. When he began the program, his weight was 288; one month later he was down to 256. His fructosamine levels dropped into normal range, from 313 at the start to 262 after one month. C-reactive protein went from 8.8 to 3.8. Total cholesterol dropped from 147 to 107, and triglyceride levels held steady at 113.

Client 2
This 25-year-old male had a medical history of hospital-diagnosed Type-1 diabetes for more than five years. His medications included Lantis 15U, and Glucophage 500mg twice/day.

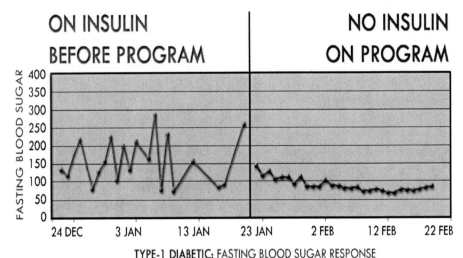

TYPE-1 DIABETIC: FASTING BLOOD SUGAR RESPONSE
TREE OF LIFE 21 DAY PLUS REVERSING DIABETES NATURALLY PROGRAM

FBS for Client 2

After just four days on the program, Client 2 was off his insulin completely, with an FBS of 88. By two weeks his FBS was consistently below 83 and remains there two years later. His fructosamine dropped from 480 to 340, within normal range, in three weeks. His glycosylated hemoglobin HgbA1c has returned to 6.0 from 11.8. Total cholesterol went from 216 to 150, and LDL cholesterol from 142 to 88, essentially eliminating him from the pool of people who tend to develop heart disease. His triglyceride level fell from 65 to 53. Weight loss was not a serious need for this client; he lost six pounds in 20 days and then gained back three pounds. To resolve the question of whether he was Type-1 or Type-2, the patient went to his local MD for further tests. His beta cell antibody titers were significantly high at 8.9 (normal is 0–1.5), strongly suggesting that he is indeed a Type-1 diabetic. His clinical history, which was a rapid and fulminating onset of diabetes, causing him to be hospitalized with a blood sugar of 1200, is consistent with a medical history of Type-1 diabetes, as contrasted with Type-2, which is characterized by a slow onset of symptoms. It is interesting, and perhaps historic in the field of diabetes research, to note that in a one-year follow-up his serum C-peptide, which is associated with a precursor to insulin, was originally less than 0.5, and is now 0.7. This suggests that the program is actually beginning to rebuild or reactivate the beta cells of the pancreas.

Client 3

This client began the program on March 27. Before she arrived, her blood sugar had hit levels as high as 465 just three weeks before the program. By her 21st day on the program, her FBS had reached 85, and weight loss was 25 pounds.

Client 4

This diabetic was 39 years old with Type-2 for five years and had a medical history of hypertension and obesity—in my estimation, a classic example of Syndrome X. At the start of the program her FBS was 400 and her weight was 352 pounds. After one month her FBS dropped as low as 109 and her weight dropped to 329 pounds. Her CRP dropped from 37.8 to 8.6. Her total cholesterol dropped from 237 to 171 and triglycerides dropped from 225 to 123 in one month.

Client 5
This client was a 55-year-old Type-2 diabetic for ten years and manifested a Syndrome X pattern. He started with an FBS of 248, and within 18 days on the program his FBS reached 83, off all medications.

Client 6
This Type-2 diabetic started with an FBS of 130 on oral diabetic medications. In one week while off all medications, her FBS dropped to 82. She also lost 13 pounds in three weeks. Her total cholesterol dropped from 217 to 140 and LDL went from 148 to 46.

Client 7
A 61-year-old female Type-2 diabetic for ten years, this client had an average FBS of 111. By the end of the program her thinking, which had been slower, became clearer and more connected to the environment. By the end of the program her FBS was 87 and has remained in the 80s for more than a year, shown at our one-year follow-up, with an HgbA1c level of 5.5.

Client 8
Type-2 diabetes was diagnosed for this 55 year old two months after her last baby was born, 35 years ago. She came to us with an average FBS of 300 and was using four doses of oral hypoglycemic medications each day. On day one, she eliminated her use of oral hypoglycemics and achieved an FBS of 105. Days two through four, her FBS was 50, and then raised to 77, 84, and 70 for days five, six, and seven, respectively. Several weeks after her green juice fast she continued to remain with an FBS of around 70 with occasional spikes up to 170 when she ate something sweet. These spikes helped convince her not to succumb to the idea of "moderation" in the Culture of Death.

Client 9
This client had Type-2 diabetes for ten years, with a history on Metformin and Glucorite for the past three years. On day one, she stopped the use of medications. Her FBS was 144 on day one, 129 on day two, and by day seven it was 102. On day eight, she achieved a non-diabetic FBS of 82.

Client 10
This Type-2 diabetic started the fasting program with an average FBS of 110–120. By day two, the FBS was 98, and by day seven, 65.

Client 11
This is an interesting case because it shows that healing does not necessarily occur completely in three to four weeks. During her one-month program, she lost

26 pounds, went from using 35 units of insulin a day to 0 units, discontinued the use of the pharmaceuticals Lantis, Byetta, Neurontin, and Monopril within four days, saw a decrease in her C-reactive protein levels from 8.4 to 2.6, lowered her total cholesterol from 210 to 136 (with LDL dropping from 142 to 85 and HDL rising from 25 to 29), and lowered her FBS from 279 to 126, for a 55 percent drop without any medications. This particular client was well on her way to a healthy reversal when she returned home.

General anti-diabetogenic Diet
The following are charts that show low-glycemic, low-insulin-score Rainbow Green food for Phases 1.0 and 1.5 of the Tree of Life cuisine program.

RAINBOW GREEN CUISINE, PHASE 1.0
- All vegetables except cooked carrots and cooked beets
- All sea vegetables
- Non-sweet fruits: tomatoes, avocados, cucumber, red pepper, lemons, limes
- Fats and oils: flax oil, hemp oil, sesame oil, walnut, almond, sunflower, and avocado, coconut (not more than 1 tablespoon per day)
- Nuts and seeds (except cashews), coconut pulp
- Superfoods: Klamath Lake blue-green algaes (E-3Live is the most active), spirulina, chlorella, Green Superfood powder mixes
- Sweeteners: stevia, cardamom, cinnamon
- Salt: Himalayan and Celtic sea salt

RAINBOW GREEN CUISINE, PHASE 1.5
(Additions to Phase 1.0)
- All vegetables: carrots (raw), beets (raw), squash (raw)
- Fruits: low-glycemic fruits—blueberries, raspberries, cherries, fresh and un-sweetened cranberries, pomegranate, goji berries, grapefruit, lemons, limes
- Condiments and sweeteners: mesquite, cacao, carob
- Bee pollen granules
- Grains: quinoa, buckwheat, millet, amaranth, spelt
- Fermented and cultured foods: apple cider vinegar, miso (non-soy), sauer-kraut, probiotic drinks

Phase 1: no grains, not sweet or fermented
Phase 1.5: grains stored less than 90 days, low-sweet fruits, and fermented food
Phase 1.5: A small amount of Phase 2 fruits and veggies in a large salad

Lifestyle habits in the Tree of Life program

Exercise
In the case of insulin-resistant or Type-2 diabetes, exercising regularly can mean the difference between pharmaceutical dependence and drug-free blood sugar control. Diabetics who exercise experience many levels of improvement. These include enhanced insulin sensitivity, and therefore less need for injecting insulin, improved glucose tolerance, reduced total cholesterol and triglycerides with in-creased HDL levels, and improved weight loss. There is no need to make exer-

cise a complicated procedure, but rather to find exercise that is enjoyable and that finds you feeling positively stimulated rather than exhausted. Jumping on a rebounder, or mini-trampoline, is possibly the best and most fun cardiovascular and lymphatic stimulating exercise, requiring the least amount of time of any exercise system. It is my favorite aerobic and lymphatic stimulating exercise.

Muscle building
When you consider that muscle tissue is responsible for 80% of blood sugar uptake following a meal, it is easy to understand why every bit of extra muscle helps. Another important benefit of muscle tissue is that, unlike fat tissue, it constantly uses energy. The more muscle tissue you have, the higher your metabolic rate will be, because while you burn a certain amount of calories during exercise, your muscle tissue will continue to burn calories hours after you exercise.

Meditation and Prayer
The Tree of Life 21-Day Plus program also includes training in meditation, as stress has been distinctly related to an increase in blood sugar secondary to an increase in epinephrine and corticosteroid secretion as well as an increase in insulin resistance. The value of meditation and yoga has been shown in such well-known programs as that of Dr. Dean Ornish, in which they were able to reverse atherosclerosis, as well as the large body of research linking meditation to general improvement in health, vitality, and longevity. It is interesting to note that researchers at the Medical University of South Carolina found that people with diabetes who regularly attend religious services had lower levels of C-reactive protein, an inflammatory risk factor for cardiovascular disease, the leading cause of death among diabetics. On a deeper level, it has been my consistent observation that those who have some sort of spiritual connection increase their ability to heal. There is never enough food for the hungry soul, and meditation and prayer feed the hungry soul.

Yoga
In addition to meditation, we also teach Kali Ray TriYoga™, which is good for decreasing physical and mental stress. Yoga in general is another form of exercise, but it has many more uses than just cardiovascular exercise. It is a total system that creates a flow of energy through the body, helps to heal the body, and stimulates the pancreas and other internal organs. Although there are certain traditional poses associated with the healing of diabetes, we prefer this system because not only does it include these diabetes-healing poses but also because the flowing system creates an energy that has a greater overall healing effect. In general, almost all forms of yoga provide a helpful tonic for the stimulation and healing of the internal organs, such as the pancreas, liver, kidneys, and adrenals. Practiced regularly, yoga can help regulate blood glucose levels, reduce stress-hormone levels, and help with weight control. Find a knowledgeable and experienced yoga teacher in your local area who feels comfortable using yoga as a means for supporting the healing of your diabetes.

Zero Point Process
One of the most important parts of the program is the Zero Point course,

a psycho-spiritual four-day training that helps people let go of their dysfunctional eating and lifestyle habits to which many diabetics, like the rest of our society, are addicted. This course also helps the diabetic let go of the allopathic myth that Type-2 diabetes is not curable and is a slow and steady downhill death march. During the course, participants open up the doors to loving themselves in a deeper way, which of course helps to facilitate healing.

This course takes place in the second week of the 21-Day Plus program. In the Zero Point process, clients receive two of the most important gifts one can receive in any healing program: first, clearing negative thought forms usually associated with the shadow of the Culture of Death, which leads to the second: allowing you to love yourself and activating the belief of your power to heal yourself.

The foundation for reversing diabetes is turning on the anti-aging genes, and turning off the expression of the diabetogenic genes.

This profoundly and positively affects the protein, lipid, and carbohydrate metabolism in diabetes. The delicious Culture of Life anti-diabetogenic cuisine at Phase 1.5 is, however, what we will always need to eat in order to maintain a healthy phenotypic expression and live a new whole way that not only prevents the onset of diabetes but also creates a healthy body, mind, and joyous spirit. The Culture of Life plant-source-only, 80% raw food diet is the primary foundation of the program, and the herbs and supplements are secondary foundations that accelerate and support the healing.

A most important key to the success of the program is its sustainability. My clinical results with the use of live foods and green juice fasting leave no doubt that we can rapidly and safely take people off insulin and oral hypoglycemics with very rapid returns to a healthy FBS. The key question that remains is the sustainability of living in the diet and lifestyle of the Culture of Life.

One advantage of the 21-Day Plus program is its rapid results, which make the point clearly that something can be done immediately to reverse the diabetic physiology back to normal. The power of the immediate results is overwhelming. This is not a compromised or "moderate" approach that slows the march to diabetic death. My observation is that it takes between one and two years to become firmly rooted in this Culture of Life diet and lifestyle. Included in our 21-Day Plus program is a one-year follow-up with a variety of support systems. A key understanding is the teaching that what the death culture euphemistically calls "moderation" actually kills. Moderation in this context kills because it reactivates the death sentence. This is why the ADA and most doctors say that diabetes is not curable or reversible, because they are prescribing moderation, which simply does not work by their own admission. It is actually a path of *immoderation*.

In the third week of the 21-Day Plus program, there is training in how to prepare Phase 1.0 plant-source-only 80-percent live foods. This is a five-day course in which we like to include the family. The focus is to empower people in the fundamentals of the Phase 1.0 Culture of Life live-food plant-source-only cuisine. A delicious anti-diabetogenic cuisine that you can joyfully live on through the years is essential for the prevention and treatment of diabetes. The Culture of Life cuisine as taught in the Tree of Life 21-Day Plus program works. The cuisine is not a diet that you go on, but rather the delightful culinary aspect of living in the Culture of Life, for your whole life. I believe that the ultimate long-term success of the program depends on the support system created through the Zero Point course, the new dietary training, and the one-year follow-up.

Summarizing thoughts

Over a period of 35 years, I have seen a variety of people heal diabetes naturally with live foods and fasting. Other live-food clinics have achieved similar results. Research reported in the literature by Dr. James Anderson, and by Dr. Neal Barnard, have validated the importance of a plant-source-only diet in the amelioration of diabetes. All we have done differently with our 21-Day plus program is to take the next logical and common sense step. As Ralph Waldo Emerson said, "Society is always taken by surprise by any new example of common sense." The common sense in this case, is that we understand the power of live foods and green juice fasting to create a genetic upgrade. We have found that by taking the next evolutionary step, supported by clinical experience and employing a diet that is based on those principles, clients move away from a phenotypic expression of diabetes to a phenotypic expression of health and well being. We have done the obvious and common sense move by making the green juice fast and live-food plant-source diet the prudent approach to healing diabetes naturally. As with all human issues of healing, one is not able to issue a 100% guarantee, but our clinical experience at this point has been that this is the case for 90% of our clients within three weeks, if they are fully attentive to the program.

It is clear that the 21-Days Plus program gives a desirable result. The big question is the human question—can people sustain themselves in the Culture of Life with a high degree of success? With highly motivated people there is a high success rate, but as this is applied to a pandemic level in many cultures and economic realities, we are looking very closely and creatively at support programs that will be desirable and thus successful for all circumstances. This will require a lot of creativity to apply this logical, common-sense breakthrough to cultures worldwide. It is one thing to develop a successful health program, but something else to create a program that is feasible for all.

The causal levels come out of the Culture of Death, which is naturally promoting a Culture of Death diet, which leads people to a place where they feel at a point of no return once the diabetes genes are activated. The sensible and important awareness is that there is always the potential of a return to health.

To make this kind of significant change requires a lifestyle and diet that is dramatically and excitingly different, resulting in powerful results in a short period of time. This requires leading a life of love, purpose, meaning, and self-value, and choosing a diet and lifestyle that reflect these values. Of course, this is the diet and lifestyle of the Culture of Life.

The essential question that is asked of participants is *"Do you love yourself enough to want to heal and save your life?"*

The healing of diabetes at the pandemic level requires the healing of the ecology of the planet and the consciousness of the people. To heal oneself requires the ability to love oneself enough to have the intention to reconnect with the Culture of Life, which is our birthright. In that way we perform an Act of Love for oneself as an individual person, and as part of the living planet. This results in the healing of the planet and all species. The healing of diabetes in this context is an Act of Love, Compassion, and Consciousness.

There Is A Cure For Diabetes, as my research document makes clear. The live-food lifestyle and cuisine is a major antidote, not only for diabetes and the 246 million diabetics currently suffering from it, but also for the imbalances in the current way of life that are overtly bringing famine, disease, war, and death to the world. It is a major gift to the world from the live-food culture and should significantly increase the awareness of the importance of live-food for healing the world, one person at a time.

About the Author:
***Gabriel Cousens**, M.D., M.D. (H) Diplomat American Board of Holistic Medicine, Diplomat Ayurveda. Dr. Cousens is an internationally celebrated healer, spiritual facilitator, peace-worker, author and lecturer. The founder and director of the Tree of Life Rejuvenation Center in Arizona, USA, Dr. Cousens is also a best-selling author whose titles include **Spiritual Nutrition, Rainbow Green Live Food Cuisine, Conscious Eating, Depression-Free for Life and There Is A Cure for Diabetes**.*

Currently the Tree of Life 21 Day program is being offered in two locations, Tree of Life US and Tree of Life by the Dead Sea.
To Reach Us in the US
For more information on our programs or for reservations, fill in the "Call-Me-Now" form at www.treeoflife.nu, or call toll-free 1-866-394-2520 (local 1-520-394-2520).
Tree of Life Rejuvenation Center
P.O. Box 778 (mail)
686 Harshaw Road (shipping)
Patagonia, AZ 85624 USA
Toll-free 1-866-394-2520; local 1-520-394-2520
E-mail: info@treeoflife.nu
Website: www.treeoflife.nu

To Reach us at The Tree of Life at the Dead Sea

Serving Israel and European communities. The Center is located thirty minutes from the holy city of Jerusalem and forty-five minutes from Tel Aviv International Airport. For further information, international air and road travel, and registration, please call Ya'ara at +972-50-226-7596.

E-mail treeoflife.israel@gmail.com.
Website at http://www.treeoflife.org.il

AFTERWORD

Getting on Track and Staying on Track

Walter Urban, PhD

The quality of your life depends largely upon what you eat. You can choose healthy raw organic food, or you can choose dead toxic food. Which do you prefer – energetic health, or disease and perhaps premature death? You can make a responsible choice starting today, or you can wait for the "wake up" crisis. The information contained in this book will give you the tools necessary to undertake the challenge to make the changes that will improve your health at any age. Open your mind, open your heart – and close your mouth to all that harms you. Join us in the adventure of a new lifestyle. If you believe you can do it, you *can* do it. You are your only obstacle. You can learn how to overcome your unhealthy food choices, and this book has been written to help educate you on how to make healthy choices.

To make healthy food choices, it helps to understand yourself and your life history. Some of us find various reasons, both conscious and unconscious, that prevent us from not only making changes, but also from looking at ourselves objectively. We can become so caught up in our pre-programmed functioning that we can't step out of our routine, because the level of consciousness that we have has not yet enabled us to do so.

From my own early life, when I was eating candy, pizza, burgers, and just about everything else from the SAD (Standard American Diet) – and was suffering from regular infections and illness – it was quite a journey to get to where I am now. I had absolutely no nutritional guidance except for what I received from school and the government. I know now that there was also an emotional side to my 2

263

former eating habits. I carried chocolate in my car for emergency feelings of loneliness, fear, and insecurities. I ate to fill my emotional emptiness, frustration, and depression.

My father died of arteriosclerosis when I was in my early 30s, and for four years before he died he took nitroglycerin pills for his chest pains when he walked. Before that he had an aorta resection due to aneurisms. I decided that the same things weren't going to happen to me. I took action, and now, at 75 years old, my blood pressure is about 118 over 68, triglycerides 46, cholesterol 180, and my hdl/ldl ration is about 2.4. I chose to live.

A look in the mirror
So now take a look at yourself. Please take this seriously, because you are dealing with your life. The statistics found in this book will make you want to embrace life rather than let it waste. Wake up before you become one of this book's negative statistics. I hope that this book's words reach and inspire you, because if they don't, the drugs and surgery you may need won't help and will surely make you worse. When you treat the symptoms rather than eliminate the cause, it's a downhill ride into the grave. This isn't meant to scare you, but rather to start the awakening process.

So what is the first step for you? Own the truth. Take a look at yourself and start an objective evaluation. Only you can start doing that; no one else can make that decision for you. It is a decision you have to make for your life, and if you delay making it, consider it as a negative one. Please don't make the usual excuses or rationalizations that have been obstacles up to now. Just make the decision to start. And you don't have to change all at once. Give yourself all the time you need to make the changes. It took me many years of little changes to get to where I am now. The key is getting on the right path and staying focused. Each minor slip or temptation will become a challenge that can strengthen you.

You can start right now by looking at yourself in the mirror. Fat and an extended abdomen are two sure signs that you need to make some changes. A complete blood analysis including homocystine would also be helpful to see if you are out of the normal range of health.

Addictions
The sugar addiction could be considered to be the biggest and most widespread addiction of all. The quick rush from sugar offers billions of people a temptation that is irresistible. There are children who are raised on cola because their parents are sugar (and caffeine) addicts and have no awareness of the effects that soft drinks have on their bodies. It's like a disease handed down from one generation to the next. I have been to 23 countries and have seen cola in every one of them. I have spoken with many people who say they know what cola does, even as they sit there slowly sipping it down! They know they're addicted, and they still have little or no capacity to challenge themselves. Many years ago I treated a patient in psychotherapy. She was depressed and angry regularly, and after two years of work with her, I found out that she drank a six-pack of

cola every day. After discovering that, I realized that I had to include nutritional information in psychotherapy!

Another unhealthy common nutritional habit that may be considered by some to be an addiction is eating meat. The uninformed believe that they need meat every day to get enough protein. I ask these people this: Where do bulls, cows, giraffes, and other herbivorous animals get their protein from if they don't eat meat and only eat greens? The milk myth for calcium is another misconception, especially for children who are taught to believe that they need milk to make their bones grow. There are many, many food addictions that are perpetuated and continue to promote unhealthy living and disease. Take that look in the mirror and ask yourself if you have any unhealthy food addictions, and then challenge yourself to change before you get the wake up call!

Emotional eating

Rather than trying to satisfy emotional issues, I believe that healthy nourishment should be a primary reason for eating. Food is a major early satisfier, as it is associated with the breast and mothering. This connection between food and comfort (and the removal of discomfort) plays a very important role in our lives. Through this association, which is repeated over and over, we develop habits that soon become automatic reactions. So when we want to comfort ourselves or get away from unpleasant feelings, we often use food as a relief device. The more we do this, the stronger the habit becomes, and we reach the point of not thinking about what or why we are eating. We just do it automatically.

If you fall into this category, even just a little bit, stop and become conscious of the connection between the discomfort and the food. Wait a few minutes before you start eating. This will give you a bit of strength to take the mountain of unhealthiness down with the first shovel of dirt.

As you become aware of your unpleasant feelings, you may discover when they occur, what initiates them, and how long they last. Try to understand the cause of these feelings and seek help if you need to. Remember that you don't fill your own cavities yourself and probably don't do your own car repairs, so getting help with negative feelings may be in order. The longer you wait to take corrective action, the stronger the habit becomes, so why not start as soon as possible?

The need for truthful public education

Most of us develop our eating habits from our family, culture, and geographic location. Very often diseases run in families because they eat the same foods. For example, if you live in Costa Rica and eat fried pork skin and other parts of the pig, you will develop a different health/disease profile than if you lived in Okinawa and ate seaweed and fish. Step back and take another look at your food history and learn how you developed tastes for certain foods. If the information in this book convinces you, then further examine, evaluate, and research the information we provide. Then you will be on the road to a healthier life.

The real need is for truthful public education rather than the corporate propaganda that has brainwashed earlier generations. Some examples of this propaganda are that you need meat for protein, milk to make your bones grow, and vitamin-enriched bread to make you healthy. There are many examples of corporate control and corruption, and one of them includes the funding of research programs. Our disease-care system costs billions, and who benefits? Elderly people are among the most vulnerable, with some taking five to ten meds a day before they have surgery. That's why I think the need for current truthful public education is crucial.

The real challenge is how we get this done. We need strength in our numbers. As green businesses continue to develop and a part of the economy becomes based on health rather than disease, we have the beginnings of change. This method may be rather slow, but it is better than no change at all. The stock prices of whole foods is an example of this growth process. The growth of a leading product called e3live, an algae from Klamath Lake, Oregon, is another example of growth taking place in the world. The fact that you have this book in your hands is a third example.

More good news is that inroads have been made in schools in California, where some raw-food teachers are giving classes in nutrition. As influence grows in various areas, the truth becomes revealed. The large number of new books about raw food is another sign of advancement. The October 2007 Raw Spirit Festival, held in Sedona, Arizona, demonstrated that there are thousands of people living a healthier lifestyle. You, too, can make those changes!

Organic farmers
The importance of organic farmers needs to be recognized. Without them, raw foodists (except for those knowledgeable enough to live on natural plant life) would not have the food supply they need. Helping these farmers is a high priority for those of us who want to stay healthy. Continued awareness, vigilance, and action is necessary to protect organic farmers from corporate and government threats to their existence.

Psychological aspects of making changes
The most important thing to remember is that you have the power and the ability to make a change in your life. When you think something is easy, you program yourself for it to be easy. When you think it's hard, you make it hard. So be sure to think that you can do anything that you want to do. Eliminate all the doubt, anxiety, and fear from your thought process. As soon as you get a negative thought, say the word "cancel" to yourself and immediately eliminate it. The more you practice this method, the easier it gets. When you practice this, you save your energy instead of wasting it on negative thoughts. You can then focus this energy on accomplishing your goals. Don't forget that you have the control over your mind and that you have the power to change.

Next, please realize that you must make a *decision* followed by a *commitment* that you are going to make a specific change. When you do that, you have taken the first step. You can then take a good look in the mirror and check-reality regarding your health. Do this with honesty rather than self-deception. The only person you would be fooling would be yourself. It is your health and your life. The mind has many ways of defending itself against discomfort or pain, so don't run from discomfort; rather, accept it as a challenge that will help you grow. Learn to believe in yourself. That is the foundation of your power. The past is over; learn from it, and strengthen your belief in yourself and the ability to accomplish your goals. When you make changes, you will open a new door to learning more about how you function. Your confidence will grow and continue to grow as you make more and more changes.

The technique for change

The following steps are suggested to learn how to accomplish change:

- Self-observation. The observing ego is used to locate the particular area in which change is desired or needed. For self-observation to take place, you have to be motivated to look at yourself. This is an easy thing to do when you're ready to look. For example, you may look at your level of physical fitness and ask whether daily exercise would enhance your condition. Or you may look at the quality of your diet and desire to enhance it. Self-observation is the necessary first step, accompanied by the motivation to change.

- Self-acceptance. Negative or self-hateful attitudes should be left behind, because only then can true self-acceptance be achieved. Understanding the how and why of a particular situation in its historical roots is helpful when brought to the consciousness. When the reasons for a thing are known, your rationality asserts itself and assists in self-acceptance. Then self-hateful attitudes that may have developed lose their power. You may have no healthy dietary program although you know the benefits of having one. You may have developed a negative attitude because you know you should eat more healthy/raw/vegan foods but for some reason haven't begun to yet. Accept this, and move forward.

- Evaluation of the current situation. Take an inventory to increase awareness of your reality. Make an evaluation of your current situation. The quality of the evaluation depends upon the amount of information you have to use as criteria. It may be a simple one, such as recognizing that you're 20 pounds overweight. Or it may be a more complex one in which a thorough physical examination is made for muscle strength, endurance, cholesterol level, heart functioning, etc. Evaluation made in the area of diet may become an ongoing evaluation as you become increasingly aware of more and new information. Making the evaluation is a necessary step that helps give you perspective and also prepares the way for goal-setting.

- New goals desired. Set appropriate new goals. Setting new goals often depends upon the amount of information that is available. The amount of effort put into step three will be useful here. However, you can gather additional information for appropriate goal-setting when sufficiently motivated and then set more sophisticated goals. Coming back to the example of physical fitness, you can set the goal of one hour of daily exercise. In the case of dietary change, you can set the goal of drinking a vegetable/green juice and eating a salad every day. To achieve this goal requires work and patience and requires the approach suggested in the following steps.

- Setting of limited goals to achieve success. The kind of limited goal that is set will guarantee success. The goal must be so limited that it is absolutely achievable. Every goal needs to be divided into its smallest sensible components. It is rare for someone to make a radical change in old habits and maintain that change for the rest of his or her life. Thus the goal of eating raw foods daily is started by adding either a vegetable juice or eating a salad three times a week. If three times a week is too much bother, then it can be reduced to two times or one time in a week. Here a new habit is being started, and repetition is vital for this step to succeed.

- Acceptance of the gradual process of change. Recognizing the gradual nature of the growth process, rather than setting high expectations, is helpful. Following our example, if you suddenly jump from one apple per day or one shot of wheatgrass once a week to being 100% vegan raw foodist, the necessary inner processes (both physiological and emotional) will not have had sufficient time to take place. Both body and mind need to change in a gradual way. Time is required for growth, and change and cannot be rushed. Accepting this concept helps in the preparation for the road ahead. After the 3-times-weekly juice, salad, or raw smoothie becomes easy to do, increasing to a daily raw food program can be done much more easily. This may take several weeks of small steps until there occurs a desire or pushing from within to increase the frequency. It is an inner process unfolding, like a seed beginning to sprout, and so is the person progressing from just one minute of exercise. There will be an inner readiness, and there will be a spontaneous desire that occurs. This concept is important and is part of staying in with yourself, as well as of using your conscious will.

- Continued effort and joy of the process. When change occurs from within, you experience the process as an integral part of your growth. The combination of these two elements – sustained efforts and an inner readiness – make for the next step forward. Each new step leads to the next one, until the sub-goals are accomplished and than finally the goal itself. You experience a sense of satisfaction as each new sub-goal is accomplished. Watching the gradual growth process that takes place brings psychological rewards, and each new increase in time reinforces the prior sub-goal. Therefore, increasing from juicing three times a week to every day is both a statement of success and a statement of continued growth. Maintaining the capacity of one minute of exercise is no longer questionable, and confidence is developed. This confidence leads to new confidence, and the recognition of how this process can be applied to other areas becomes part of the personality. Sustained effort is necessary for change. It takes time and repetition for a new change to become integrated, but the process of change can be joyful rather than a struggle.

- Allowing for regressions. During the course of changing, regressions may occur. They must be accepted lightly rather than allowed to become destructive. After any regression occurs, repeat step seven. You need to allow for a natural part of the growth process: namely, those times when something does not proceed according to plan. This may occur for various reasons and interrupt the steady progress. For example, feeling depressed, being ill, or having an emergency may cause you to miss making vegetable juice on one day. This is okay and will probably occur. However, do not expend unnecessary energy on that one missed day – simply continue the program the next day.

When you apply these eight steps, change will occur for you. As you achieve success in making a change, your capacity for making change increases. You'll develop confidence both in the process and in yourself, and with a greater confidence, you'll come to experience a far greater level of personal freedom and health.

About the Author:

Dr. Walter J. Urban is a Research Psychoanalyst registered with the medical Board of California. He is the founder and Director and Visionary of the Energy of Life Institute in Costa Rica and consultant to the Dance of Life Massage School. Dr. Urban is the author of Do You Have the Courage to Change: The 12 Reasons Why People Don't Change and How You Can and of Integrative Therapy: Foundations of Holistic and Self Healing, published in 1978. This was the first book published on Integrative therapy. He was a consultant on a National Institute of Mental Health Grant from the US Government and Director of the Theodor Reik consultation center of New York and the director and owner of the El Reposo Health Spa in Desert Hot Springs, CA.

Please refer to www.drwalterurban.com for more information. 'When I was asked who I am, my answer is, love, compassion, spirit, and part of nature."

Someone Implored Me to Eat Venison for Breakfast

One vivacious venison pranced and gamboled into a grove of thousands of venerable

white aspen trees

disappearing into a shaft of dawn

when another beatific bit of meat

gazed into my eyes, then shyly lowered her head

as we dined together, she and i, beside the brook

surrounded by aspens

beside the brook

across the flowers

at a respectable distance

on raspberries, shrubbery and yarrow

and shared a giant green plate

of miners' lettuce

just standing there, mutually mesmerized

on our six legs

crunching and chewing together

occasionally twitching our ears

while listening to the stream

singing beside our ankles

for an undefinable time

Poem by
Happy Oasis

Raw Spirit Festival

In a gorgeous, natural yet comfortable locations,
participants discover ancient wisdom and the latest findings
from the greatest minds in healthy living.
Features include: 100+ Fascinating Health Seminars,
World Class Vegetarian Musicians,
A Vast Eclectic Array of Raw-Eco-Educational Booths,
Electric Cars, Rickshaws and Bicycles,
Raw Chocolate Emporium, Speed Dating Game,
Creative Children's Program, Raw-Eco-Peace Job Fair,
Teenagers Table, Investors-Meet-Entrepreneurs Forum,
Raw Restaurant Food Court, Raw Vegan Demos & Tasting Parties,
Outdoor and Indoor Main Stages (generally),
Eco-Architecture, Interactive Discovery Dome Workshops,
Raw Business Leaders Forum, Art Garden,
Music, Dancing, Poetry, Theatre,
Sacred Exercise Area Yoga, Meditation Circle, Open Mike,
Hug Patrol, Leadership Sharing Circle, Peace & Harmony Services,
Nature Trails, Fantastic Foods and Fabulous Friends!

*"This is more than a raw vegan food festival. Our vision is to
integrate Healthy Living, Eco-Sustainable Solutions and
World Peace because together these comprise a comprehensive
strategy for addressing current global challenges.
We feel that our Raw Spirit Fest non-profit organization belongs
to the entire ever-expanding, international community."*
— Happy Oasis, Chief Visionary Officer

Santa Barbara, CA at Live Oak Campground
June 5–7 2009

Washington, DC at a Beautiful Park in Maryland
August 29–30 2009

Prescott, AZ in the Gorgeous Granite Dells
September 26–27, 2009

——— RawSpiritFest.com ———

About the Co-ordinating Editor

Diana Store was born in Belfast in 1973 and was brought up in Ireland's countryside and England's suburbs. She has had a lifelong interest in harmonious living and being close to nature. Diana decided to be vegetarian at the age of seven after naming all the cows in the local fields and then finding out they were being taken away to be killed so that they could be eaten. Being told it was not possible for a child to be vegetarian and not believing it led her on a quest for (dietary) truth. Diana became vegetarian at 14 and vegan and interested in raw foods at the age of 22.

Diana's formal education includes diplomas in art and design and a first-class honors degree and post-graduate qualifications in landscape architecture. She started visiting the Netherlands in 1998, first for an internship, and then returning to live and work. In 2000, she won an ideas competition for sustainable urban design, which led to employment for 18 months in 2001 and 2002, working on the future planning of Amsterdam City. In 2000 Diana also became a "100% raw foodist" consequent to living on the land for three months at a vegan, raw foods, permaculture community in Spain. She has never eaten a cooked meal since!

After experiencing first-hand the multitude of benefits associated with a diet high in raw foods, including better sleep, clearer thinking, increased immunity from common illnesses, and a lot more energy, Diana became inspired to do "whatever it takes" to stimulate a raw-food culture in her adopted country of Holland. This led to establishing a business in 2004 on the organic farmers market in Amsterdam, offering wheatgrass, books, information, raw snacks, ingredients, superfoods, and equipment to support others in embracing a raw food diet and lifestyle. This enterprise has gone from strength to strength, and Diana's company, Raw Superfoods, now sends raw food products all over Europe.

Since 2003 Diana has also hosted many public events and given her own workshops in Holland as well as Spain, Austria, Belgium, Hungary and the USA. In 2006 and 2007, Diana participated in the first two International Living Foods Summits held at West Palm Beach in Florida, USA, a global meeting of raw-food teachers, held to establish common principles of optimal dietary practice. The Summit Statements and participants of these meetings together formed the basis for this book.

Diana's website: www.rawsuperfoods.com

Lightning Source UK Ltd.
Milton Keynes UK
18 August 2009

142789UK00001B/133/P